SPORT SCIENCE AND STUDIES IN ASIA

Issues, Reflections and Emergent Solutions

SPORT SCIENCE AND STUDIES IN ASIA

Issues, Reflections and Emergent Solutions

editors

Michael Chia

Nanyang Technological University, Singapore

Jasson Chiang

Chinese Culture University, Taiwan

World Scientific

NEW JERSEY • LONDON • SINGAPORE • BEIJING • SHANGHAI • HONG KONG • TAIPEI • CHENNAI

Published by

World Scientific Publishing Co. Pte. Ltd.
5 Toh Tuck Link, Singapore 596224
USA office: 27 Warren Street, Suite 401-402, Hackensack, NJ 07601
UK office: 57 Shelton Street, Covent Garden, London WC2H 9HE

British Library Cataloguing-in-Publication Data
A catalogue record for this book is available from the British Library.

SPORT SCIENCE AND STUDIES IN ASIA
Issues, Reflections and Emergent Solutions
Proceedings of the 2008 ACESS Conference in Sports Science

Desk Editor: Tjan Kwang Wei

ISBN-13 978-981-4304-08-5
ISBN-10 981-4304-08-5

Printed in Singapore by World Scientific Printers.

FOREWORD

First and foremost, I congratulate Michael Chia and Jasson Chiang for their foresight in galvanising the enlightened minds of sport scientists, academic intellectuals and young researchers of sport from Asia and encouraging their expert contribution to this sport science and studies tome, which represents, apparently a first foray into sport science by the international publishing house. This is indeed an important milestone for sport in Asia. Sport in Asia is experiencing an unparallel *renaissance* of sorts with the Olympic Games held in Beijing, China in 2008, the World Student Games hosted in Kaohsiung, Taiwan in 2009 and the Inaugural Youth Olympic Games anchored in Singapore in 2010, just to name a few.

Sport science and studies encompasses the disciplines of sport or exercise physiology, psychology, motor control, biomechanics, medicine, management, history, sociology and philosophy. International comparisons of elite sport performance provides persuasive evidence, which suggest that the use of sport science and studies knowledge at all levels of training, competition and recovery, improves medal tallies and promotes the understanding of universal issues in sport, exercise or health. Sport is multi-faceted and is used by governments of many countries in many contexts- as a people builder in nation building, as a neutral medium to forge relations among different races and cultures, as an avenue for the population to adopt healthy lifestyles throughout the lifespan and of course as a celebration of human physical talents.

Scientific wisdoms suggest that sport science and studies information can also be employed at the recreational and health-promoting levels so that all can better reap the benefits of their sporting engagements and stay sport-injury-free, thereby enjoying a better quality of life all round. As more people enjoy sport as leisure, there are also opportunities for sport science and studies to contribute to the economic well-being of nations and to generate jobs, thereby providing another dimension for sport science and studies in society.

Whilst sport science and studies is more established in the West, because of a longer sport history, the transfer of sport science and studies knowledge from West to East is fraught with challenges and difficulties because of the diversity of cultures, languages, ethos and environments. Since many of the chapter contributors are sport scholars based in Asia with regular academic sojourns to the West, they are in a unique position to juxtapose research findings, and blend the best knowledge from the East and the West. This is a key and unique characteristic of *Sport Science and Studies in Asia* that differentiates it from others. *Sport Science and Studies in Asia* brings sport and sporting issues in the region to a sharper focus.

Professor Lee Sing Kong
Director
National Institute of Education
Singapore

PREFACE

MICHAEL CHIA (NANYANG TECHNOLOGICAL UNIVERSITY, SINGAPORE)
AND JASSON CHIANG (CHINESE CULTURE UNIVERSITY, TAIWAN)

Dr Michael Chia and Dr Jasson Chiang lead and galvanise an international group of luminary researchers, academicians and young scientists in tackling current issues in sport, exercise and health from the perspectives of sport science and studies as seen through a set of 'asian lenses'. The first fruit of their toil and effort is a collection of essays that is *diverse* in associated topics, *devoted* to strong beliefs and *developed* in a manner that undergraduate, post graduate and in general, people with an interest in sport, will find interestingly and useful.

This timely tome comes at an opportune time when the business of sport in the Asia Pacific Region is booming, in the midst of economic uncertainty. [1]An independent management consulting firm estimates that the sports industry is worth $17 billion Singapore dollars in 2009 and is set increase many-fold in the years to come. Sports science support, management consultancy services and sports-related knowledge services are identified as the key growth areas in dire need of development to meet this explosion of interest and engagement in sport and healthy lifestyles.

Each contributor addresses a topic that is grounded in a particular country's context or circumstance but nonetheless have wider regional implications and applications. Almost all the contributors had academic sojourns in sport outside of their native countries and outside of Asia. However all share a commonality- each contributed chapter represents the distilled crystallised thoughts of a global outlook of an issue that is grounded in local actions.

The book aims to challenge readers to be reflective practitioners- as students or researchers, or thinkers of sport, to be independent seekers of future sport knowledge, and yet mindful and grounded in a full knowledge and awareness of the social, cultural and country-specific nuances of sport. It invites discussion and debate on a diversity of topics covered, and is therefore is a suitable text for undergraduate and graduate study of sport in Asia and the editors' hope is that this will light the fuse that ignites an explosion of sport-associated outcomes-fostered collaborative research, heightened and more enlightened sport interest, more discerning consumers of sport, greater spin-offs in sport innovation in terms of new training approaches and sport products, and a greater appreciation that sport and human kind are inseparable.

Dr Michael Chia is Head of Physical Education and Sports Science at the National Institute of Education In Singapore. Dr Jasson Chiang is a Professor at the Graduate Institute of Sports Coaching Science at the Chinese Culture University in Taiwan. Both are vice-presidents of the Asian Council of Exercise and Sports Sciences, a regional think-tank for the sport intelligentsia of Asia.

Reference

1. Singapore Sports Council website http://www.ssc.gov.sg/publish/Corporate/en/industry.html. Accessed 17 September 2009.

LIST OF CONTRIBUTORS

Dr Michael Chia is Head and Associate Professor of Physical Education and Sports Science (PESS) at the National Institute of Education (NIE), Nanyang Technological University (NTU) in Singapore. He completed his PhD studies at Exeter University in the United Kingdom on academic staff scholarships from Nanyang Technological University and The Association of Commonwealth Universities, United Kingdom in 1998. He was Visiting Professor to the Chinese Culture University, Taipei, Taiwan and Visiting Research Scientist to Chukyo University, Nagoya, Japan in 2008 and 2009, respectively. He is also a British Association of Sport and Exercise Science (BASES)-accredited sports scientist (Physiology Research) and an American College of Sport Medicine (ACSM) Health and Fitness Director, and the Vice-President of the Educational Research Association of Singapore and Vice-President of the Asian Council of Exercise and Sports Science. As a teacher of physical education teachers, he received three Commendation Awards from the NIE for Excellence in Teaching in years 2003-2005. He successfully supervised 10 graduate students to the attainment of Master and PhD degrees in NIE/NTU. He is on the Editorial Boards of the International Journal of Sports Science and Coaching, Acta Kinesiologica, International Journal of Sports Science, Asian Journal of Exercise and Sports Science and The Open Education Journal. He published more than 180 journal papers, book chapters, books, monographs and articles in print and on the internet and gave more than 75 keynote and invited presentations on sport, exercise, fitness and health issues in youth and adults to national and international audiences. His research expertise is in paediatric exercise physiology and health, physical education, personal training and health education. He is listed in the USA Marquis 2009 publication of Who's Who in Medicine and Healthcare.

Dr Jasson Chiang is a Professor at the Graduate Institute of Sports Coaching Science, Chinese Culture University, Taiwan. He earned his M.S. Degree in athletic training, and PhD Degree in exercise physiology from Oregon State University, USA. He was invited by Dr Chang Ching-Hu - Chairman of the Board of Trustees, Chinese Culture University, to be the Head of the Department of Physical Education in 1983. Under stewardship, the master and doctoral programmes were established in 1993 and 2004, respectively. Dr Chiang was appointed as the Head Coach of the Track and Field team of the Kingdom of Swaziland, from 1980-1981, and the Secretary General of Chinese Taipei Track and Field Association from 1992 to 1998. He is currently the Director of the Sports Center at the Chinese Culture University, and member of the Sports Medicine Commission of the Chinese Taipei Olympic Committee. He is one of the founders and is the Vice-President of the Asian Council of Exercise and Sport Science. His research interests are in exercise physiology, and training pedagogy. His publications can be found in journals of exercise immunology and other refereed journals.

Dr Chang-Zern Hong is medical doctor and a Professor at the Department of Physical Medicine and Rehabilitation, University of California-Irvine, Irvine, California, USA and also a Research Professor at the Department of Physical Therapy Hungkuang Technical University, in Sa-Lu, Tai-Jong in Taiwan.

Dr Chow Jia Yi is an Assistant Professor in Physical Education and Sports Science of the National Institute of Education (NIE) in Singapore. He taught Physical Education in Singapore schools upon his graduation with an honours degree in Physical Education from NIE, Nanyang Technological University. Jia Yi was subsequently awarded an Overseas Graduate Scholarship from NIE to undertake a PhD study with University of Otago, New Zealand in 2004. His area of specialisation is in examining multi-articular human movement and learning from a theoretical perspective grounded in Dynamical Systems Theory. Particularly, he is proficient in the use of 3D motion analysis systems to examine coordination of complex movements in sports such as soccer and table-tennis. His specific research interests includes the investigation of the functional role in movement pattern variability, transitions between movement patterns and coordination changes as a function of skill level as well as practice. He also adopts a Nonlinear Pedagogical approach to understand how the dynamic interaction among constraints in a learning environment can inform practitioners and researchers about practice, instructions and feedback for learning game skills. He has published his works in internationally peer review impactful journals in the area of motor control and learning as well as in Education such as Journal of Motor Behavior, Motor Control, Human Movement Science, Acta Psychologica and Review of Educational Research.

Dr Do Young Pyun is an Assistant Professor and member of the faculty in the field of Sport Management in the National Institute of Education, Nanyang Technological University in Singapore. He teaches several sport management-related courses in undergraduate and graduate levels. Dr Pyun conducted a variety of research on consumers' psychometric properties on advertising through sport, effectiveness of virtual signage, brand globalness, brand extensions, perceived locus of causality, and competitive balance in professional leagues, coaching leadership, organizational citizenship behaviour, and burnout. He is interested in scale development; selection and construction of required measurement or assessment instruments. Dr Pyun published in various journals including the Personality and Individual Differences, the Journal of Teaching in Physical Education, the International Journal of Sport Communication, the International Journal of Sport Management, Journal of Sport Consumer, Journal of Sport Leisure Studies, Journal of Leisure and Recreation Studies, and the Korean Journal of Sport Management. Dr Pyun received his PhD in Sport Management from the Florida State University and both MSc in PE as well as BSc in Sport and Leisure Studies from Yonsei University, South Korea.

Dr Govindasamy Balasekaran did his Post Doctoral Fellowship in molecular genetics with a renowned genetics professor at the University of Pittsburgh, USA. He is an Associate Professor with the Physical Education and Sports Science, National Institute of Education, Nanyang Technological University, in Singapore. His research projects include physiological responses in exercise and adaptations to health and sports performance. The influence of genetic factors on exercise related outcomes are also investigated. Dr Balasekaran obtained his PhD from the University of Pittsburgh, USA through an overseas government scholarship. He is a certified American College of Sports Medicine (ACSM) Health/Fitness Director. He also has a strong interest in coaching and holds the level one and level two International Amateur Athletic Federation (IAAF) coaching certificates. As a keen runner and a former competitor, he had represented Singapore in long distance running events and had won medals in various international meets. He had also qualified and raced in the prestigious National Collegiate Athletic Association (NCAA) cross-country championships where American athletes are often selected to represent the USA at elite international events, such as the Olympics.

Dr James Russell is a senior researcher and a doctor of vascular medicine and is the Head of the Section for Cell Biology and Signal Transduction, National Institute of Child Health and Human Development, National Institutes of Health, in Bethesda, Maryland in the USA.

Dr Jamie Mervyn Lim is a Deputy Director at Tan Tock Seng Hospital in Singapore. He graduated with a BSc (Hons) from King's College London, University of London, under a Singapore Government Public Service Commission scholarship and was also awarded the Joe Jeans Memorial Fund for clinical internship during the final year of his study. In 2002, Jamie was awarded the Young Investigator Award by the Singapore General Hospital for his work on the Effects of EDTA on Plasma Creatine Kinase in Rat's Skeletal muscle after Eccentric Contractions. He subsequently went on to complete his doctoral studies with the National Institute of Education, Nanyang Technological University, Singapore in 2006. His area of research for his PhD is in Exercise Physiology. He studied the impact of work-to-rest ratios, gender difference and the use of allometric scaling to analyse peak exercise performance.

Dr John Wang is an Associate Professor in Physical Education and Sports Science Academic Group, National Institute of Education, Nanyang Technological University in Singapore. He is also an accredited sport psychologist by the British Association of Sport and Exercise Science (Sport Psychology-Support and Research). His areas of research have been on sport ability beliefs, achievement goal theory, self-determination theory, intrinsic motivation, emotion, self-esteem, outdoor adventure, and project work. He is currently lecturing in sport psychology, research methods, measurement and evaluation and various sport modules. He also works with teachers, coaches, and athletes in mental preparation for peak performance. Recently, he wrote a book titled Mental Skills for Peak Performance: An Athletes' Guide with Co-Curricular Activities Branch, Ministry of Education. This book is disseminated to all schools in Singapore. He has also written book chapters on National Education and Project Work.

Dr Joseph Lin graduated from the physical education department at College of Chinese Culture in Taiwan. He then went to University of Wisconsin,

St. George's University and Yuin University for his Master's, Doctor of medicine, and Doctor of philosophy degrees. He received his professional trainings at Harvard, Stanford, UCLA, Northwestern, and University of Wisconsin. He is a certified Fitness Instructor from American College of Sports Medicine, and is board certified by American Board of Physical Medicine and Rehabilitation; American Academy of Pain Management; American Association of Integrative Medicine; American Board of Forensic Examiners; American Board of Forensic Medicine; and National Board for Certified Clinical Hypnotherapists. Dr Lin was a Medical Officer at National Institutes of Health; an Adjunct Professor in Sports Medicine at University of Maryland; and a Consultant to the White House Athletic Center. He was the Attending Team Physician at the Vince Lombardi International Cup for the American and USSR Olympic Volleyball Teams shortly before the 1988 Summer Olympic Games. He is currently the Medical Director of Physical Medicine and Treatment Center in Gaithersburg, Maryland and is a researcher at National Institutes of Health. Dr Lin was selected as "Physician of The Year" in 2002 and 2003 by the National Republican Congressional Committee's Physician's Advisory Board, in Recognition of The Top Medical Leaders in the United States. He was the Honorary Chairman of the National Republican Congressional Committee's Physician's Advisory Board in 2003, and was selected by the Consumer's Research Council of America as one of the America's Top Physicians.

Dr Junko Tahara is Professor at the Faculty of Physical Education, Kokushikan University, in Tokyo, Japan. She taught in the areas of sport history, ethical perspectives in sport, and physical education at Chukyo Women's University, Kokushikan University, and other educational institutions after receiving a PhD in health and sport sciences from Chukyo University in 1994. She was a visiting academic at the School of Human Movement Studies and also the Olympic Studies Centre in the University of Queensland, Australia in 2002. Her primary research includes history of the Olympic Movement in Japan and the international community; Olympism and Olympic Education; and gender issues in sport and physical education. Professor Tahara was a board member of the Japan Olympic Academy (JOA) since 2000, a board member of the Japan Society for Sport and Gender Studies since 2001, an associate member of the Science Council of Japan since 2006, and chair of the Japan Pierre de Coubertin Committee since 2007. Internationally, she was a council member of the International Pierre de Coubertin Committee since 2006 and is a Board Member of the Asian Council of Exercise and Sports Science since 2007. She attended sessions of the International Olympic Academy representing the NOA of Japan between 1985 and 2005. In the field of the Olympic Movement and Olympic Education, Professor Tahara contributed as editor-in-chief and a contributing author of the Pocket-Size Olympic Dictionary: The Comprehensive Guide to the Olympic Movement published by the Japan Olympic Academy (2008) and the "JOA Times," annual reports of the JOA. She also served as one of the authors of Olympic Readers for elementary school, junior high school and senior high school students published by the Tokyo Metropolitan Government, the Japanese Olympic Committee, and the TOKYO 2016 Bid Committee in 2008. Professor Tahara had a competitive sport career in lawn bowls and participated in several World Women's Bowls Championships, Asia-Pacific Bowls Championships, and Champion of Champions Tournaments as a representative player and/or manager of the Japanese lawn bowls team between1995 and 2006.

Dr Kaoru Kitagawa is Professor of Exercise and Sport Physiology at Chukyo University. He received his PhD from The University of Tokyo. Concurrently, he is also the President of Chukyo University and also held previous administrative appointments as the Dean of the School of Health and Sport Sciences and was also the Director of the International Center at Chukyo University. He is the Vice-President of the Japan Society of Physical Education, Health and Sport Sciences and is a Fellow of American College of Sports Medicine for over 25 years. His international contributions include stints as a research physiologist at the University of California at Santa Barbara, Institute of Environmental Stress and also as a Sports Science Expert at the Ministry of Education, Department of Physical Education in Thailand. His research foci are on the assessment of body composition, the effect of exercise and nutrition on body composition, athletic performance in relation to age, sports physiology and biomechanics of golf, skiing, swimming and soccer. His publications include five books on physical fitness, obesity, weight control, health and programming for land- and water-based exercise, and more than 120 journal papers in international and Japanese journals.

Dr Karen Philomena Nonis is Associate Professor of Early Childhood and Special Needs (ECSE) at the NIE, NTU, Singapore. Graduating from The University of Western Australia, Perth, she has published and presented at various conferences locally and internationally in the areas of Motor Control, Development and Learning and Special Needs. As a former Principal in a local

Special School, she has a firm foundation in the applied field of Special Needs. She is board member for the International Association for Special Education, USA and is the External Consulting Editor for the Journal of IASE, USA. She is panel resource member for AWWA TEACH ME Services, Singapore.

Dr Keiko Miyauchi Ikeda is an Associate Professor at the Faculty of Education, Yamaguchi University in Japan. She was a visiting fellow of Centre for the Study of Social History, The University of Warwick, UK, during March 1997 to January 1998. She has been a corresponding member of ISHPES Council since September 2005, a member of the board of ACESS since December 2007, a member of the board of directors for JSSH since December 2006 and a member of the board of the Historical Research Section of Japanese Society of Physical Education, Health and Sport Sciences since May 2007. She is the author of Pre-Victorian Sport: Pierce Egan's 'Sporting World' (Tokyo: Fumaido Publishing Co., 1996) and other books and articles on both Pre-Victorian British popular sports and Radicals, and Japanese sport history of the nineteenth and twentieth centuries.

Dr Swarup Mukherjee has a PhD in Exercise Physiology, is a graduate in medicine and a post-graduate in Sports Medicine. He is also a graduate in Physical Education. Dr Mukherjee is an International Sports Medicine Federation certified Team Physician, World Health Organization certified trainer in disability prevention and rehabilitation and a International Society for the Advancement of Kinanthropometry (ISAK) accredited Level 2 Anthropometrist. He is a lecturer in Physical Education and Sports Science. He is also the member of Youth Development and Scientific committees of the Singapore Hockey Federation and the Football Association. He has served as the sports scientist and the Fitness coach for the National Football Academy, Football Association of Singapore. Dr Swarup Mukherjee is active in research, especially in the areas of youth intermittent team games players. He has publications in international journals, a book, book chapters, a monograph, conference papers and newspaper articles to his credit. His focus of research is in exercise physiology specifically in the area of the functional bases of the capability to perform repeated high-intensity exercise in youth intermittent team games players. His area of research interest also includes training and testing of intermittent team games players. Dr Mukherjee's research interest also includes growth and motor development, talent identification and development, kinananthropometry, exercise, nutrition, health and fitness in school children and the general population.

Dr Takeru Kato graduated from the Nippon Sport Science University in 1989 with a degree in Sports Science and Physical Education. He gained a PhD from Chukyo University in the field of Exercise Physiology and Sports Biomechanics, where his PhD research focused on underwater walking and running. He also worked as a Research Assistant in the Faculty of Health Science at Suzuka University of Medical Science. Associate Professor Takeru's main research interests are developing exercise programmes to strengthen bone in order to prevent osteoporosis.

Dr Tsung-Min Hung received his doctoral degree from the University of Maryland, College Park in 1996. He is a Professor in the Department of Physical Education at the National Taiwan Normal University (Taiwan) with an area of expertise in psychophysiology of sport and exercise. He has been the sport psychology consultant for Taiwan's elite athletes for the past 10 years. Dr Hung's research interests include psychophysiological signature of optimal sport performance and psychophysiological consequences of physical activity. He has published more than 60 articles in peer-reviewed journals or book chapters and made more than 90 presentations at international conferences. Dr Hung is serving as the President of the Society for Sport and Exercise Psychology of Taiwan (2008-2009). He is also a member of the managing council and the treasurer for the International Society of Sport Psychology (ISSP), a committee member for the Society for Psychophysiological Research (SPR) and the Sport Science Committee of the International Table Tennis Federation.

Dr Tzyy-Yuang Shiang received his PhD degree from the Pennsylvania State University in Mechanical Engineering (majoring in Biomechanics) in 1993. He was also a Postdoctoral Researcher at the Center for Locomotion Studies, Pennsylvania State University. From 1994 to 1995, he was a research scientist and was Head of the Sports Science Department at the National Sport Training Center in Taiwan. From 1995 to 2000, he was a faculty member of the Institute of Coaching Science at the National College of Physical Education and Sports. From 2000-2004 he served as the Head of the Center for Exercise and Sports Science at the Taipei Physical Education College, where he established the Graduate Institute of Sports Equipment Technology and served as the first chairman of the institute till 2007. He is at present a professor in the Graduate Institute of Exercise & Sport Science at the National Taiwan Normal University. He was appointed head of the biomechanics division for the Chinese Taipei National Team for the Olympic Games. He is currently the President of the Taiwanese Society of Biomechanics. His research interests are devoted to various aspects of Biomechanics, Biomedical Engineering and Sports Equipment Design.

Dr Visvasuresh Victor Govindaswamy has a PhD and Master of Science in computer science and engineering with a Bachelor of Science in electrical and computer engineering from University of Texas in Arlington and University of Texas at Austin, USA respectively. He is an Assistant Professor and is presently teaching at Texas A&M University at Texarkana, USA. He has worked on a number of research projects and a notable one is in the area of Preparing Dependable, Dynamic Real-Time Application Systems for an Adaptive Resource Management Environment which was sponsored by DARPA (Defense Advanced Research Projects Agency USA - the central research and development organization for the Department of Defense (DoD) and NASA. Dr Victor has a strong interest in physiological research and has collaborated on a number of projects. He is also an avid runner and has participated in a number of races during his school and varsity days.

Dr Yoshihisa Umemura is a Professor at the School of Health and Sport Sciences, Chukyo University in Japan. He completed his PhD studies at The University of Tokyo in 1989. His research expertise is in exercise physiology and bone metabolism.

Dr Yvonne Wang received her medical degree from Fu Dan University in Shanghai, China with special training in public health. She pursued a Master degree in science with the Nanyang Technological University in Singapore from 2005 to 2008. Her focus areas are exercise physiology and health promotion and she is a certified exercise specialist by American College of Sports Medicine. She was running an exercise rehabilitation programme for patients with kidney failure and other complications for 4 years with the National Kidney Foundation in Singapore and then pursued her career with the National University of Singapore and other organizations in healthcare sector.

Professor Peter Chen is a Visiting Professor at the School of Health, Physical Education and Leisure Services, University of Northern Iowa, USA since 2005 and was a Professor at the Graduate Institute of Sport Coaching Science, Chinese Culture University, Taipei, Taiwan from 1993 to 2008. He was also a Professor, on a part-time basis at The National Taiwan Normal University. He is also Visiting Professor to the National Hsinchu University of Education, Taiwan from February to June 2010. Professor Chen is an Emeritus Principal Lecturer of the Dunedin College of Education, now merged with the University of Otago in New Zealand. His university experience reflected 25 years of service in the West and 26 years in the East, teaching in the areas of coaching leadership, training methodology, pedagogy in physical education, philosophical perspectives in physical education and philosophical perspectives between the East and the West. He was the 1964 Tokyo Olympic and 1968 Mexico Olympic Games Coach for gymnastics, for the Republic of China. He was also an International Gymnastics Judge for the International Gymnastics Federation from 1965 to 1980. He served as a New Zealand National Coach for 1974 World Gymnastics Championship in Verna, Bulgaria and the manager of the New Zealand Gymnastics Team for 1978 Commonwealth Games in Edmonton, Canada. He was appointed as the President of the New Zealand Gymnastics Association in 1978 and the Principal of the National Gymnastics School from 1978 to 1995. He was a Member of Scientific Committee for the Chinese Taipei Olympics Team to the 2000 Sydney Olympic Games. His awards and honours include an Outstanding Teacher's Award, Chinese Culture University; The Biennial Distinguished Scholar Award, International Council of Health, Physical Education, Recreation, Sport and Dance; Distinguished Visiting Professor, University of Northern Iowa, USA and an Outstanding Alumnus Award, National Taiwan Normal University. Among his recent books are Leadership in Teaching Physical Education Beyond 2000; Wisdom Formulas in Action; Evolution, Education and Physical Education; Wisdom of Eastern and Western Thoughts; Unlimited Challenges; Powerful Inspiration; and 50 Years of Teaching Between East and West. Professor Chen serves as a member of the Board of Directors of the World Leisure Organization; an International Advisor; Asian Council of Exercise and Sports Science; and also served as Vice President for Oceania from 2002 to 2005, and again from 2009 to 2013 for the International Council of Health, Physical Education, Recreation, Sport and Dance. Recently he received an award as a Senior Fellow of American Leisure Academy on 6 October 2008 in Quebec City, Canada.

Mr Alan Ch'ng was an academic staff of the Physical Education and Sports Science (PESS) Academic Group and an Associate Dean of PE and Special Programmes of the National Institute of Education (NIE) in Singapore. He taught courses in Sport Management, Organisation and Administration of Physical Education, Health and Wellness, and Exercise Physiology. He is also involved in consultancies in areas of coach and sport administrators' education, leadership development, and character building through sports. Prior to joining the NIE, he has taught in schools and a junior college where he served as the Head of Physical Education. Currently, he is a member of NIE's management in corporate planning and development.

Mr Eugene Chew Wai Cheong has a Bachelor of Physical Education (First Class Honours) from the University of Calgary, Canada is a member of the Physical Education & Sports Science faculty at the National Institute of Education, Nanyang Technological University in Singapore. A trained physical educator, his wide teaching experience ranges from secondary school, junior college, to polytechnic levels. He has a particular interest in character development and was part of the team in Temasek Polytechnic that developed the Character Education Programme. Eugene was a member of the senior management of the Singapore Sports Council responsible for charting the direction for sport development and driving the sporting vision for Singapore. He was also Singapore's representative in the International Council for Coach Education. For his close involvement in coach education and having implemented various policies and initiatives that brought about progressive changes, he was invited to share his experience at conferences by foreign governmental sport agencies. Having worked at various levels in the sport industry for more than eight years, Eugene's extensive corporate experience in sport management and sport development enables him to view the theory and practice of sport and physical activities from a fresh insightful perspective. Currently, pursuing his post-graduate studies, his research foci centre on motivation, parental influence, and physical activity in youths.

Ms Jernice Tan Sing Yee holds a Master of Education (Early Childhood). She is a PhD candidate holding the NTU Research Scholarship in Early Childhood and Special Needs Education, National Institute of Education in Singapore. Her research interest includes motor control, learning and development during early childhood, inclusion experiences of children with special needs education, motor learning and development of hearing impaired children and effective inclusion in physical and outdoor education. She has also had her maiden paper presented in a national conference as well as she has published in an international journal.

Ms Nidhi Gupta did her post graduation from Lakshmibai National Institute of Physical Education (LNIPE), Gwalior, Madhya Pradesh, India and secured first rank in under-graduation and post-graduation studies. She was a recipient of Junior Research Fellowship (JRF), India and Institute Merit Scholarship, LNIPE, Gwalior India. Nidhi Gupta has represented her university in many games and participated in school games federations of India (SGFI). Currently, Nidhi Gupta is PhD scholar with the Physical Education and Sports Science, National Institute of Education, Nanyang Technological University, in Singapore and working towards her PhD degree under the tutelage of Associate Professor Balasekaran.

CONTENTS

SPORT
SCIENCE

THE NATURE AND PROMOTION OF PHYSICAL ACTIVITY IN SINGAPOREAN YOUTHS

MICHAEL CHIA

Physical Education and Sports Science, National Institute of Education, Nanyang Technological University, Singapore

The conveniences of modern living for work and for play pose serious challenges for young people in school and outside of school, to be physically active on a daily basis. Physical play offers many benefits for the holistic development-cognitive, physical, psychomotor and affective domains- of young people. Physical activity guidelines for young persons and youths reveal that they should be accumulate at least 90 minutes or more of at least moderate intensity activity on a daily basis for health benefits to accrue in terms of having a positive metabolic profile. Girls should accumulate at least 12 000 steps or 120 minutes and boys, 15 000 steps or 150 minutes of physical activity daily. These guidelines are established for cohorts that are from the West and should be tested and validated against cohorts from the East. Physical activity and physical inactivity behaviours is complex and are resistant to simplistic explanations such as hours of computer use and/or television viewing. Instead clusters of cohorts, with different characteristics, such as venerability to being overweight and physically inactive and should be identified. No singular factor strongly predicts either behaviour; rather the behaviours are based upon a basket of factors and the interplay among the factors of the physically active or physically inactive person. Intervention programmes that target the holistic development of young people can be successful and sustainable when there is whole school acceptance of the programme, a strong trust between the school management, stakeholders (school, parents, and MOE) and the researchers, when the interventions are multifaceted- before, during and after school programmes, active recess, an extended recess, tuck-shop or canteen nutritional programme, the availability of safe equipment and facilities, parental involvement, school events and school partnerships with the community. The use of electronic gadgets such as PDAs, mobile phones and new technology monitors, coupled with youth-friendly software programs can help increase awareness of the need for a healthy lifestyle among youths in Singapore.

1. Introduction

Physical activity is the natural inclination of all young people, regardless of race, language or religion in Singapore. Physical activity is the capstone for the growth and development of toddlers, children, adolescents and young adults. Among toddlers and young children, physical activity through physical play offers ample opportunities for holistic development. Child-directed play fosters creativity, problem-solving, social interaction, motor development, physical fitness and enhances parent-child relationships (Chia, 2007). Conversely, a serious deprivation or restriction of physical activity may impair or retard physical, social, mental and emotional development of young children.

Among adolescent and young adults, physical activity through sports and games provide opportunities to build a sport-loving culture, for social intercourse, for stress-release and for the pursuit of a healthy lifestyle. However, there is a compelling attractiveness in embracing lives of convenience and sedentary forms of entertainment with the advancement of technology and innovation. In Singapore, young people are at a very young age 'socialised' into study, transport and leisure habits and activities that require minimal amounts of physical exertion and energy expenditure. This is exacerbated by the ease high-calorie convenience foods via food delivery services and lifestyle choices for study, work and leisure that are mostly sedentary.

Indeed physical inactivity appears to be better tracked over time than physical activity from childhood to adolescence to adulthood (Raitakan et al, 1994).This means that it is easier for sedentary habits or the cycle of very little physical activity in daily life to be entrenched than it is for active physical activity habits to take root. Modern-day technological conveniences include the television, computers, the cell phones, elevators and lifts, forms of vehicular transport (cars, buses, and trains), and all forms of labour-saving electrical appliances (e.g. washing machines and vacuum cleaners). Reduced daily and total energy expenditure, coupled with an over-consumption of calories in childhood and adolescence, increases the likelihood of heart-disease, stroke and some forms of cancers in adulthood. This threatens both life-span and the quality of life of youths. In the USA, there are already projected warning signs that the lifespan of the present population of youths could be shorter than those of their parents because of a 'tsunami of obesity' that affects the USA (Ludwig, 2007). Singapore, a first-world nation must not go down this route and must instead make haste and exercise a resolute determination to take on the road less travelled, where the youths morph into physically active, sport-loving and healthy adults.

The cardinal purpose of this chapter is to provide information about the nature of physical activity among Singaporean youths and some innovative approaches at promoting physical activity among school-going youths in Singapore. The purpose of the overview is to provide a firm foundation for school administrators, physical activity, play and sport advocates and school teachers to justify, plan and craft beneficial programmes for the advancement of holistic health among youths in Singapore.

2. Benefits of physical activity through physical play

Research informs that physical play is beneficial to the holistic development of young children and that the benefits of physical play out-weigh the disincentives of physical play such as accidents and physical injuries (Chia, 2008). Play is natural and is a simple joy that is a most cherished part of childhood. Play fosters creativity, promotes imagination, practices dexterity and encourages emotional, cognitive and physical strength. Indeed, play is important for the healthy development of the brain (Tamis-LeMonda et al, 2004). Through play, children can explore the world, interact and engage with peers and adults, practising mastery and resiliency and acquiring competencies that will help them to face future uncertainty (Chia, 2008).

Play that is undirected by adults, allows children to learn to share, to care, to negotiate, to get along in groups, to resolve conflicts and also to learn self-advocacy skills (Hurwitz, 2003). When play is child-directed, children practise decision-making, move at their own, discover their own interests and children ultimately engage in the passions that they wish to pursue. When play is adult-directed, which is common, children acquiesce to adult standards and this sometimes compromises creativity, leadership and group skills (MacDonald, 1993). This should be a cautionary reminder that adult-based interventions should be tampered to allow for a greater licence for children to freely mingle and interact, rather than to inhibit physical activity without intent.

Play builds active and healthy bodies and encouraging unstructured play every day of the week that is interspersed throughout the day could increase the habitual physical activity of children and help ameliorate childhood obesity or delay it, helps with stress alleviation and allows for 'good mood' hormones, which are released into the circulation when physical activity thresholds are achieved, to take effect (Chia & Wang, 2002).

Parents who spend time at play with young children get a glimpse of the world through the 'child's eyes' and apart from opportunities to offer gentle and nurturing guidance, the interactions also promote enduring relationships between the child and parent (Smith, 1995). Interestingly, play is also used to foster academic and social-emotional learning. Play helps children to adjust to the school environment, heightens children's readiness to learn, enhances positive learning behaviours and fine-tunes problem-solving skills (Fisher, 1992).

Apparently, no other medium apart from physical play allows for so much gain for so little investment. Persuasive anecdotal evidence garnered from the parents of pre-school children who make their transition into primary school and from principals of primary schools show that young pupils miss the daily opportunities for physical play in their pre-schooling years that become limited and more restrictive once enter primary school. Researchers, education specialists and physical activity protagonists should re-energise their efforts in exploring intervention programmes that can facilitate increased daily physical activity engagement through play, either through expanded physical education sessions, in terms of duration and frequency, co-curricular sport and game activities conducted during and after-school hours and other events that 'regularise' physical activity.

This will buttress the notion that daily physical play is fundamental and a pre-cursor requirement for the holistic development of young persons, without and without disabilities. Our data suggest that youths with disabilities have reduced functional performance capabilities and perhaps reduced daily physical activity compared to their normal peers and therefore it is important that youths will special needs are accorded special attention and provided with opportunities for play or development remediation (Chia, 2002). In the cited study, Chia reported that in the 16 adolescent boys with moderate intellectual disability, peak power and mean power in the Wingate Anaerobic Test and the subsequent post-blood lactate concentrations were markedly lower (i.e. up to 35 % lower) than that of age-matched peers, using a similar test methodology.

Importantly, the mindset that physical play is most important will become entrenched and pervasive and provide a clear societal mirror that Singapore recognises and enshrines the right of children to play as espoused by the United Nations High Commission for Human Rights (General Assembly Resolution 44/25, 1989).

3. Consequences of physical activity insufficiency and associated conditions

Extended periods of physical inactivity once entrenched as a daily habit may result in adult ailments like cardiovascular disease and altered glucose metabolism, which are documented to begin in infancy and childhood (Williams et al, 2002). Other paediatric conditions arising from severe physical activity insufficiency include obesity, orthopaedic problems such as joint pains in the feet, knees and hip, which are exacerbated by excessive body weight, and disrupted sleep due to obstruction of the airflow because of too much fat around the neck (Kimm & Obarzanek, 2002). Obese and overweight children, including those in pre-schools experience weight-teasing by peers and they are bothered by the teasing episodes (Chia, 2006). Bruche (1975) summarises the deleterious psychological impact of obesity in the young:-

"The lot of fat children is a sad one. They are bashful & ashamed of their shapeless figures yet unable to conceal them. Wherever they go, they attract attention...Obesity is a serious handicap in the social life of the child... Obesity does not have the dignity of other diseases, and is not often taken seriously by adults". (pp. 95).

Weight-teasing in schools is associated with disordered eating behaviours that may place overweight children at risk for weight gain. In a survey of 4746 young people in the USA, 63 % of the very overweight girls and 58 % of the very overweight boys reported being teased by their peers, while weight teasing by family members was reported by 47 % by these girls and 34 % by these boys (Neumark-Sztainer et al., 2002)

In an eight-year retrospective prevalence study on eating disorders (anorexia nervosa) in Singapore, Lee et al (2005) reported a six-fold increase in patient referrals, between 1994 and 2002, to the Child Guidance Eating Disorder Clinic at the Institute of Mental Health. The following results are instructive: the mean age of onset of the disorder was at 15.5±3.9 years; 91 % were female, 94 % were Chinese and 74 % of the patients were of school-going age with 47 % coming from all-girl schools; the mean BMI at diagnosis was 15.6; 25 % suffered from depression and the 27 % identified the triggers as weight teasing and comments from others, with 11 % having been members of the Trim and Fit (TAF) Scheme in schools. These results highlighted that perceived weight teasing was significantly associated with disordered eating behaviours among overweight and non-overweight boys and girls (Neumark-Sztainer et al, 2002), echoing in the Straits Times on eating disorders in all-girl-school in Singapore (Davie, 2006).

The TAF scheme was launched in 1992 and was successful in reducing national school rates of overweight from about 15 % in 1991 to about 10 % in 1998 and has largely stayed about 10 % since year 2000 (Chia, via personal communication with MOE, PE Unit, 2007). Chia (1998) in his published discourse on rethinking TAF programme strategies raised concerns about some of the deleterious effects that the programme may have on some vulnerable school students and also furnished suggestions about engaging overweight youths with forms of physical activity and exercise that are more suited and personalised to the conditions of overweight youths.

The MOE reviewed the TAF scheme and with the MOH launched a nationwide holistic health framework for schools in 2000, (CHERISH; Championing Effort Resulting in Improved School Health) which targets the holistic development of students, which included a healthy maintenance of body weight for all students, not just those who are under-weight weight or over-weight. Importantly CHERISH echoes the WHO's Health Promoting Schools concept, adopted by many countries.

In 2003, Chia and Wang published survey results among primary school children that showed that a sizeable proportion of children of normal body weight voiced the intention to lose body weight, rather than to gain body weight. In the study that involved 518 pupils in a primary school in Singapore, where the relationships between weight-for-height classifications, body weight satisfaction, perceived physical self-worth and physical fitness among 275 boys and 243 girls aged between nine and 13 years were examined, results revealed that across the three weight-for-height classifications, more pupils intended to want to lose body weight than to gain body weight. Underweight pupils were the most satisfied with their body weight, were the most physically fit and had the highest rating for perceived physical self-worth than the healthy weight and overweight groupings. It is noteworthy that girls and boys had similar ratings for perceived physical self-worth but younger pupils had higher perceived physical self-worth than older pupils.

These data suggest that programme leaders in physical activity, exercise and sport must practise sensitivity and care by not perpetuating negative stereotypes about body weight. Concomitantly, education and awareness of the dangers of body image disorders among school youths particularly in all-girl schools and in young secondary school students should be stepped up. Apart from health and physical ailments, other social and emotional and disciplinary deficiencies are also likely to accrue, as the opportunities and outlets for stress-alleviation through exercise and physical play become limited. However, such an assertion awaits research validation among Singaporean youths. This is a fertile area for future research.

In Singapore, paediatric growth charts had to be revised in the late 1990s to take into account the increased body mass of children aged 1 to 6 years, where there was an average increase of half a kilogram in of body mass for all ages without any corresponding increase in stature. These changes were attributed to increased energy storage because of better nutrition but equally could be attributed to reduced energy expenditure at the paediatric ages. Research informs that in the USA, young people within the 95 % percentile for BMI are likely to remain obese and overweight in adulthood and also suffer from obesity-related ailments (Williams et al, 2002). Therefore it seems prudent to monitor young people's BMI when they appear to be on an upward trend so as to ameliorate large groups of young people become overweight and obese in adulthood.

Another indirect consequence of the lack of activity in childhood is also one of the highest incidence rates of adult-onset diabetes in the world among Singaporeans. Since the 1990s, heart disease and stroke continues to be the leading cause of premature death in Singaporean adults (Singapore Heart Foundation, 2006). Yet, against this backdrop, regular physical activity in youth has a strong and effective preventative role in the onset of Type II diabetes (Chia, 2002).

Singapore apparently also has one of the highest rates of childhood and juvenile myopia in the world and many youths suffer from myopia at a younger age than before. In 2001, 34 % of Primary 1 students were myopic. This increased to 66 % for Primary 6 students and 68 % for Secondary 4 students (Teo, 2001). Cogent data suggest a negative relationship between the rates of myopia and the amounts of physical activity, sports and outdoor activity. In a longitudinal study of 514 children from 1989 to 2001, Jones et al (2007) reported that the chances of children with parents without myopia becoming myopic were lowest in the children with the largest amounts of sports and outdoor activities. These health conditions among young Singaporeans are a wake-up call for action that much more needs to be done to motivate our young towards an active lifestyle imbued with regular physical activity. Research data in the Singaporean context are urgently needed to verify if these observations are also valid in our youths.

4. Physical activity guidelines for young persons and youths

There are apparently no universally accepted guidelines for physical activity that are promoted or accepted by all countries for toddlers, young children and youths. This is not surprising since there is a dearth of relevant, reliable and adequate data on dose-response benefit of physical activity (i.e. amount of activity engaged with corresponding results in health benefits) for these age groups. Moreover, the nature and context of physical activity among different communities in different countries are likely to be dissimilar.

The National Association for Sport and Physical Education (NASPE, 2002) in the USA enunciated physical activity guidelines for toddlers and young children. The guidelines were articulated based upon the premise that adopting a physically active lifestyle early in life increases the likelihood that infants and young children will learn to move skillfully.

The NASPE physical activity guidelines for toddlers (persons between 2 and 5 years old) are:

1. Toddlers should accumulate at least 30 minutes daily of structured physical activity and pre-school children, at least 60 minutes.
2. Toddlers and pre-school children should engage in at least 60 minutes & up to several hours per day of unstructured physical activity and should not be sedentary for more than 60 minutes at a time except when sleeping.
3. Toddlers and pre-school children should have indoor and outdoor areas that meet or exceed recommended safety standards for performing large muscle group activities.
4. Individuals responsible for the well-being of toddlers and pre-school children should be aware of the importance of physical activity & facilitate the child's movement skills.

For persons older than 5 years of age to adolescence, the current physical activity guidelines for the promotion of lifelong physical activity, the improvement in current health, physical fitness and well-being are:

1. Children should accumulate at least 60 minutes and up to several hours of age-appropriate physical activity on all or most days of the week. The daily accumulation should include moderate-to-vigorous physical activity of which the majority being intermittent in nature. Brisk walking is considered as moderate intensity. Continuous vigorous physical activity should not be expected for most children, nor should it be a condition for meeting the guideline.
2. Children should participate in several bouts of physical activity lasting 15 minutes or more. The majority of children's physical activity will be

intermittent in nature. For optimal benefits to accrue, 50 % of the accumulation should be in bouts of 15 minutes or more. These bouts can take place during recess, physical education, play or sport practices. Bouts of activities typically include activity time interspersed with rest or recovery periods.

3. Children should participate each day in a variety or age-appropriate physical activities designed to achieve optimal health, wellness, fitness and performance benefits.

A study by Anderson et al (2006) showed that a daily accumulation of least 90 minutes of moderate-to-vigorous intensity exercise or physical activity would be necessary in European children (Danish, Estonian and Portuguese) to prevent insulin resistance and to avoid a clustering of cardiovascular risk factors in European 9- and 15-year-old children (N=1156 girls and N=1045 boys). However the guideline for a minimum of 90 minutes of moderate-to-vigorous intensity exercise or physical activity is not well-publicized and has not yet gained widespread acceptance. These dose-response relationships for physical activity and disease antecedents in young people require further research and validation in the Singaporean context and should be pursued.

In Singapore, the Ministries of Community Development, Youth and Sport (MCYS), and the Ministry of Education (MOE) have apparently not articulated equivalent physical activity guidelines and in pre-schools, though physical activity sessions are encouraged, there is at the present time, no requirement for specialist physical education teachers to be deployed in pre-schools and in primary schools. All things considered, specialist PE teachers are better equipped to provide physical activities that are gainful and positive, and exercise and sport experiences that help children develop holistically.

The Ministry of Health (MOH) published New Dietary Guidelines for Children and Teenagers in 2007, which articulated the following guidelines for physical activity: Children and teenagers should engage in at least 60 minutes of at least moderate physical activity for at least 5 days of the week. PE time counts towards the 60 minutes. The guideline should be reinforced, practised and reiterated frequently and resolutely by school leaders. In terms of aggregated daily step count, researchers propose guidelines that are based are based upon tangible health outcomes. For instance, Tudor-Locke et al (2004) studied pedometer steps accumulated in 995 girls and 959 boys aged between 6 and 12 years, from the USA, Australia, and Sweden, in relation to weight status based on international cut-offs for normal and overweight in relation to BMI. They recommended a median cut-off of 12 000 steps for girls and 15 000 steps for boys. The researchers reported that boys taking less than 15 000 steps and girls less than 12 000 steps a day were more likely to be classified as overweight or obese based on their BMI, which is a measure of relative fatness. Accordingly, this translates to 120 minutes per day of activity for girls and 150 minutes per day for boys (Welk et al, 2000). As the total daily step count recommendations furnished by Tudor-Locke et al (2004) are based on BMI of children from the West, the recommended total daily pedometer step counts should be validated in Asian or Singaporean children in relation to Asian standards of BMI. This represents another fertile area for research.

5. Prevalence of physically active and physically inactive behaviours

Physical activity measurement is complex and there are many instruments that are used to quantify amounts of physical activity (PA) - self report or proxy methods include the use of validated and age-appropriate PA questionnaires, physical activity diaries and logs, direct observation and associated computer software, doubly labeled water, mechanical devices such heart-rate monitors, pedometers and accelerometers and associated computer software. These measurement tools measure associated but non-identical aspects of PA and the merits and demerits of use in young persons and youths are reviewed elsewhere (e.g. Oliver et al, 2007; Reilly et al, 2008). The cited reviews are instructive and researchers must select the most appropriate measurement tool (s) based on validity, reliability, feasibility, human ethics and the availability of research resources and the objectives of the research.

6. Physical activity in pre-primary school pupils (toddlers)

There are apparently no data on the physical activity of pre-primary school children in Singapore. Baseline studies are particularly important. This area represents a compelling area for future research.

7. Physical activity in primary school pupils (children)

In a 1995 study, Gilbey and Gilbey examined the physical activity patterns of Singapore school children (43 boys and 53 girls) aged 9-10 years assessed by continuous heart rate monitoring over three 14-hour periods on week days and a single period on a Saturday. Only 13 children (11.4 %) experienced a daily 10-min period of continuous activity at a heart rate >140 bpm. Twenty percent of the boys and more than 50 % of the girls never achieved a single 10-minute period >140 bpm. Boys achieved more periods of moderately intense activity ($p<.01$) than girls on weekdays. Lean girls were more active ($p <.05$) than the obese girls during weekdays. No differences were detected between activity levels on weekdays or on Saturday. The results indicate that school children in Singapore rarely experience the quantity or quality of physical activity needed for maintenance and development of cardiovascular health and cardiopulmonary fitness, articulated by the ACSM for adults. No physical activity guidelines for children were available then.

A study conducted by Chia et al (2002), using heart rate (HR) monitors in 120 boys and girls aged 10-11 years showed that they were mainly sedentary on a weekday (a median of 86 % of time spent at a heart rate intensity of less than 120 beats per minute and on a weekend day (a median of 96% of time spent at a heart rate intensity of less than 120 beats per minute). It is of interest that they were no sex significant difference in physical activity in this cohort of primary school pupils who were all of normal body weight (90-110 % for weight-for-height classification). However, primary school pupils were significantly more active than the secondary school students at HR thresholds that are described as light (120-139 bpm), moderate (140-159 bpm) and vigorous (>160 pbm) for both the week days and the week end day.

Wang, Chia, Quek and Liu (2006) used accelerometer-validated pedometers to examine in-school and out-of-school step count of 160 Primary 5 pupils from four schools. In-school step count was not significantly different from out-of-school step count (5364 vs 3805, $p>.05$) and the mean daily step count was 9169 ± 4551. The daily total accumulated step count translated to 76 % and 61 % (12000 for girls and 15 000 for boys; Tudor Locke et al, 2004) of the daily recommended step count of girls and boys, respectively.

8. Physical activity in secondary school students (adolescents)

In the above cited study, HR monitors used to monitor PA intensity over 3 week days and the week end day (Saturday) revealed that for secondary school students, aged between 14-15 years, the median time spent at HR intensity<120 bmp were 94 % and 99.5 % for the week day and the week end day respectively. It is of interest that they were no sex significant difference in physical activity in this cohort of secondary school students who were all of normal body weight (90-110 % for weight-for-height classification).

Lee and Trost (2006) examined the physical activity patterns of 105 adolescent boys and 116 adolescent girls, aged 14.5 ± 1.1 years, using a 3-day recall questionnaire on physical activity and pedometers. Results showed that boys reported higher overall mean activity (METs) and significantly higher level of vigorous activity blocks than girls but boys and girls reported similar number of blocks of moderate activity as the boys. Both boys and girls had similar mean total daily step counts over the average of three week days (boys-girls: 12134±2574 vs 11714±2339, p>.05) and on the week end day (Saturday) (boys-girls; 11662±2476 vs 11603±3009, p>.05). Though not reported in the study it appears that physical activity in adolescent boys and girls were not significantly different between week days and week end days as assessed using pedometers.

9. Explanations for physical inactivity among youths in Singapore

Emergent data suggest that it is the entire basket of physical inactive behaviours (e.g. reading and writing, doing homework, chatting with friends on the phone, listening to music, etc) rather than singular factors such as television viewing, video gaming activities and/or computer use that are responsible for youths being physically inactive.

For instance, Chia et al (2002) examined the associations between hours of computer use, physical activity using HR monitors and physical fitness among 120 primary school pupils aged 10.6 years and 120 secondary school students aged 14.8 years of normal body weight (80-110 % of weight-for-height charts). They reported no meaningful associations between hours of computer use, physical activity and physical fitness in secondary school students, and a significant positive correlation between hours of computer use and physical activity for primary school pupils (r=0.23, p<.05). However, the shared variance (i.e. coefficient of determination) was less than 6 %. Even so, the association was a positive one (as the hours of computer use increased, so did the level of physical activity) in primary school pupils.

Wang et al (2006) examined the physical activity and sedentary behaviours of a sample of 780 children aged between 10 and 14 years using a 7-day recall questionnaire. Results of one-way MANOVA showed that boys and girls had significant different patterns of physical activity and sedentary behaviours. Three distinct clusters were found for each sex using cluster analysis. 36 % of the boys spent much of their sedentary time in technology-based entertainment (e.g. computer/internet), and 38 % of them reported substantial amount of time spent studying and doing homework. The rest of the boys spent their time being physical active but they also played a lot of video games. Among the girls, time spent socialising with friends, studying as well as engaged in physical activity amounted to 57.3 %. 15 % of the girls reported spending most of their time studying and doing homework. A group of girls reported little study time, little socialisation as well as low engagement in physical activity (27.8 %) compared to their peers.

These data suggested that activity programme interventions should aim at increasing physical activity behaviours and not simply reducing sedentary behaviours. Interventions aimed at increasing the perceptions of competence, autonomy, and incremental beliefs may also be influential at increasing physical activity engagement among Singaporean school children.

10. Innovative school-based interventions to increase physical activity and reduce physical inactivity

10.1. *HealthTrek Information Tracking System- a tool for building a health-enabling environment in schools*

NIE researchers juxtaposed the use of information and computer programming technology to create the world's first HealthTrek Information Tracking System (HITS) housed in a Personal Digital Device (PDA) (Quek, 2003). HITS, allows an individual to appraise his/her current body weight, food intake, physical activity patterns and mood status over time. Importantly, the system is able to prescribe suggestions for remediation based upon recommendations enunciated by the Health Promotion Board of Singapore. Highlights of the HITS' features include an age and a sex-specific weight gain/weight loss calculator, for safe weight gain or weight loss, a food planner that gives a breakdown of key nutrients in foods that are selected and a physical activity planner that gives the rates of energy expenditure for different activities selected. The food database encompasses over 2000 local and non-local food items, while the physical activity database has more than 800 specific activity-types. The mood gauge allows a person to track negative or positive feelings over time.

The attractiveness of HITS is that it offered real-time data of participants, overcoming the need for recall, which can be used on its own or pooled as group data in providing individualised evidence based data so that specific lifestyle changes can be made. The effectiveness of HITS for monitoring individualised physical activity and food consumption and mood states was evaluated in 37 primary school pupils, aged 9-10 years (Wang et al, 2005). Participants kept track of their daily food intake, physical activity consumption and mood state for seven days, by keying in the relevant data required as soon as they consumed food or engaged in physical activity while data on mood was keyed in immediately before and after food and/or physical activity consumption. Results affirmed the researchers' assertions that in IT-savvy primary school pupils, the use of HITS housed in a PDA, provided an excellent means for the transmission of individualised and real time data that effected positive intentions and increased awareness for a healthy lifestyle- 92 % of pupils felt that HITS made them more discerning of their food choices and 95 % of the pupils reported that HITS made them more conscious of their daily energy expenditure and for a healthy lifestyle. Nearly 100 % of the pupils surveyed reported that they wished to continue using HITS and also continue to raise their levels of daily physical activity. At present, HITS is no longer available for use due to cost factors but its utility and effectiveness (real-time localised and holistic data- food, physical activity consumption and mood) as a health-enabling device can be further explored, when the cost of its implementation becomes more affordable.

10.2. *PRIDE for PLAY- personal responsibility in daily effort for participation in lifetime activity for youths*

PRIDE for PLAY is an acronym for Personal Responsibility in Daily Effort for Participation in Lifelong Activity for Youths (Chia, 2006). MOE advocates that schools should emphasize holistic development of pupils- this means paying sufficient and appropriate attention to the mental, physical, emotional, social and environmental development of all pupils and students.

Weekly compulsory physical education classes of 70 minutes in schools and the associated sports activities after classes are inadequate to meet emergent physical activity guidelines of a daily accumulation of at least 90 minutes of physical activity of at least moderate intensity.

Daily play sessions that are exclusive of an active daily recess, physical education classes taught by trained specialists and after-school sport sessions, can provide many developmental and holistic health benefits that may carry over into adulthood. A school environment that is play-encouraging, play-enabling and play-inviting can help a useful, innovative and natural way of inculcating a love for movement and help redress a serious trend of physical activity insufficiency while youngsters engage electronic gaming activities.

Pilot initiatives in two primary schools for the PRIDE for PLAY programme were conducted (Chia et al, 2007). This involved working closely with the school leaders and all teachers involved to forge a strong partnership for action and subsequent evaluation. The pilot study involved an infusion daily physical play of between 20 to 45 minutes during curriculum hours, either as stand-alone additional play and physical activity sessions or as part of an extended recess. Outcome deliverables like pre-and post school-based physical activity, assessed using pedometers, social-emotional outcomes among pupils, assessed using age-modified questionnaires and indicators of academic achievement were garnered. For one pilot school that involved 270 Primary 2 pupils, daily step count in school was significantly increased by 24 % from 3742 to 4642. In the other pilot school that involved 225 Primary 2 pupils, daily step count in school increased by 10 % from 4520 to 4984. These amounted to achieving 39-42 % of the daily recommended step count for girls and 31-33 % of the recommended step count step count for boys (Tudor-Locke et al, 2004).

Social emotional learning outcomes of the pupils involved with the PRIDE for PLAY programme were also significantly improved with no compromise to academic standards. The principals of both schools raised the following points that are instructive for the success of PRIDE for PLAY- the programme had the support and buy-in from the key stakeholders- school management, teachers, parents and the pupils themselves. Other schools have translated, customised and adapted the PRDIE for PLAY programme into daily physical education. Further research directions associated with PRIDE for PLAY include establishing holistic or social-emotional learning outcomes as a result of programme implementation in a wider spectrum of schools in Singapore.

10.3. *Every step counts- how an active recess can help to buttress physical activity achieved during physical education lessons*

Wangye and Chia (2008), embarked on a study to evaluate the step rate of 125 boys and girls from Primary 2 and Primary 6, using the Omron HJ-005 pedometers during four 30-minute PE lessons, taught by specialist PE teachers with games-based activities, rope skipping, throwing, jogging and shuttle-run based activities and during an 30-minute unstructured recess where pupils were free to play with games equipment. Results revealed that the average number of steps achieved in a typical 30-minute PE lesson was 1660±535 steps with a step rate of 55.4±17.8 steps/min. Steps accumulated during daily recess averaged 1208±526 steps or a step rate of 40.3±17.5 steps/min. There was no significant sex difference ($p>0.05$) in steps accumulated or step rate among the four structured PE lessons. However, the boys were significantly more physically active than girls ($p<0.05$) during unstructured daily recess.

The difference in steps accumulated between Primary 2 and Primary 6 pupils was not significant during daily recess ($p>.05$). Aggregated step count or step rate during PE and recess among Primary school pupils in Singapore are within the range of findings documented elsewhere (e.g. Scruggs et al., 2005; Tudor-Locke et al., 2006). When the steps were aggregated for PE and recess, girls achieved 24 % and boys achieved 19 % of the daily recommended steps

(Tudor-Locke et al, 2004). Primary school girls were just as physically active as the boys during school structured PE, but boys were significantly more active during the unstructured daily recess. Primary 6 pupils were just as physically active as Primary 2 pupils during the daily recess periods and the results of the present study did not support the view that physical activity declines with age, (e.g. Trost et al, 2002) at least not during the daily recess periods, a finding that finds agreement with Ridgers et al (2005).

Schools should capitalise on young pupils' natural inclination for play and the availability of qualified PE teachers and games equipment during recess to chalk-up as many steps as possible so that more youths are able to meet the daily recommended step count of 12 000 for girls and 15 000 steps for boys (Tudor-Locke et al, 2004).

11. Conclusion

The nature of modern living poses serious challenges for young people to remain physical active on a daily basis. Yet the merits of daily physical activity through play and sporting activity in formal and informal settings in the holistic development of young people should not be underestimated and discounted. Physically active and physically inactive behaviours are different constructs are worthy for further research so that more appropriate programmes can be implemented to improve the current situation where habitual physical inactivity is more the norm than the exception among Singaporean youths. Current evidence suggest that Singaporean young people are not physically active on a daily basis and more should be done in integrating strategies for the promotion of physical activity at the school, home and community fronts

References

1. Andersen, L.B., Andersen, S.A., Harro, M., et al (2006). Physical activity and clustered cardiovascular risk in children: a cross sectional study (The European Youth Heart Study). *The Lancet, 368,* 299-304.
2. Bruche, H. (1975). Emotional aspects of obesity in children. *Pediatric Annals, 4,* 91-99.
3. Chia, M. & Wang, J. (2002). Physical activity, exercise & health of the mind in young people. *Journal of Physical Education and Recreation, 8,* 64-67.
4. Chia, M. & Wang, J. (2003). Fat, unfit and dissatisfied: relationships among perceived physical self-worth, body weight satisfaction and physical fitness among primary school children. *ACHPER Healthy Lifestyles Journal, 50,* 14-19.

5. Chia, M. (1998). Rethinking Trim and Fit programme strategies...weighing in the scientific evidence. *Review of Educational Research and Advances for Classroom Teachers, 2,* 37-42.
6. Chia, M. (2002). Role of exercise in the management of Type II diabetes. *Journal of Physical Education and Recreation, 8,* 80-82.
7. Chia, M. (2002). Using the Wingate Anaerobic Test for measuring the maximal lower limb power of boys with Intellectual Disability. *Advances in Exercise and Sports Physiology, 8,* 51-56.
8. Chia, M. (2007). PRIDE for PLAY: personal responsibility in daily effort for participation in lifelong activity for youths. A Singaporean context. *Journal of Sports Science and Medicine, 6,* 374-379.
9. Chia, M. (2008). Physical inactivity among children and adolescents in Singapore- a paradoxical issue. *Acta Kinesiologica, 2,* 7-15.
10. Chia, M. (2007). Fit to play: enabling play and physical activity in children. In: *The Power of Movement–Enhancing Children's Cognitive, Social & Emotional and Physical Development through Movement.* (pp. 112-128). K. Nonis and S. Daswani (Eds). Pearson Education Asia, Singapore.
11. Chia, M., Quek J.J. & Wang J. (2009). Should we promote physical activity or physical fitness? In: *Perspectives on Physical Education and Sports Science in Singapore: An Eye on the Youth Olympic Games 2010.* Aplin Nicholas (Ed). Singapore: McGraw Hill.
12. Chia, M., Wang J., Teo-Koh, S.M., et al. (2002). Relationships between hours of computer use, physical activity and physical fitness among children and adolescents. *European Journal of Physical Education, 7,* 136-155.
13. Chia, M., Wang, J. & Quek, J.J. (2005). Measures of reliability and validity of school-based pedometer step count of Singaporean children. *Asian Journal of Exercise and Sports Science, 1,* 17-24.
14. Davie, S. (2006). Eating disorders on the rise in teenage girls. *The Straits Times*, 23 May.
15. Fisher, E.P. (1992). The impact of play on development: a meta-analysis. *Play Culture, 5,* 159.
16. Gilbey, H., & Gilbey, M. (1995). The physical activity of Singapore primary school children as estimated by heart rate monitoring. *Pediatric Exercise Science, 7,* 26-35.
17. Hurwitz, S.C. (2003). To be successful-let them play. *Child Education, 79,* 101-102.
18. Kimm, S.Y.S., & Obarzanek, E. (2002). Childhood obesity: a new pandemic of the new millennium. *Pediatrics, 110,* 1003-1007.
19. Lee, H.Y., Lee, E.L., Pathy, P., & Chan, H.Y. (2005). Anorexia in Singapore: An eight year retrospective study in Singapore. *Singapore Medical Journal, 46,* 275-281.

20. Lee, K.S. & Trost, S.G. (2006). The physical activity patterns of Singaporean adolescents. *Pediatric Exercise Science, 18,* 400-414.
21. Ludwig, D.S. (2007). Childhood obesity- The shape of things to come. *New England Journal of Medicine, 357,* 2325-2327,
22. MacDonald, K.B. (1993). *Parent-Child Play: Descriptions and Implications*. Albany, NY: State University Press.
23. Ministry of Health (2007). *Dietary guidelines for children and teenagers.* Singapore.
24. National Association for Sport and Physical Education (NAPE 2002) website. http://www.naspe.com. Accessed 30 August 2006.
25. Neumark-Sztainer, D., Falkner, N., Story, M., Perry, C., Hannan, P.J. & Mulert, S. (2002). Weight-teasing among adolescents: correlations with weight status and disordered eating behaviours. *International Journal of Obesity and Related Metabolic Disorders, 26,* 123-131.
26. Oliver, M., Schofield, G. M., & Kolt, G. S. (2007). Physical activity in preschoolers: Understanding prevalence and measurement issues. *Sports Medicine, 37,* 1045 – 1070.
27. Quek, T. (2002, 3 May, pp. H3). Software invention: get weekly tips on your PDA. *The Straits Times.*
28. Raitakan, O.T, Kimmo, V.K., Porkka, S.T., et al. (1994). Effects of persistent physical activity and inactivity on coronary risk factors in children and young adults: The cardiovascular risk in young Finns study. *American Journal of Epidemiology, 140* (3), 195-205.
29. Reilly, J.J., Penpraze, V., Hislop, J., et al. (2008). Objective measurement of physical activity and sedentary behaviour: review with new data. *Archives of Disease in Childhood, 93,* 614-619.
30. Ridgers, N.D., Stratton, G., & Fairclough, S.J. (2005). Assessing physical activity during recess using accelerometry. *Preventive Medicine, 41,* 102-07.
31. Scruggs, P.W., Beveridge, S. K., Watson, D.L., et al. (2005). Quantifying physical activity in first-through fourth-grade physical education via pedometry. *Research Quarterly for Exercise and Sport, 76,* 166-175.
32. Singapore Heart Foundation website. Retrieved 30, August, 2006 from http://www.shf.org.sg.
33. Smith, D. (1995). How play influences children's development at home and in school. *Journal of Physical Education and Dance, 66,* 19-23.
34. Teo, C.H. (2001). Speech by Minister for Education at the Inaugural CHERISH Award Presentation Ceremony at The Grand Hyatt Hotel. Singapore. 24 August.
35. Trost, S.G., Pate, R.R., Sallis, J.F., Freedson, P.S., et al. (2002). Age and gender differences in objectively measured physical activity in youth. *Medicine and Science in Sports and Exercise, 34,*350-355

36. Tudor-Locke, C., Lee, S.M., Morgan, C.F., Beighle, A, & Pangrazi, R.P. (2006). Children's pedometer-determined physical activity during the segmented school day. *Medicine and Science in Sports and Exercise, 38,* 1732-1738.
37. Tudor-Locke, C., Pangrazi, R.P., Corbin, C.B., et al. (2004). BMI-referenced standards for recommended pedometer-determined steps/day in children. *Preventive Medicine, 38,* 857–864.
38. United Nations High Commission for Human Rights General Assembly Resolution 44/25, 1989.
39. Wang J., Quek, J.J., Chia, M., et al. (2005). HealthTrek Information Tracking System (HITS): Examining the effectiveness of a portable health-enabling device in adults and children. *Journal of Asian Society for Physical Education & Sport, 2,* 53-57.
40. Wang, J., Chia, M., Quek, J.J., et al. (2006). Patterns of Physical Activity, Sedentary Behaviours and Psychological Determinants of Physical Activity among Singaporean School Children. *Journal of Sport and Exercise Psychology, 4,* 227-249.
41. Wangye, Y. & Chia, M. (2008). Every step counts: school physical activity during physical education and recess in a primary school in Singapore. In: *Innovative Physical Education and Sports Case Studies in Asia* (pp. 81-100). Lenie De Vries (Ed). Asia-Pacific Programme of Educational Innovation for Development (APEID), UNESCO Bangkok.
42. Welk, G., Differding, J., Thompson, R., Blair, S., Dziura, J. & Hart, P. (2000). The utility of the Digi-Walker step counter to assess daily physical activity patterns. *Medicine & Science in Sports and Exercise, 32,* S481–S488
43. Williams, D.P., Going, B., Lohman, T.G., et al. (1992). Body fatness and risk for elevated blood pressure, total cholesterol and serum lipoprotein ratios in children and adolescents. *Amsterdam Journal of Public Health, 82,* 358-363.

VALIDITY AND RELIABILITY OF OMRON HJ-005 PEDOMETER IN QUANTIFYING FIELD-BASED PHYSICAL ACTIVITY AMONG SINGAPOREAN CHILDREN

YVONNE WANG YE

National University of Singapore, Singapore

MICHAEL CHIA

Physical Education and Sports Science, National Institute of Education, Nanyang Technological University

The purpose of the study was to examine the validity and reliability of the OMRON HJ-005 pedometer in quantifying pupils' physical activity (PA) under ecological school settings. One hundred and twenty-five Primary 2 and 6 children from a primary school in Singapore participated in the study. In the first part of the study, 15 boys and 19 girls were recruited and were randomly allocated to a validity or a reliability group, All subjects were instructed to perform slow walking (4 km/h), brisk walking (6 km/h) and slow jogging (8km/h) on a 240-m athletic track. In the second part of the study, all 125 subjects were randomly assigned to a validity group or a reliability group and physical activity (PA) during a 30-min school physical education (PE) and 30-min recess was evaluated. The validity of the Omron HJ-005 was examined using Pearson correlation, R between pedometer step counts and GT1M ActiGraph accelerometer outcomes. The reliability of the pedometer was calculated by computing intra-class correlation coefficient (ICC) between the two units worn at the waist, on the left and right sides of the body. Pearson correlation, R from the study was 0.850, 0.829 and 0.685, respectively, under 4km/h, 6km/h and 8km/h speed-controlled conditions, 0.819 during PE and 0.703 during recess (all $p<.05$). Reliability ICC was 0.918, 0.812, and 0.876, individually, under 4km/h, 6km/h and 8km/h controlled speed, 0.923 during PE and 0.936 during recess (all $p<.05$). The OMRON HJ-005 pedometer demonstrated promise as a reliable and valid measurement tool for assessing school-based PA in Singaporean children.

1. Introduction

Although most research has focused on adults, it is also well accepted that regular physical activity benefits children and adolescents (Bar-Or, 1995; CDC, 1997; NASPE, 2004). Adequate participation in physical activity during childhood and adolescence is considered essential for good health and for normal growth and development (USDHHS, 1996 & 2000). Research evidence indicates that, among youth, regular physical activity is inversely related to an array of negative health outcomes, including obesity, elevated blood lipids, hypertension, and cigarette smoking, whereas it is positively related to favorable health outcomes such as increased cardiorespiratory fitness, elevated high-density lipoprotein (HDL) cholesterol, increased bone mass, and improved psychological well-being (Boreham & Riddoch, 2001; USDHHS, 1996 & 2000).

Given the potential role of childhood physical activity on health-related fitness phenotypes (Casperson, 1989) and children's normal growth and maturation (Cooper, 1994), there is considerable interest in assessing physical activity in children (Kohl, Fulton, & Casperson, 2000; Welk, Corbin, & Dale, 2000). But methodological issues always require further examination (Montoye, 2000), particularly in children (Welk, Corbin, & Dale, 2000). A variety of methods are used to evaluate PA in children including self-report, behavioral observation, electronic sensors, and indirect measures such as heart rate and physical fitness. There are advantages and disadvantages for each method. Most large-scale, population-based research studies employ self-report measures of physical activity. But self-report measures have limitations as young children are unable to accurately self-report their physical activity (Sirard & Pate, 2001), and many surrogate reports by parents have limited validity (Sallis & Saelens, 2000). Observation has the potential for the most accuracy but the least feasibility as it incurs high cost and may have low acceptability. Indirect measures such as physical fitness correlate to levels of physical activity but do not provide detailed information related to the frequency, intensity, type and duration of physical activity. Heart rate monitoring is also used to measure daily physical activity of children. Its usefulness is limited, however, because factors other than physical activity can cause the heart rate to be elevated such as high temperature or emotional stress (Freedson, 1992; Rowlands, Eston, & Ingledew, 1997).

Electronic motion sensors, namely accelerometers and pedometers have gained international support as a measure for the assessment of physical activity levels of children (Rowlands et al., 1997; Trost, 2001). Compared to accelerometers, pedometers are more popular in children due to their low cost and feasibility and are shown to be reliable and valid in children (Eston, Rowlands, & Ingledew, 1998; Vincent & Sidman, 2003). Pedometers record physical activity as a simple and raw measure of ambulatory movement that is the number of steps taken. Studies using pedometers on children often report that daily steps among children are within a range of 11000 and 16000 (Rowlands, Eston, & Ingledew, 1999).

With the promotion of regular physical activity as a public health priority, it is important that researchers and practitioners have access to precise, yet practical instruments for measuring physical activity in children. Bassett and colleagues (1996) reported that the Yamax DW-500 to be the most accurate pedometer among commercially available instruments, which recorded 100.7% and 100.6% of actual steps under controlled conditions. The Yamax DW-500 is commonly used in applied research (Le Masurier & Tudor-Locke, 2003; Moreau et al., 2001; Swartz et al., 2003; Tudor-Locke, Ainsworth, Thompson, & Matthews, 2002) and its precision is reported as high due to good quality control by the manufacturer. However, the cited brand of pedometer is apparently discontinued. A reasonably-priced pedometer that is available in Singapore is the Omron HJ-005 STEP Pedometer.

The reliability and validity of the electronic pedometer (Omron HJ-005) for the use among Singaporean children within the school context is in need of investigation. To date, there are apparently no relevant data on the application of the cited model of pedometer (Omron HJ-005) in local schools. Therefore, the purpose of this study was to verify whether this model of pedometer (OMRON HJ-005) provided a valid, reliable and objective measure of physical activity among Singaporean pupils in primary school.

2. Method

2.1. *Participants*

In the first part of the study, 15 boys and 19 girls were recruited and randomly allocated to a validity or a reliability group, and were instructed to perform slow walking (4 km/h), brisk walking (6 km/h) and slow jogging (8km/h) on a 240m athletic track. Sixteen of them were from Primary 2 (8 years old) and eighteen were from Primary 6 (12 years old). In the second part of the study, all subjects (n=125) were randomly assigned to a validity group or a reliability group and PA during the 30-min school PE and a 30-min recess were evaluated. The 125 pupils were from two Primary 2 classes (2A & 2C) and two Primary 6 classes (6B & 6D). Ethical approval on experimental and theoretical aspects of the research was sought and was granted from the Ethics Review Committee, Physical Education and Sports Science (PESS) at the National Institute of Education (NIE), Nanyang Technological University (NTU) of Singapore.

2.2. *Data collection*

Before the data collection, ActiLife Software used with the ActiGraph GT1M was initialized and set parameters were adjusted to collect data. A two-second epoch was programmed for the study. Given that children typically perform activity intermittently in short bursts lasting several seconds, traditional 1-min time intervals may be inappropriate and may result in an underestimation of moderate-to-vigorous physical activity (MVPA) (Strath, Brage, & Ekelund, 2005). In recent research using the ActiGraph as a motion sensor among pre-schoolers (Pfeiffer, McIver, Dowda, Almeida, & Pate, 2006) and pre-pubertal children (Baquet et al., 2007), shorter epoch durations were employed and were set at 15 seconds and 2 seconds, respectively. The high-frequency sampling method allowed for valid data collection that is commensurate with primary school pupil's natural physical activity behavior during PE lessons and during recess.

Pupils from the validity group were provided with one pedometer (Omron HJ-005) and one accelerometer (ActiGraph GT1M) and children from the reliability group were given two pedometers (Omron HJ-005). Pedometer(s) bore the same label number as the pupils' school registration number for recording convenience. For the validity group, the Omron HJ-005 pedometer was clipped on the right side of pupil's PE shorts and the accelerometer was secured onto the left side of the shorts, at the waistband. For the reliability group, the two pedometers were clipped on the right and left sides at the shorts at the waistband. All motion sensors were adjusted to be in line with the midline of the left and right thigh. Prior to the distribution, all pedometers were reset to zero and checked for functionality and then sealed to prevent accidental resetting and behavior modification due to feedback. The sensitivity switch remained in the middle (neutral) position at all times. There is no ON/OFF button or screen for reading on the ActiGraph GT1M.

Anthropometric measurements of standing height (SH) and body mass (BM) were measured during a PE session one week prior to the data collection. For the speed-controlled test group, selected pupils were instructed to walk or jog around an athletic track where a distance of 240 m was measured and marked out before the study using marker cones. The study began with participants walking one round of the marked out distance at a pace of 4 km/h, which is equivalent to 3.0 METS or described as moderate-intensity physical activity. Participants then briskly walked for another 240 m at 6 km/h, or equivalent to 5.0 METS and described as moderate-to-vigorous physical activity, before jogging for another 240 m at 8 km/h, which is equivalent to 8.0 METS and described as vigorous intensity physical activity (Ainsworth et al., 2000). Three trained research assistants acted as pacers for each group throughout the three rounds and ensured that the participants maintained the desired steady speed at all times.

During the PE data collection period, and a typical PE lesson was conducted in accordance to the PE curriculum of the school. The activities performed by the pupils during the PE lessons did not require a high level of physical skill and no water sports were included. Table 1 outlines the different contexts of the four PE lessons, when the PA data were collected.

Table 1: Content of PE classes during formal data collection

Class	Lesson content of Physical Education
2A	Ball games and rope skipping
2C	Throwing activity
6B	1.8 km jog or walk
6D	Shuttle run practice

During the 30-min recess, no instructions were given to the children and they were free to play outdoors within the school premises. Rackets, balls and skipping ropes were provided for pupils to use, if they chose to. At the end of each activity, pupils were instructed to sit down and place the pedometers/or accelerometer on the ground. The pedometers were collected by the research assistants, unsealed and the step data were recorded. As this model of ActiGraph GT1M does not bear the ON/OFF button, the start and end time of the data collection period were noted. The readings for each 2-second epoch from the ActiGraph GT1M accelerometer were later downloaded onto a computer and the total readings during the activity were summarized.

2.3. *Statistical analyses*

All analyses were performed using SPSS 13.0 for Windows (SPSS, Inc., Chicago, IL).

The validity of pedometer step counts was assessed by examining the relationship between the Omron HJ-005 and the ActiGraph GT1M output and by inter-class correlations (Pearson Product Moment correlation coefficient). Cohen's guidelines (Cohen, 1988) were used for interpretation purposes, where 0.5 is large, 0.3 is moderate and 0.1 is small. Coefficient of variation (CV) and intra-class correlation coefficient (ICC) were used to indicate the reliability of the two pedometer outputs. In accordance with the standards for evaluating ICC (Baumgartner, Jackson, Mahar, & Rowe, 2003), the following guidelines were used to determine the level of agreement of the ICC calculated for each comparison: a) 0.60-0.79 is low agreement; b) 0.80–0.89 is moderate agreement; and c) ≥0.90 is high agreement.

Bland-Altman plots were used to graphically show the variability in pedometer error scores. In this manner, the mean error score can be illustrated, and the 95 % prediction interval (i.e., 95 % confidence interval for the individual observations) is shown. Individual error scores that have a tight prediction interval around zero signify a more accurate device.

3. Results

The physical characteristics of the primary school pupils were found to be within the normal ranges for Singaporean children using the height-weight chart developed by Ministry of Health and School Health Service of the Ministry of Education. Table 2 presents the physical characteristics for each age and sex of the participants.

There was no statistically significant sex differences in height and body mass ($p>.05$) for each age cohort or Primary level. Based on a two-tailed t-test, there was also no significant difference ($p>.05$) in anthropometric measures between speed-controlled group and all other participants. Thus, the speed-controlled group was considered representative of the total participants with regard to height and body mass.

Throughout the three controlled-speed activities led by the researchers (4km/h normal walking, 6km/h brisk walking and 8km/h jogging), the number of steps detected by the Ormon HJ-005 pedometer at the 3 different speeds was significantly correlated to accelerometer readings (Table 4).

Table 5 shows that pedometer steps (right) in comparison with pedometer steps (left) and the correlations were moderate to high across all controlled speeds ($ICC \geq 0.812$). Paired t-test was used to determine whether there was any large systematic bias in the number of pedometer counts recorded between two motion sensors. There was no statistical difference between two pedometers output ($p=0.457$). Hence, the mean of right and left pedometer output were used for further analysis.

The correlation between pedometer and accelerometer became weaker as the walking/jogging speed increased. The correlations were considered 'Large' using Cohen's guideline to examine the relationship using Pearson Product Moment. The reliability between the right and left pedometer output was less consistent, in relation to when there was an increase in locomotion speed. Normal walking (4km/h) achieved the highest correlations, while jogging was slightly higher than brisk walking. The reliability of the pedometer under 4km/h walking was considered high and the other two speeds were categorized as moderate using Cronbach's alpha cutoffs (Baumgartner et al., 2003).

Interclass correlation coefficient was 0.819 for 56 validity group participants during PE and 0.703 for 55 during recess. Both were considered statistically significant (see Table 6). Correlation during the PE lesson was slightly higher than during recess.

Table 7 shows that pedometer steps (right) in comparison with pedometer steps (left) were in high agreement during PE and recess ($ICC \geq 0.923$). Paired t-test indicated no significant side-to-side differences during PE and during recess ($p>.05$), so the means of left and right data were used to evaluate steps from the reliability group (which have two pedometers) during PE and during recess. The Coefficient of Variation (CV) during PE was 28.20 % (1766.26±498.12) and the CV during recess was 39.38 % (1269.39±499.84). Hence there was larger variation in step counts during children's activity at recess compared to at PE.

Table 2: Physical characteristics of the participants (N = 125). Data are Mean ± SD

	Primary 2		Primary 6		Combined	
	Boys (N=30)	Girls (N=28)	Boys (N=30)	Girls (N=37)	Primary 2	Primary 6
Stature (cm)	122.63±4.90	122.25±7.08	146.60±8.25	148.43±7.53	122.45±6.00	147.61±7.85
Body mass (kg)	26.65±6.72	24.25±5.30	42.33±12.57	41.49±12.41	25.49±6.14	41.86±12.39

The 34 pupils who were randomly selected from the 125 pupils to form the controlled-speed group have their height and body mass summarized in Table 3.

Table 3: Physical characteristics of speed-controlled group (N =34). Data are Mean ± SD

	Primary 2		Primary 6		Combined	
	Boys (N=7)	Girls (N=9)	Boys (N=8)	Girls (N=10)	P 2 (N=16)	P 6 (N=18)
Height (cm)	123.86±2.67	120.44±4.28	143.38±8.52	147.70±7.93	121.94±3.96	145.78±8.25
Body mass (kg)	2501±3.93	22.41±3.36	35.14±10.02	38.99±9.52	23.55±3.74	37.28±9.65

Table 4: Pearson Correlation between pedometer steps and accelerometer recorded counts during speed-controlled activities

Speed (km/h)	N	Pedometer steps (Mean ±S.D.)	Accelerometer counts (Mean ±S.D.)	R of correlation (N=17)	P
4	17	460.00±60.99	9374.06±1899.24	0.850	<0.05
6	17	361.53±28.99	9875.47±2316.04	0.829	<0.05
8	17	303.94±26.69	11774.65±1807.15	0.685	<0.05

Table 5: Intraclass correlation coefficient (ICC) and dependent t-test for pedometers (right & left) during speed-controlled test

Speed (km/h)	N	Pedometer right (Mean±S.D.)	Pedometer left (Mean±S.D.)	Mean steps of right and left (Mean±S.D.)	ICC (N=17) (95% CI)	P of ICC	P of paired t test (right vs. left)
4	17	440.65±64.60	442.65±66.38	441.65±62.96	0.918 (0.773-0.970)	<0.05	0.822
6	17	363.59±31.13	373.76±48.14	368.68±31.18	0.812 (0.480-0.932)	<0.05	0.212
8	17	284.53±33.89	281.88±28.24	283.21±29.42	0.876 (0.658-0.955)	<0.05	0.605

Table 6: Pearson Correlation between pedometer steps and accelerometer recorded counts during PE & recess

Content	Pearson Correlation		
	N	r	P
PE	56	0.819	<0.05
Recess	55	0.703	<0.05

Table 7: Intra-class correlation coefficient and dependent t-test for pedometers (right & left) during 30-min PE &30-min recess

Content	N	Pedometer right (Mean±S.D.)	Pedometer left (Mean±S.D.)	Mean steps of the right and left (Mean±S.D.)	CV% (S.D./ Mean)	R (N=17) (95% CI)	P	P of paired t test (right vs. left)
PE	52	1747.33±511.53	1814.04±544.18	1766.26±498.12	28.20%	0.923 (0.866-0.956)	<0.05	0.397
Recess	58	1278.64±488.19	1260.14±541.62	1269.39±499.84	39.38%	0.936 (0.892-0.962)	<0.05	0.580

Figures 1-5 display Bland-Altman plots depicting the reliability of the Omron HJ-005 pedometer under different walking/jogging speed or under PE and recess conditions. The mean difference between right and left pedometer (P1 & P2) and the confidence level (95 % CI) set the limit on the vertical axis against the average of two ratings on the horizontal axis. The solid horizontal line is the mean difference score, and dashed lines represent the 95 % prediction intervals. Table 8 provides descriptive data for the Bland-Altman plots. Among three speed-controlled activities, the pedometer reliability under 4km/h normal walking showed the tightest prediction around mean and thus the highest agreement was demonstrated. Reliability indicators showed similar plot distribution under free-living conditions compared to speed-controlled.

Table 8: Descriptive data for Bland-Altman plots

Speed or conditions	(Right+Left)/2	Mean of (Right-Left)	S. D of (Right-Left)	95% Confidence Intervals of mean difference
4km/h	441.65	-2.00	36.13	(-74.26, 70.26)
6km/h	368.68	-10.18	32.28	(-74.74, 54.38)
8km/h	283.21	2.65	20.71	(-38.77, 44.07)
PE	1780.68	-66.71	282.55	(-631.81,498.39)
Recess	1269.39	18.5	252.96	(-487.42, 524.42)

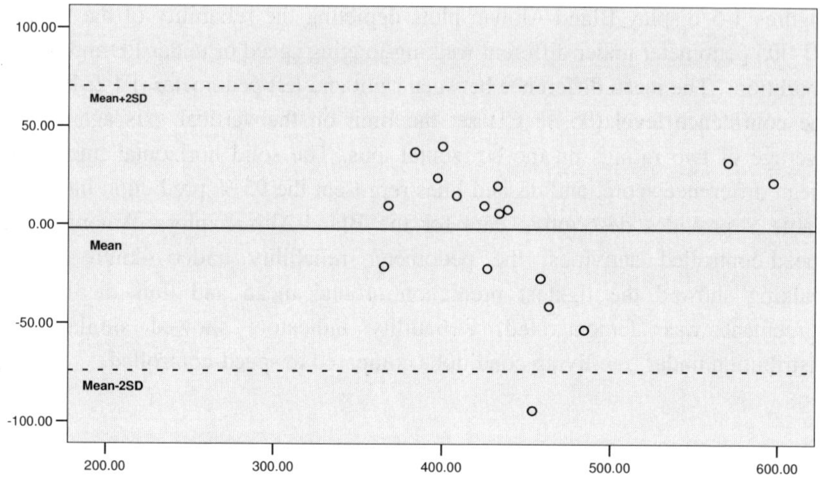

Figure 1: Bland-Altman plots for Omron HJ-005 pedometers with speed of 4km/h

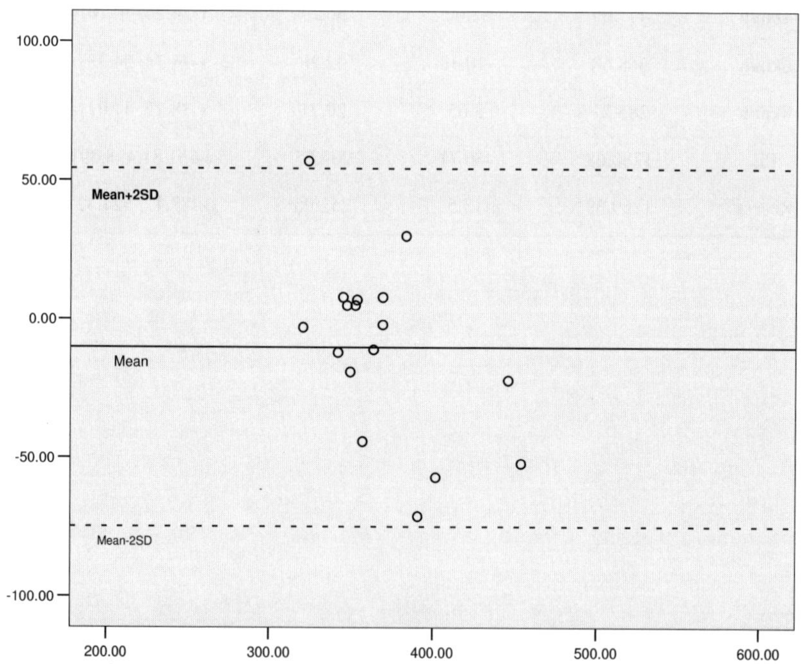

Figure 2: Bland-Altman plots for Omron HJ-005 pedometers with speed of 6km/h

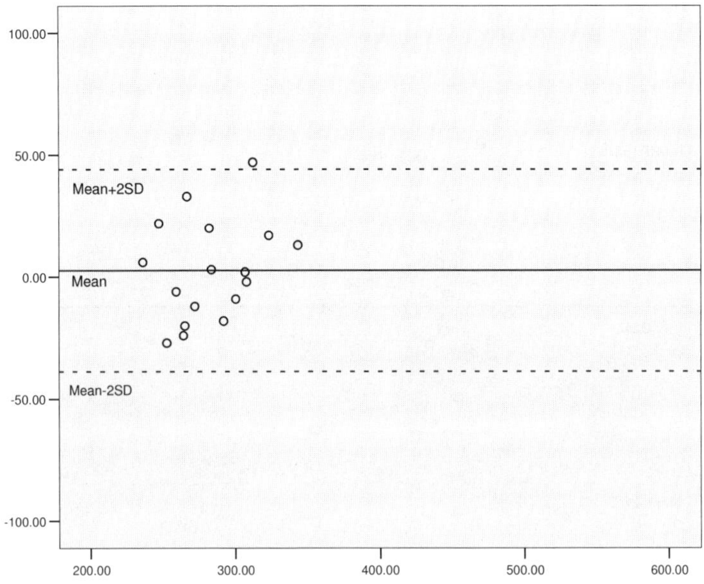

Figure 3: Bland-Altman plots for Omron HJ-005 pedometers with speed of 8km/h

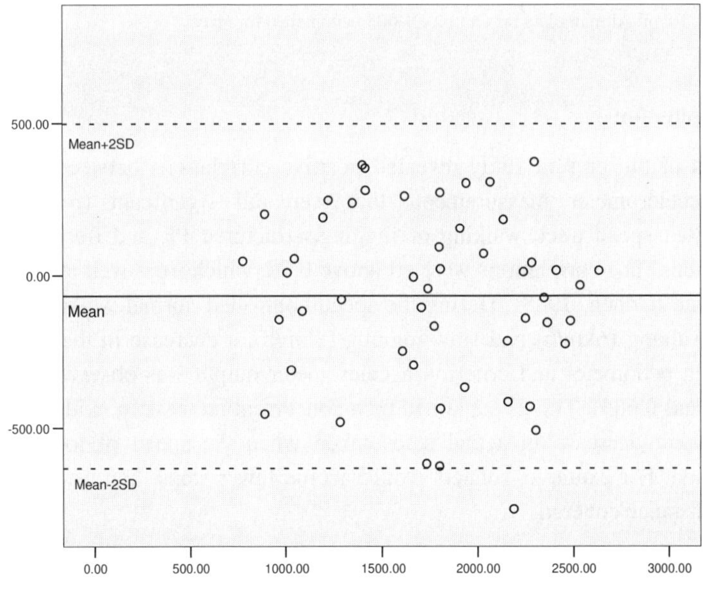

Figure 4: Bland-Altman plots for Omron HJ-005 pedometers for PE

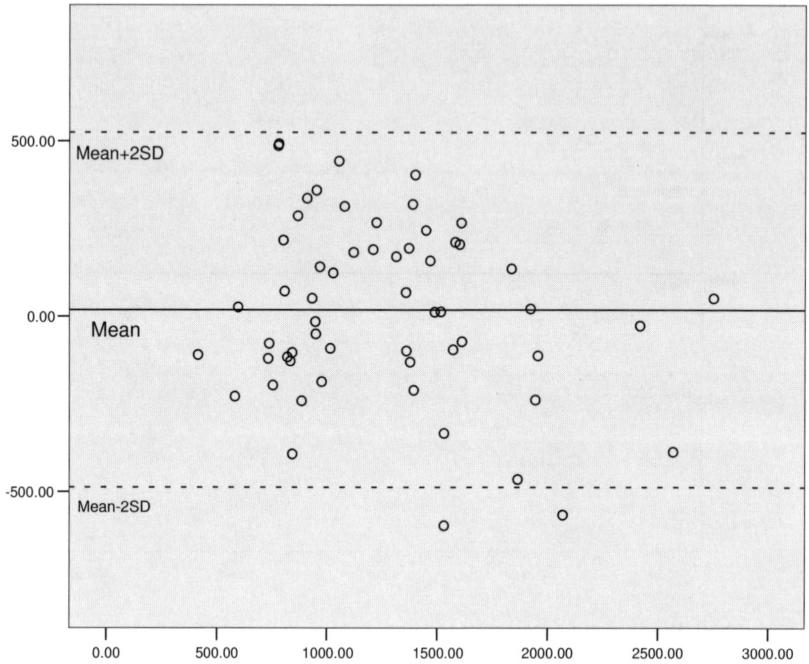

Figure 5: Bland-Altman plots for Omron HJ-005 pedometers for recess

4. Discussion

Results of the present study revealed positive correlations between pedometer and accelerometer measurements that were all significant ($p<.05$) under controlled speed track walking or jogging, structured PE and free-play recess conditions. The correlations were all above 0.70, which were well above the 0.5 guideline (Cohen, 1988). During the speed-controlled normal walking (4km/h), brisk walking (6km/h) and slow jogging (8km/h), a decrease in the association between pedometer and criterion accelerometer output was observed (r=0.850, 0.829 and 0.685). This is explained by a concurrent increase in stride length and subsequent decrease in actual steps taken when the speed of locomotion is increased. For example, runners would accrue fewer steps than walkers for the same distance covered.

Pedometers are designed to register steps in the vertical direction and thus fewer steps are expected if the speed increases. However, the accelerometer is designed to capture body movements in terms of acceleration, which is directly proportional to the muscular forces generated and is related to energy expenditure (Melanson & Freedson, 1996; Montoye et al., 1996). Accelerometer output tends to increase as physical activity become more vigorous.

The results of the speed-controlled walk/jog showed that pedometer steps correlates better with accelerometer counts under moderate intensity activity (normal walking or brisk walking) than with vigorous activity (jogging). There is apparently little field-based speed-controlled validity research. In Jago's et al. (2006) study which involved a similar age-group subjects (10-15 years old boys) and under a similar pacing conditions (4.83 km/h normal walking, equivalent to 3 METs; 6.44 km/h brisk walking, equivalent to 5 METs; 8km/h running, equivalent to 8 METs), New Lifestyles Digiwalker (SW-200) demonstrated a positive association (r=0.60) with the MTI Actigraph when an ordinary least squares regression model was used. As different statistical methodologies were employed across the cited study and the present one, a direct comparison of the two study results is not convenient.

In the second part of the validity study, results showed that the relationship between accelerometer and pedometer was similar during taught PE (r=0.819) but were much lower during recess (r=0.703). The activity patterns for most children during their recess is irregular with brief bursts of moderate or high intensity physical activity in combination with periods of low intensity activity or sedentary activity (Gilliam, Freedson, Geenen & Shahraray, 1981; Sallo & Silla, 1997). Direct observation by the research assistants confirmed the statements cited. A likely explanation for the relative inaccuracy of the magnetic-levered pedometers is that at low intensity or sedentary activity during recess, the vertical movement at the hip may be insufficient in magnitude to cause the glass cylinder to touch the level, which will normally result in a step being counted. For example, Tudor-Locke et al. (2002) recently demonstrated that the Yamax SW-2000, which requires a force of 0.35 g to register a step, significantly under-counted steps, as compared to an accelerometer with a sensitivity of 0.30 g. Hence, it is probable that the lever-arm pedometers may not be detecting steps taken at lower intensity activity due to a reduced level of sensitivity compared to accelerometers. The present results are consistent with other investigation in free-living conditions (Bassett, 2000; Chia, 2005; Leenders et al., 2000; Rowlands & Easton, 2005; Treuth et al., 2003; Tudor-Locke, Williams, Reis, & Pluto, 2002), the relationship between accelerometer and pedometer values was in the range of reported values (from 0.47 to 0.90).

The present result showed that pedometer had a substantial degree of internal consistency reliability with strong intra-class correlations between two units of the same model on the right and left side of the body. Under controlled speed-conditions, ICC across the three activities was from 0.812 to 0.918, consistent with the results of a similar study by Jago et al. (2006). In agreement with the findings of Jago et al. (2006), the present study showed that there were minor differences between walking and running. This is in contrast with the results of Beets et al. (2005)'s study, which showed that agreement between right and left placements of motion sensors increased as treadmill speed increased. Moreover a calibration study with a larger number of subjects is required to confirm the association with increasing speed and output reliability. Compared to other studies using Omron products on a motor-driven treadmill where the ICC was reported as 0.83 for Omron HJ-105 at various walking speeds (3.2km/h, 4km/h, 4.8 km/h, 5.6km/h and 6.4 km/h) (Crouter et al., 2003) and 0.991 for HJ-105 with self-paced walking (averaged speed of 5.8 km/h) (Schneider et al., 2003), the established reliability of step counts derived by the Omron HJ-005 is more than satisfactory.

During PE and recess (free-living and variable conditions), the reliability coefficients between the right and left hip were similar and were as high as when they were established under the controlled speed condition. This supports the results published by Barfield et al. (2004) where they studied elementary (3rd through 5th grade) pupils under classroom, recess and PE conditions. They reported high reliability indicators (above 0.92) and also no obvious differences observed in reliability between structured (PE) and unstructured (recess) activity mode in terms of ICC. The findings of the present study therefore reinforce the reliability of the pedometer output across varying intensity levels.

5. Conclusion

Validity and reliability are theoretical concepts used to describe the quality of a measurement instrument. Researchers and practitioners require evidence of both to justify measurement approaches for surveillance, screening, programme evaluation, and intervention. The first part of the study was designed under speed-controlled walk or jog conditions on a school outdoor track and the second part was conducted during school PE and recess conditions. The high correlation between the pedometer and the accelerometer and between two pedometers on the opposite sides of the body indicated that the Omron HJ-005 is an accurate and reliable measurement tool that can be used to quantify children's physical activity during speed-controlled walk/jog, structured PE and unstructured recess conditions. Importantly, the validity and reliability measures were taken in the context of normal school-based activities, thereby heightening the ecological validity and reliability of the study. Additional research is needed with larger sample sizes and across more varied school conditions to ensure the generalizability of the results to other populations, increase the power of the statistical analyses, and improve the stability of the correlations.

References

1. Ainsworth, B.E., Bassett, D.R. Jr, Strath, S.J., Swartz, A.M., O'Brien, W.L., Thompson, R.W. et al. (2000). Comparison of three methods for measuring the time spent in physical activity. *Medicine& Science in Sport & Exercise, 32*(9 suppl): S457-464.
2. Baquet, G., Stratton, G., Van Praagh, E., & Berthoin, S. (2007). Improving physical activity assessment in prepubertal children with high-frequency accelerometry monitoring: A methodological issue. *Preventive Medicine, 44*:143-147.
3. Bar-Or, O. (1995). Health benefits of physical activity during childhood and adolescence. *President's Council on Physical Fitness and Sports Research Digest, 2*(4): 1-5.
4. Barfield, J.P., Rowe, D.A., & Michael, T.J. (2004). Interinstrument consistency of the Yamax Digi-Walker pedometer in elementary school-aged children. *Measurement in Physical Education and Exercise Science, 8*(2): 109-116.
5. Bassett, D.R. Jr. et al. (1996). Accuracy of five electronic pedometers for measuring distance walked. *Medicine& Science in Sports & Exercise, 28*(8): 1071-1077.
6. Bassett, D.R. Jr., Cureton, A.L., & Ainsworth, B.E. (2000). Measurement of daily walking distance-questionnaire versus pedometer. *Medicine& Science in Sports & Exercise, 32*(5):1018-1023.
7. Baumgartner, T. A., Jackson, A. S., Mahar, M. T., & Rowe, D. A. (2003). *Measurement for evaluation. in physical education and exercise science* (7th ed.). Boston: McGraw-Hill.
8. Beets, M.W., Patton, M.M., & Edwards, S. (2005). The accuracy of pedometer steps and time during walking in children. *Medicine & Science in Sports & Exercise, 37*(3): 513-520.
9. Boreham, C. & Riddoch, C. (2001). The physical activity, fitness and health of children. *Journal of Sports Science, 19*: 915-929.

10. Caspersen, C.J. (1989). Physical activity epidemiology: concepts, methods, and applications to exercise science. *Exercise Science and Sport Science Reviews, 17*:423-473.
11. Centers for disease control and prevention. (1996). *Guidelines for nutrition for adolescents.* Atlanta.
12. Chia, Y.H.M., Wang, J. & Quek, J.J. (2005). Measures of reliability and validity of school-based pedometer step count of Singaporean children. *Asian Journal of Exercise & Sports Sciences, 1* (2), 17-24.
13. Cohen, J. (1988). *Statistical power analysis for the behavioral sciences.* (3rd ed.). New York: Academic Press.
14. Cooper, D.M. (1994). Evidence for and mechanisms of exercise modulation of growth: an overview. *Medicine & Science in Sports & Exercise, 26*(6):733-740.
15. Crouter, S.E., Schneider, P.L., Karabulut, M., & Bassett, D.R. Jr (2003). Validity of 10 electronic pedometers for measuring steps, distance, and energy cost. *Medicine& Science in Sports & Exercise, 35*(8): 1455-1460.
16. Eston, R.G., Rowlands, A.V., & Ingledew, D.K. (1998). Validity of heart rate, pedometry, and accelerometry for predicting the energy cost of children's activity. *Journal of Applied Physiology, 84*(1): 362-371.
17. Freedson, P.S. (1992). Physical activity among children and youth. *Canadian journal of Sports Science, 17*(4): 280-283.
18. Gilliam, T.B., Freedson, P.S., Geenen, D.L., & Shahraray, B. (1981). Physical activity patterns determined by heart rate monitoring in 6-7-year-old children. *Medicine & Science in Sports & Exercise, 13*:65-67.
19. Jago, R., Watson, K., Baranowski, T., Zakeri, I., Yoo, S., Baranowski, J., et al. (2006). Pedometer reliability, validity and daily activity targets among 10- to 15-year-old boys. *Journal of Sports Science, 24*(3):241-251.
20. Kohl, H.W., Fulton, J.E., & Casperson, C.J. (2000). Assessment of physical activity among children and adolescents: a review and synthesis. *Preventive Medicine, 31*(2):S54-S76.
21. Le Masurier, G.C., & Tudor-Locke, C. (2003). Comparison of pedometer and accelerometer accuracy under controlled conditions. *Medicine& Science in Sports & Exercise, 35*(5): 867-871.
22. Leenders, N.Y., Sherman, W.M., & Nagaraja, H.N. (2000). Comparisons of four methods of estimating physical activity in adult women. *Medicine & Science in Sports & Exercise, 32*(7):1320-1326.
23. Melanson, E.L. Jr, & Freedson, P.S. (1996). Physical activity assessment: a review of methods. *Critical Review in Food Science and Nutrition, 36*(5): 385-396.
24. Montoye, H.J. (2000). Introduction: evaluation of some measurements of physical activity and energy expenditure. *Medicine & Science in Sports & Exercise, 32* (suppl 9): S439-S441.

25. Montoye, H.J., Kemper, H.C.G., Saris, W.H.M., et al. (1996). *Measuring physical activity and energy expenditure*. Champaign (IL): Human Kinetics.
26. Moreau, K.L., Degarmo, R., Langley, J., McMahon, C., Howley, E.T., Bassett, D.R. Jr, et al. (2001). Increasing daily walking lowers blood pressure in postmenopausal women. *Medicine& Science in Sports & Exercise, 33*(11): 1825-1831.
27. National Association for Sports and Physical Education. (2004). *Guidelines for Appropriate Physical Activity for Elementary School Children: Update 2004*. Reston, VA: National Association of Physical Education and Sports.
28. Pfeiffer, K.A., McIver, K.L., Dowda, M., Almeida, M.J., Pate, R.R. (2006). Validation and calibration of the Actical accelerometer in preschool children. *Medince & Science in Sports & Exercise, 38*(1):152-157.
29. Rowlands, A.V., & Eston, R.G. (2005). Comparison of accelerometer and pedometer measures of physical activity in boys and girls, ages 8-10 years. *Research Quarterly for Exercise and Sport, 76*(3):251-257.
30. Rowlands, A.V., Eston, R.G., & Ingledew, D.K. (1997). Measurement of physical activity in children with particular reference to the use of heart rate and pedometry. *Sports Medicine, 24*(4):258-272.
31. Rowlands, A.V., Eston, R.G., & Ingledew, D.K. (1999). Relationship between activity levels, aerobic fitness, and body fat in 8- to 10-yr-old children. *Journal of Applied Physiology, 86*(4):1428-1435.
32. Sallis, J.F., & Saelens, B.E. (2000). Assessment of physical activity by self-reports: status, limitations, and future directions. Research *Quarterly for Exercise and Sport, 71*(2 Suppl):S1-14.
33. Sallo, M., & Silla, R. (1997). Physical activity with moderate to vigorous. intensity in preschool and first grade schoolchildren. *Pediatric Exercise Science, 4*:44-54.
34. Schneider, P.L., Crouter, S.E., Lukajic, O., & Bassett, D.R. Jr. (2003). Accuracy and reliability of 10 pedometers for measuring steps over a 400-m walk. *Medicine& Science in Sports & Exercise, 35* (10): 1779-1784.
35. Sirard, J.R., & Pate, R.R. (2001). Physical activity assessment in children and adolescents. *Sports Medicine, 31*(6):439-454.
36. Strath, S.J., Brage, S., & Ekelund, U. (2005). Integration of physiological and accelerometer data to improve physical activity assessment. *Medicine & Science in Sports & Exercise, 37*(11 Suppl):S563-571.
37. Swartz, A.M., Strath, S.J., Bassett, D.R., Moore, J.B., Redwine, B.A., Groer, M., et al. (2003). Increasing daily walking improved glucose tolerance in overweight women. *Preventive Medicine, 37*(4):356-362.
38. Treuth, M.S., Sherwood, N.E., Baranowski, T., Butte, N.F., Jacobs, D.R. Jr, McClanahan, B., et al. (2003). Validity and reliability of activity measures in African-American girls for GEMS. *Medicine& Science in Sports & Exercise, 35*(3): 532-539.

39. Trost, S.G. (2001). Objective measurement of physical activity in youth: current issues, future directions. *Exercise and Sports Science Review, 29*(1): 32-36.
40. Tudor-Locke, C., Jones, R., Myers, A.M., Paterson, D.H., & Ecclestone, N.A. (2002). Contribution of structured exercise class participation and informal walking for exercise to daily physical activity in community-dwelling older adults. *Research Quarterly for Exercise and Sport, 73*(3):350-356.
41. Tudor-Locke, C., Williams, J.E., Reis, J.P., & Pluto, D. (2002). Utility of pedometers for assessing physical activity: convergent validity. *Sports Medicine, 32*(12):795-808.
42. U. S. Department of Health and Human Services. (1996). *Physical activity and health: a report of the Surgeon General.National Center for Chronic Disease Prevention,* Atlanta.
43. U. S. Department of Health and Human Services. (2000). *Healthy people 2010: National health promotion and disease prevention objectives.* Washington, DC: Author.
44. Vincent, S.D., & Sidman, C.L. (2003). Determining measurement error in digital pedometers. *Measurement in Physical Education and Exercise Science, 7*: 19-24.
45. Welk, G.J., Corbin, C.B., & Dale, D. (2000). Measurement issues in the assessment of physical activity in children. *Research Quarterly for Exercise and Sport, 71* (2 Suppl):S59-S73.

YOUNG CHILDREN'S MOTOR SKILL DEVELOPMENT IN OUTDOOR EXPERIENCES

KAREN PHILOMENA NONIS

Early Childhood and Special Needs Education, National Institute of Education, Nanyang Technological University, Singapore

JERNICE TAN SING YEE

National Institute of Education, Nanyang Technological University, Singapore

Many studies show how physical activities can affect fundamental motor skills as well as how fundamental motor performance can also influence the participation of sports and physical activities. Parents' and/or guardians' perception of motor skills development is equally important for the interest and participation in sports and physical activities by young children. This chapter provides an overview of the development of motor skills of young children in the Asia-Pacific region with a focus on recent research in Singapore. A portion of the paper addresses research on preference and performance, and how these affect young children's motor performance. The importance of outdoor physical experiences and the constraints of space, and the implications for children's sports and physical experiences in Singapore are discussed.

1. Introduction

It is not new to early childhood educators that the learning and development of motor skills develops the young child holistically from the cognitive, the social and emotional to the physical phases of development (Bjorklund & Brown, 1998; Diamond, 2000; Nonis & Daswani, 2007). While the majority of young children develop the fundamental motor skills such as running, skipping and hopping, it is becoming more apparent that some of them do not show mastery of these skills as they get older (Tan & Nonis, 2008; Wong & Cheung, 2006). Consequently, researchers recommend that motor skills be included into the overall repertoire of young children's movement programmes at the early nursery classes so that more children can have increased opportunities for motor skills development at an earlier age (Gabbard, 2000; Nonis, Parker & Larkin, 2004).

The lack of daily physical activities as part of the young child's daily routine is linked to the higher occurrence of childhood obesity seen in children in the past 10 years and the incidence of childhood overfatness continues to threaten the future health of the nation (Chia, 2007ab; Chua, 2001). Chua (2001), for example, reported that in 1997, 12% of Singapore children aged six to 16 years were obese based on a weight-for-height chart. The advantages of physical activities are not limited to fitness and health-related benefits alone. Young children's active involvement in daily physical activities at a young age allows them to explore not only their movement abilities but also the interactions allow them to develop new friendships that sometimes last over a lifetime. Through physical play, children are exposed to opportunities to enhance their motor skills which promote physical growth (Gallahue & Donnelly, 2003; Gallahue & Ozmun, 2006). Further, young children learn socially acceptable behaviours. In this way, the young child develops positive self esteem, pro-social attitudes and behaviours, problem solving skills and discipline. Developing social and emotional competence equip the young child to cope with lifelong challenges (Mackenzie, 2007).

Physical growth and motor behaviour form a significant part of developing the child as a whole. Whole child development encompasses cognitive, physical, language, social and emotional domains. The following sections will discuss whole child development from the perspective of the physical.

2. The importance of motor and physical development to whole child development

Adults visualise movements of infants and toddlers as non-verbal communication and can use this communication channel to monitor their progress in developmental milestones. This is especially so for infants who often cannot express themselves accurately or clearly through verbal communication but use movements as their primary means of communication (Wang, 2004). The sensitive learning period during fundamental motor stage is important as it establishes the foundation for specialized movement abilities in later years (Gabbard, 2000; Payne & Isaacs, 1995). Without the mastery of fundamental motor skills, young children may fail to participate in physical activities actively due to their inability to perform skills such as jumping and hopping. Therefore, providing foundation for fundamental motor skills is essential to maximize their potential and/or future participation in sports (Benelli & Yongue, 1995; Ignico, 1994; Nonis, 2005; Wang, 2004).

While some motor development theorists believe that young children will progress and improve their motor skills based on individual differences or physical maturation (Gesell, 1928; McGraw, 1935), modern theorists (Gallahue & Ozmun, 2006; Thelen & Smith, 1994) and researchers (Benelli & Yongue, 1995; Fisher, et al., 2005; Garcia & Garcia, 2006; Ignico, 1994; Nonis, 2005; Wang, 2004) emphasize the importance of mastering fundamental motor skills through environmental stimulation such as movement education and/or sports activities during early childhood to nurture children's full potential in motor performance. Both individual maturation and movement stimulation are important factors affecting motor performance.

The traditional view of how the brain and muscles worked was simply the body responded to the brain's instructions (Lockman & Thelen, 1993). Development of motor skills was thought to be primarily a result of maturation (Bushnell & Boudreau, 1993). However, Diamond's study (2000) examining motor and cognitive development suggests that they may be interrelated. Through movement, young children learn about their bodies and movement capabilities and develop fine and gross motor skills which then facilitate cognitive growth. While Piaget (1952) believed that cognitive abilities were developed through the interaction with the environment, Diamond (2000) further explained that the overall cognitive development can be established through the coordination of bodily movements and brain synapses.

When young children play alone or with friends, they develop personality traits described as spontaneous, humorous, curious, active and imaginative. Language, social and cognitive skills tend to develop next as they are involved in divergent play and critical thinking. Research show that playfulness and motor creativity are interconnected as movement during preschool age is the primary way of action, expression, learning and development (Trevlas, Matsouka & Zachopoulou, 2003). In this way, the young child develops positive self esteem, pro-social attitudes and behaviours, problem solving skills and discipline. In addition, through play, young children will develop social and emotional competence to equip the young child to cope with lifelong challenges (Mackenzie, 2007).

3. The development of children's fundamental motor skills

Infant independent walking can be expected between the ages of nine *and* 15 months (Gallahue & Ozmun, 2006). Observed during the Rudimentary Movement Phase (RMP, 0 – 2 years old), independent walking continues along the development of other fundamental motor skills during the Fundamental Motor Phase (FMP, 2 – 7 years old) with increasing proficiency, which is described as a well-coordinated gait in independent walking observed at the mature stage (Hennessy, Dixon & Simon, 1984). As the young child approaches two years old, she moves into what is called the FMP (Gallahue & Ozmun, 2006). Unlike in RMP, the young child makes voluntary movements in response to various stimuli in the environment during the FMP. The FMP is considered as building blocks to later more specialise movement skills for future sports participation.

The quality of fundamental motor skills such as running, galloping, hopping, jumping, single leg hopping, skipping throwing, catching, rolling and bouncing a ball can be seen developing along a range of stages within the FMP (Gallahue & Donnelly, 2003; Gallahue & Ozmun, 2006). For example, at the initial stage of running, the young child will often fall, which gradually improves as they move into the elementary stage with better balance control and coordination. By the mature stage, young children can be expected to run skilfully such that they are able to anticipate obstacles (Tan & Nonis, 2008; Wong & Cheung, 2006).

In Wong & Cheung's study (2006) of Hong Kong Chinese young children (692 boys, 559 girls) aged three to 10 years using the Test of Gross Motor Development, Version 2 (TGMD-2, Ulrich, 2000; Locomotor skills: hop, slide, gallop, jump, leap, run; Object Control skills: dribble, kick, catch, throw, roll, strike) revealed that there was a gradual increase in scores with age for both males and females for both tests. Further, these young children attained mastery levels in the run and kicking task as they attained full marks. The researchers reported that the skill of hopping was the most underdeveloped locomotor skill and that young children found throwing as the most difficult upper limb task (Wong & Cheung, 2006).

This is similar to other research on young children's hopping (Choi Tsu, 2004; Nonis et al., 2004; Parker, Monson & Larkin, 1993; Williams, 1983). The task of single leg hopping is a difficult task that requires the young child to take off and land on the same foot with a good control of dynamic balance. Similar to Wong and Cheung (2006), Nonis et al. (2004) study of 40 girls (4.5 – 7.5 years, and adults) hopping on the preferred and non-preferred limbs showed that as age increased, not all components of actions (leg and arm actions, balance control, trunk lean and foot landing style) had regressions to lower proficiency levels when hopping on the non-preferred leg. Younger children were at lower developmental levels while older children were at higher developmental levels, on the hopping task. Further, adults were significantly different from the youngest children (4.5 year olds) in the proficiency of leg and arm actions and trunk lean. The majority of the 4.5 year olds had the least balance control ("uncontrolled", Nonis et al., 2004).

When referring to baby walker users (BWU), Tan and Nonis (2008) reported that young children, within a Singapore population sampled (N = 14; Mean age = 49 months), did not attain the mastery of hop and leap skills. Leaping is another fundamental motor skill that requires balance control. When children leap they need to transfer their weight from one foot to the other while being in mid-air (flight; Nonis, 2007). When compared with the TGMD-2 norm population (Ulrich, 2000), toddlers continued to show poorer overall performance for leap and hop tasks only (Tan & Nonis, 2008). The authors suggest that the performance criteria of the TGMD-2 requires the participant to hop three consecutive times on both right and left foot and may be related to the proficiency of limb performance and preference suggested in other research (Armitage & Larkin, 1993; Nonis, Larkin & Parker, 2006; Nonis & Parker, 2005; Nonis et al., 2004).

More recently, a mixed-longitudinal study, tracing the development of Singapore-born young children of age range from four to six years (N = 65; Nonis, Chia & Quek, manuscript in preparation, 2010abc; Nonis & Chia, 2008) using the TGMD-2, revealed that there was a wide gap between children's Gross Motor Quotient (GMQ) at age three years. The GMQ is an indicator of young children's overall motor performance. It is the derived summation of the standard scores for both locomotor and object control TGMD-2 subtests (Ulrich, 2000). The authors reported that while the majority of young children in the 3-year-old age group showed overall motor performance ranging from average to very superior (Average = 15%, n = 10; Above average = 11%, n = 7; Superior = 37%, n = 24; Very superior = 25%, n = 16 respectively), seven children performed between below average to very poor performance (Nonis & Chia, 2008). This is not an alarming response given the young age of the children. In relation to the mastery of skills, significantly poorer skill masteries in hop, leap and catch but significantly better skill masteries in horizontal jump, slide, strike a stationary ball, stationary dribble, kick, overhand throw and underhand roll were revealed in the study. Zero mastery in leap and catch was observed in all three age groups (Nonis, Chia & Quek, manuscript in preparation, 2010abc). At age five years, overall young children had made significant progress to higher levels of performance with the largest percentage of Singapore-born young children at Very Superior and Superior (57%, n = 37; 22%, n = 14 respectively; Nonis et al., manuscript in preparation, 2010abc; Nonis & Chia, 2008).

4. Preference and performance in motor skills

From the numerous studies investigating fundamental motor skills, researchers have suggested that young children have a preferred side or limb that they choose to perform motor skills (Armitage & Larkin, 1993; Nonis et al., 2006; Nonis & Parker, 2005; Nonis et al., 2004). How is it that young children come to do this? What underlying neuromuscular systems govern such "natural selection" and in this case, limb selection to perform a given task? Many theories have been proposed to explain the preference and performance of young children's movements and how movement is controlled (Annette, 1991; Bakan, 1971; Corbalis & Beale, 1976; Didia & Nyenwe, 1988; McManus et al., 1988; Peters, 1990; Vanden-Abeele, 1980). The continued interest in how movement is controlled lies in the question if movement specialist should leave young children to use their first choice in their limb selection to perform a task? In the event that young children are left to choose their preferred limb, what would their performance be?

Preference (or Handedness and Footedness) is usually referred to as the limb dominance or sidedness. As a definition, preference is the limb chosen by the child to perform a specific task using the upper or lower limb. While limb preference in adults is established for most tasks, the research shows that young children's limb preference is both task specific and age-dependent (Nonis et al., 2004). For example, a young child may use his or her "chosen hand" to use a fork to eat vegetables, this chosen hand may be the right or the left. The preferred side gradually develops for some tasks while in others such as kicking appears to be established at an early stage of a young child's motor development (Armitage & Larkin, 1993; Nonis, Larkin & Parker, 1996).

Preference can be assessed in terms of the direction (right or left or mixed) or the strength (the consistency of the choice of the limb made to perform any one task). Direction of preference is measured as a right or left on a single trial as in the case of the use of the fork. Research shows that children tend to use their right foot for kicking task when the direction of preference was used (Belmont & Birch, 1963; Nonis, Larkin & Parker, 2006a). However, tasks that involve a large component of balance control tend to somewhat challenge the theoretical support for a right-preferred-world. For example, in hopping, left preference seems to be more common in young children (Larkin & Revie, 1995; Nonis et al., 1996). When two or more trials are used to assess preference, the option to change the direction of preference is thus given to the young child. This measures the consistency of the preference over time (repeated sessions or trials). Assume the task of eating vegetables with a fork that have been placed on a plate in a three-trial-observation, a 17-month-old young child may use his right hand to eat vegetables closer to his right side and swop over to his left hand and then back, to use his right hand. Depending on the criteria established for this observation, the hand preference would be mixed with a tendency to use the right hand (2/3 trials) for the task of holding a fork.

The key word is consistency. The methodology used to classify preference varies and this poses problems when comparisons are made with other studies on limb preference (Coren, 1993; Nonis, 1996). In addition, where the strength of preference is considered, the observations become more complex with increased sessions or trials accorded for each task (Peters & Petrie, 1979; Provins, 1992). The observable change in preference over time (as in the consistency or stability of preference) conducted with repeated sessions in comparison with single session design, suggests that the strength of preference differs from the direction of preference (Gabbard & Hart, 1995). Nonis, Larkin and Parker (2006b), study of 51 girls within the age range of three to six years, showed that strength of preference changed according to the task performed. However, girls consistently used their right leg to kick a stationary and moving ball over time. By comparison, girls changed their preference for the in-place hopping task (Nonis et al., 2006b). Interestingly, the results also showed that there were task groupings. These groupings for the strength of preference demonstrated that kicking (stationary and rolling ball) were similar to pick up (shells) task, pick-up, step-up (bench) and hopping formed another group but separated from balance task as a group. The strength of preference for the balance task was also similar to step-up and hopping tasks (Nonis et al., 2006b). Performance measures in deciding preference is directly linked to the skill level of the task. In this case, the proficiency of the limb performance of the preferred and non-preferred limb is taken into consideration (Nonis et al., 2004; Nonis & Parker, 2005; Nonis & Daswani, 2007).

5. Task affecting preference and performance in children's motor skills

Different motor skills have different demands on young children and as such, may influence preference. Research suggests that given the varying functional demands of each task, young children may perform and express different preference (Peters, 1990; Vanden-Abeele, 1980). This has implications on assessments for not only preference but the overall motor development of young children. Task difficulty would demand different neuromuscular inputs from the young child. Steingrueber (1975) wrote that in a three-level task complexity of dotting to tap-on-squares, left-handedness increased from 6% to 16% as the task became more difficult for the 310 girls and boys tested, aged nine and 10 years. Since functional asymmetries has been hypothesised to underlie foot preference patterns (Peters & Petrie, 1979; Vanden-Abeele, 1980), Nonis et al. (1996) explored the patterns of preference of an operant task – kicking and a postural task – single leg static balance. Over the four sessions, the three-year-olds used their right leg for kicking and 79% of the four-year-olds were right-footed (21% left-footed). The five- and six-year-olds girls (80%) were also right-footed for kicking with 13% of mixed preference (changed their preference). In the postural control task of static balance control, mixed preference was predominantly demonstrated by the three- and four-year-olds girls although a large percentage of the five-and six-year-olds were also mixed preference (67% & 60% respectively, Nonis et al., 1996). These data support the idea that patterns of preference are affected by task and in this case, the operant task (kicking) showed strong right preference while no clear right or left preference was shown for the postural task (single leg static balance).

Limb preference plays an important role at the different stages of motor development as it determines the different levels of motor proficiency as the child grows (Bakan, 1971; Corbalis & Beale, 1976; Didia & Nyenwe, 1988; McManus et al., 1988; Peters, 1990; Vanden-Abeele, 1980). While it is essential to understand how limb preference can influence the individual constraints of young children (Nonis et al., 2004; Nonis & Parker, 2005; Nonis & Daswani, 2007), others stress the environmental influences such as early movement programmes can do for young children's motor skills development (Gabbard, 2000; Nonis, 2005) which highlights the importance of providing for physical play space.

6. Space for children's movement experiences

In recent years, the Government of Singapore has been very active in promoting birth policies. Given the increasing number of live births in the past three years in Singapore (2005 = 37,492; 2006 = 38,317; 2007 = 39,490, Yearbook of Statistics, 2008), the need to provide space for young children's motor development is becoming increasingly urgent. The ideal for whole child development is to provide diverse and varied stimulus to the young child. Thus, outdoor play and physical space are important influential factors in the development of motor control and learning affecting children's potential participation in sports.

Natural landscapes provide young children with opportunities to play hide-and-seek in bushes, climbing slopes, rocky areas and trees, navigating through the outback as in Australia, and trekking on the uneven terrains. Researchers suggest that there is a significant relationship between the diversity of the landscape and its affordances for play (Fjørtoft & Segeie, 2000). This is to say that when young children perceive a high functionality that the environment can offer for play; it does have a functional impact on young children's play behaviour and performance. This physical diversity then increases the opportunities for learning and development, which promotes motor performance and motor fitness. Further, Fjørtoft (2001) suggested that the relationship between versatile play in the natural environment and the impact of motor fitness in young children were found in balance and coordination abilities of the experimental group compared to the control group.

In early childhood education, the outdoor environment is a significant component influencing curriculum design and planning for young children. It allows extended potential to foster whole child development, particularly in physical and motor development. Further, the research suggests that outdoor environments give young children more positive effects such as greater sense of freedom, more creative play and fun (Fjørtoft, 2001), compared to indoor movement experiences in early education settings. Young children can also experience and appreciate nature and interact with the natural elements such as insects, animals and plants during outdoor play (Fjørtoft, 2001).

According to a survey conducted in July 2004 by the Singapore Sports Council (SSC), although 98% (N = 5,467; n = 5,357) of Singaporean parents and/or guardians encouraged their young children (preschoolers aged 3 to 6 years old) to participate in some form of physical activity, 92% (N = 5,283; n = 4,860) and 84 % (N = 5,283; n = 4,437) spent their typical days watching television and playing indoors respectively. The top three reasons for not encouraging children's involvement in physical activities included: afraid of hurting themselves (45.7%), too young to participate (41.9%) and a lack of time to bring them out (41.0%). Given that the survey shows that parents and/or guardians are not predisposed towards nurturing their young children with the outdoors, can we then expect kindergartens and or schools to act differently and to support outdoor play? In general, three-to-six-year-olds schooled in Singapore can be expected to spend approximately thirty minutes in daily outdoor play. In addition, some young children may have two thirty-minute sessions on separate days per week for indoor gym and water play. Whether this is sufficient daily play time for young developing children remains uncertain.

More young children are spending time in sedentary activities such as watching television programmes and playing computer games instead of engaging in physical outdoor activities. Tandy (1999) reported that young Australian children were facing diminishing play spaces not only due to home-based leisure such as computer games, but surprisingly, parents prefer children to stay at home. In comparison, Singapore has fewer natural environments for young children to explore. Further, there is limited physical space within the school for young children to play freely. According to the guidelines given by the Ministry of Education (2008), a minimum of 30 m^2 of indoor physical activity area is allocated for every 10 children.

7. Children's involvement in sports

Given that many researchers support the "sensitive learning period" for the emergence of fundamental motor skills, which builds the foundation for more complex movement abilities in later years (Gabbard, 2000; Gabbard, 2004; Gallahue & Donnelly, 2003; Gallahue & Ozmun, 2006; Payne & Isaacs, 1995), the urgency of children's involvement in movement programmes is apparent. Missing the sensitive learning opportunities may not achieve positive and optimum improvement in motor learning and sports performance. Without the mastery of fundamental motor skills, young children may fail to participate adequately in physical activities. This would inevitably affect motor development during their fundamental stage as well as the later stages of sports performance. Therefore, providing the foundation for fundamental motor skills is essential to maximize children's potential and/or future participation in sports (Benelli & Yongue, 1995; Ignico, 1994; Nonis, 2005; Nonis et al., manuscript in preparation 2010abc; Wang, 2004).

Since gaining independency in 1965, Singapore, a multicultural country, has increasingly put sports as an important role in nation building (Aplin, 2005). To date, many medal-winning athletes who are nurtured in Singapore are not born locally. In supporting youth sports, the Singapore Olympic Academy– the educational arm of the Singapore National Olympic Council (SNOC), organizes annual sessions for trainee teachers of physical education. In addition, hosting international sporting events becomes an important pillar in developing a sporting culture (Aplin, 2005).

In 2010, the first Youth Olympic Games (YOG) will be held in Singapore. In preparation, the Ministry of Community Development, Youth and Sports (MCYS) formed the Singapore2010 team to work with the SNOC. The Singapore2010 set up YOG learning centre for young Singaporeans to discover and experience the spirit of Olympism and to trace Singapore's journey in hosting the first YOG (Singapore2010, 2009). The Singapore Sports Council also plays a role in nurturing a young sporting nation by transforming the way Singaporeans view sports. These include outreach sport programmes, healthy lifestyle marketing, sports promotion and collaborating with other public agencies and private organisations in upgrading sports facilities and making sports as inclusive as it could be (Singapore Sports Council, 2009). In the year 2010, we can expect Singapore to emerge as a vibrant and sport-seeking nation. In doing so, we remain hopeful of the long term effect that YOG will have on parents and/or guardians' and educators' perception toward outdoor activities and sports participation of all young Singaporeans.

8. Conclusion

Early childhood educators and researchers recognize that the learning and development of motor skills educate the young child holistically from the cognitive, the social and emotional to the physical domains (Bjorklund & Brown, 1998; Diamond, 2000; Nonis & Daswani, 2007). Physical growth and motor development provide visible indicators of how the young child is developing through the lifespan. Attention must be paid to limb preference and performance at the different stages of motor development, which show different levels of motor proficiency as the young child grows (Bakan, 1971; Corbalis & Beale, 1976; Didia & Nyenwe, 1988; McManus et al., 1988; Peters, 1990; Vanden-Abeele, 1980). While some theories support the acquisition of motor skills based on maturation (Gesell, 1928; McGraw, 1935), others stress the influence that the environment, and consequently what early movement programmes can do for children's motor skills development (Gabbard, 2000; Nonis, 2005). These include the introduction of versatile outdoor play (Fjørtoft,

2001) in attaining competence and mastery of motor skills, which can enhance more specialised motor movements and/or sport performance in later years. There is a need to educate parents' and/or guardians' and educators' perception of the development of motor skills in promoting young children's participation in sports and physical activities, with an emphasis on the outdoors.

References

1. Annette, M. (1991). Annotation: Laterality and cerebral dominance. *Journal of Child Psychology Psychiatry, 32,* 219-232.
2. Aplin, N. (2005, June 4). Singapore. *Berkshire Encyclopedia of World Sport, 4,* 1376-1378. Retrieved February 6, 2009, from SPORTDiscus with Full Text database.
3. Armitage, M. & Larkin, D. (1993). Laterality, motor asymmetry and clumsiness in children. *Human Movement Science, 12,* 155-177.
4. Bakan, P. (1971). Handedness and birth order. *Nature, 229,* 195.
5. Belmont, L. & Birch, H. G. (1963). Lateral dominance and right-left awareness in normal children. *Child Development, 34,* 257-270.
6. Benelli, C. & Yongue, B. (1995). Supporting young children's motor skill development. *Childhood Education, 71*(4), 217-220.
7. Bjorklund, D. F. & Brown, R. D. (1998). Physical play and cognitive development: Integrating activity, cognitive, and education. *Children Development, 69*(3), 604-606.
8. Bushnell, E. W. & Boudreau, J. P. (1993). Motor development and the mind: The potential role of motor abilities as a determinant of aspects of perceptual development. *Child Development, 64*(4), 1005-1021.
9. Chia, M. (2007a). PRIDE for PLAY: personal responsibility in daily effort for participation in lifelong activity for youths. A Singaporean context. *Journal of Sports Science and Medicine, 6,* 374-379.
10. Chia, M. (2007b). Fit to Play: Enabling Play and Physical Activity in Childhood. In K. P. Nonis and S. Daswani (Eds), *The Power of Movement – Enhancing Children's Cognitive, Social and Emotional and Physical Development through Movement* (pp. 112-128). Singapore: Pearson Education, South Asia.
11. Choi Tse, K. (2004). A preliminary study on gross motor performance of Hong Kong children aged 6-8 years. *Journal of Physical Education & Recreation (Hong Kong), 10*(2), 67-72.
12. Chua, C. (2001). Chubby kids grow up to be chubby adults unless... *K. K. Women's and Children's Hospital, K.K. Juniors Club, 128,* 1-5.
13. Corbalis, M. C. & Beale, I. L. (1976). *The psychology of the left and right.* Hillsdale, NJ: Lawrence Erlbaun Associates.

14. Coren, S. (1993). The lateral preference inventory for measurement of handedness, footedness, eyedness and earedness: Norms for young adults. *Bulletin of the Psychonomic Society, 31*(1), 1-3.
15. Diamond, A. (2000). Close interrelation of motor development and cognitive development and of the cerebellum and prefrontal cortex. *Child Development, 71*(1), 44-56.
16. Didia, B. C. & Nyenwe, B. (1988). Foot breadth in children- Its relationship to limb dominance and age. *American Orthopaedic Foot and Ankle Society, 8*(4), 198-211.
17. Fisher, A., Reilly, J., Kelly, L., Montgomery, C., Williamson, A., Paton, J., et al. (2005). Fundamental movement skills and habitual physical activity in young children. *Medicine & Science in Sports & Exercise, 37*(4), 684-688.
18. Fjørtoft, I. (2001). The natural environment as a playground for children: The impact of outdoor play activities in pre-primary school children. *Early Childhood Education Journal, 29*(2), 111-117.
19. Fjørtoft, I. & Sageie, J. (2000). The natural environment as a playground for children. Landscape description and analyses of a natural landscape. *Landscape and urban planning, 48,* 83-97.
20. Gabbard, C. P. (2000). Outcome-based preschool physical education. *International Journal of Physical Education, 37*(1), 17-23.
21. Gabbard, C. P. (2004). *Lifelong motor development* (4th ed.). San Francisco: Pearson Benjamin Cummings.
22. Gabbard, C. & Hart, S. (1995). Foot performance of right- and left-handers: A question of environmental influence. *Perceptual and Motor Skills, 80,* 671-674.
23. Gallahue, D. L. & Donnelly, F. C. (2003). *Developmental physical education for all children* (4th ed.). IL: Human Kinematics.
24. Gallahue, D. L. & Ozmun, J. C. (2006). *Understanding motor development infants, children, adolescents, adults* (6th ed.). NY: McGraw-Hill.
25. Garcia, C. & Garcia, L. (2006) A motor development and motor-learning perspective. *Journal of Physical Education, Recreation & Dance, 77*(8), 31-33.
26. Gesell, A. (1928). *Infancy and human growth.* NY: Macmillan.
27. Hennessy, M. J., Dixon, S. D. & Simon, S. R. (1984). The development of gait: A study in African children ages one to five. *Child Development, 55*(3), 844-853.
28. Ignico, A. (1994). Early childhood physical education: Providing the foundation. *Journal of Physical Education, Recreation & Dance, 65*(6), 28-30.
29. Larkin, D. & Revie, G. (1995). *Foot preference and skill in children.* Poster presented at the International Neuropsychological Society and Australian

Society for the Study of Brain Impairment 2nd Pacific Rim Conference, Cairns, Queensland, Australia.
30. Lockman, J. & Thelen, E. (1993). Developmental biodynamics: Brain, body, behavior connections. *Child Development, 64*(4), 953-959.
31. Mackenzie, B. (2007). Developing Social and Emotional Skills through Movement. In K. P. Nonis & S. Daswani (Eds), *The Power of Movement – Enhancing Children's Cognitive, Social and Emotional and Physical Development through Movement* (pp. 112-128). Singapore: Pearson Education, South Asia.
32. McGraw, M. (1935). *Growth: A study of Johnny and Jimmy*. NY: Appleton-Century-Crofts.
33. McManus, I. C., Sik, G., Cole, D. R., Mellon, A. F., Wong, J. & Kloss, J. (1988). The development of handedness in children. *British Journal of Developmental Psychology, 6,* 257-273.
34. Ministry of Education, Singapore. (2008). *Registration of New Kindergartens*. Retrieved January 26, 2009, from www.moe.gov.sg/education/preschool/files/presch-registration-geninfo.doc.
35. Nonis. K. P. (1996). *The Mixed Longitudinal Study of the Development of Lower Limb Preference and Hopping Performance in Girls.* Unpublished Doctoral Thesis, The University of Western Australia, Perth, Western Australia.
36. Nonis, K. P. (2005). Kindergarten teachers' views about the importance of preschoolers' participation in sports in Singapore. *Early Child Development and Care, 175*(7 & 8), 719-742.
37. Nonis, K. P. (2007). Developing a Basic Understanding of Children's Movement. In K. P. Nonis & S. Daswani (Eds), *The Power of Movement – Enhancing Children's Cognitive, Social and Emotional and Physical Development through Movement* (pp. 38-66). Singapore: Pearson Education, South Asia.
38. Nonis, K. P. & Chia, M. (2008). *Tracing the development of pre-schoolers fundamental motor skills in Singapore* (pp. 1-22). Executive Academic Research Summary Report, The National Institute of Education, Nanyang Technological University, Singapore.
39. Nonis, K. P., Chia, M. & Quek, J. J. (2010a). The development of fundamental motor skills of Singaporean born children of Malay Ethnic Decent – A Longitudinal Investigation. Manuscript in preparation.
40. Nonis, K. P., Chia, M. & Quek, J. J. (2010b). The development of fundamental motor skills of Singaporean born children of Indian Ethnic Decent – A Longitudinal Investigation. Manuscript in preparation.
41. Nonis, K. P., Chia, M. & Quek, J. J. (2010c). The development of fundamental motor skills of Singaporean born children of Chinese Ethnic Decent – A Longitudinal Investigation. Manuscript in preparation.

42. Nonis, K. P. & Daswani, S. (2007). Which Hand, Which Leg do I use? Concerns about Preference and Performance in Movement. In K. P. Nonis & S. Daswani (Eds), *The Power of Movement – Enhancing Children's Cognitive, Social and Emotional and Physical Development through Movement* (pp. 129-145). Singapore: Pearson Education, South Asia.
43. Nonis, K. P., Larkin, D. & Parker, H. E. (1996). Patterns of Preference: A contrast between kicking and balance tasks. *Abstracts for the 1996 Australian Psychology Conferences, 48,* 19.
44. Nonis, K. P., Larkin, D. & Parker, H. E. (2006a). Preference in girls' lower limb Tasks. *Journal of Physical Education & Recreation (Hong Kong), 12*(1), 39-47.
45. Nonis, K. P., Larkin, D. & Parker, H. E. (2006b). The Strength of Preference in Girls' Lower Limb Tasks. *Journal of Physical Education & Recreation (Hong Kong), 12*(2), 7-12.
46. Nonis, K. P. & Parker, H. E. (2005). Lateral Preference and Performance Asymmetry in Girls' Hopping Skills. *The Asian Journal of Exercise and Sports Science, 1*(2) 55-60.
47. Nonis, K. P. Parker, H. & Larkin, D. (2004). The development of Hopping: An Observation Checklist for Educators. *Journal of Physical Education and Recreation (Hong Kong), 10*(1), 8-18.
48. Parker, H. E., Monson, K. P. & Larkin, D. (1993). Symmetrical and asymmetrical motor control in children: Bipedal and unipedal hopping. *Human Movement Science, 12,* 129-143.
49. Payne, V. G. & Isaacs, L. D. (1995). *Human motor development: A lifespan approach* (3rd ed.). CA: Mayfield.
50. Peters, M. (1990). Neuropsychological Identification of Motor Problems: Can we learn something from the feet to legs that hands and arms will not tell us? *Neuropscyhology Review,* (1 & 2) 165-183.
51. Peters, M. & Petrie, B. F. (1979). Functional Asymmetries in the stepping reflex of human neonates. *Canadian Journal of Psychology 33*, 198-200.
52. Piaget, J. (1952). *The origins of intelligence in children.* NY: International Universities Press.
53. Provins, K. A. (1992). Early Infant motor asymmetries and Handedness: A critical evaluation of the evidence. *Developmental Neuropsychology, 8*(4), 325-365.
54. Singapore2010. (2009). *Youth Olympic Games (YOG) Learning Centre.* Retrieved May 20, 2009, from http://www.singapore2010.sg/about_us/yog_learning_centre.
55. Singapore Sports Council. (2004). *Parents'/Guardians' perception of motor skills development in pre-school children.* Singapore Sports Council. (2009). *An Overview.* Retrieved May 20, 2009, from

http://www.ssc.gov.sg/publish/Corporate/en/about/Sporting_Singapore_An_Overview.html

56. Steingrueber, H. J. (1975). Handedness as a function of test complexity. *Perceptual and Motor Skills, 40,* 263-266.
57. Tan, S. Y. J. & Nonis, K. P. (2008). The influence of the Use of Baby Walkers on Toddler Locomotor Skills in Singapore. *Journal of Physical Education and Recreation (Hong Kong), 14*(2), 49-57.
58. Tandy, C. A. (1999). Children's diminishing play space: A study of inter-generational change in children's use of neighbourhoods. *Australian Geographical Studies, 37*(2), 154-164.
59. Thelen, E. & Smith, L. B. (1994). *A dynamic systems approach to the development of cognition and action.* MA: The MIT Press.
60. Trevlas, E., Matsouka, O. & Zachopoulou, E. (2003). Relationship between Playfulness and Motor Creativity in Preschool Children. *Early Child Development and Care, 173*(5), 535-543.
61. Ulrich, D. A. (2000). *Test of Gross Motor Development (2nd Ed).* TX: Pro-Ed Inc.
62. Vanden-Abeele, J. (1980). Comments on the functional asymmetries of the lower extremities. *Cortex, 16,* 325-329.
63. Wang, J. (2004). A study of gross motor skills of preschool children. *Journal of Research in Childhood Education, 19*(1), 32-43.
64. Williams, H. G. (1983). *Perceptual and motor development.* Englewoods Cliffs, N. J. Prentice Hall.
65. Wong, A. & Cheung, S. Y. (2006). Gross motor skills performance of Hong Kong Chinese children. *Journal of Physical Education & Recreation (Hong Kong), 12*(2), 23-29.
66. Yearbook of Statistics, Singapore (2008). *Demography 3.6.* Retrieved May 20, 2009, from http://www.singstat.gov.sg/pubn/reference/yos/statsT-demography.pdf.

INSIGHTS FROM AN EMERGING THEORETICAL PERSPECTIVE IN MOTOR LEARNING FOR PHYSICAL EDUCATION

CHOW JIA YI

Physical Education and Sports Science, National Institute of Education, Nanyang Technological University, Singapore

Research in motor learning and pedagogy has advanced tremendously over the last two decades. However, there seems to be very little synergy in the transfer of knowledge between the two disciplines. It would be sensible and even necessary for researchers in motor learning and pedagogy to work collaboratively to explore and advance knowledge on how game skills can be acquired. Certainly, the area of motor learning, with strong theoretical grounding from motor control, can augment critical pedagogical approaches in the applied setting for practitioners to improve teaching and learning of game skills. Specifically, a discussion on a pedagogical approach based on concepts from nonlinear dynamics in motor learning is shared in this chapter to explore how pedagogical practices can be refined and adapted to more effectively engage learners. With increasing wealth and economic development in the East over the last decade, sport and health awareness as well as physical education have also gained greater prominence among populations in these countries. Undoubtedly, there is a greater need to understand and develop sound pedagogical practices to help equip the population with the relevant game skills to be effectively involved in playing games that will reap critical health, emotional and social benefits. The introduction focuses on some of the historical background on motor learning and its contributions to pedagogy research. Subsequently, key concepts pertaining to how movement behaviors self-organize as a consequence of dynamic interactions among constraints (performer, task and environment) from a systems perspective is shared. Key discussions are undertaken to highlight the relevance of an embodied approach to understand learning. The role of perception-action coupling is also presented to emphasize how movement solutions can continuously be adjusted in real-time with little influence by conscious cognitive processing. Movement variability, often seen as a phenomenon that is undesirable can have a positive role in assisting learners to transit from one movement behavior to a new functional movement behavior. Empirical work from the motor learning and control literature is shared to provide evidence of these theoretical principles that underlie the ideas for a nonlinear pedagogical approach. Such an approach emphasizes the role of the teacher or coach as a facilitator, who manipulates the relevant constraints in learning contexts, to channel learners to search for functional movement solutions within the myriad of movement possibilities. Practical implications relating to how these key nonlinear concepts can inform the teaching and learning are discussed. Such practical implications can have positive effect on how physical education is structured in our schools to allow for a more explorative and facilitative approach to learn game skills that may be less prevalent at the moment in our Eastern societies.

1. Introduction

Motor learning and physical education pedagogy research share many common content strands related to teaching and learning skills. It would seem logical that there should be huge amount of opportunities for synergetic flow of knowledge between motor learning and pedagogy. However, as pointed out by McMorris (1998), there seems to be a lack of contribution from the motor learning literature in informing the pedagogical practices in physical education. The lack of sharing of content knowledge does not bode well for development of theoretical and applied knowledge in both motor learning and physical education pedagogy.

This gap between motor learning and physical education was in fact, first brought to attention in the early 90s with the publication of a special issue in *Quest*. It was specifically pointed out that research in motor learning did not lead to large scale adaptation of empirically tested practical implications in the schools for the purpose of improving skill learning (see Hoffman, 1990; Locke, 1990). Hoffman (1990) went further to discuss how motor learning research focused on the development of major learning theories with little relevance to the practical setting while research in physical education were seen by motor learning specialists to be overly narrow to specific contexts and lacked any value in generalization.

Most recently, Renshaw, Chow, Davids and Hammond (in press) further reiterated the critical need to make clear and relevant connections between motor learning and physical education to help both areas grow further, that is, making connections between theory and practice. It was recognized that there needs to be a shift away from physical education research based heavily on socially constructed critical discourse to an interdisciplinary based approach to understand relationships between information and movement as well as adopt an ecological perspective to examining the acquisition of coordination (Renshaw et al., in press). While some researchers in physical education pedagogy (e.g., Kirk & McPhail, 2002; Rovegno & Kirk, 1995; Rovegno, Nevett & Babiarz, 2001; Rovegno, 2006), had previously shared some ideas on a 'situated' learning approach, where understanding of learning should be envisaged within the learning setting, there has been very little adaptation of those ideas by the majority of pedagogists.

The development and emergence of systems-based approaches built on theoretical concepts in nonlinear dynamics within the motor learning literature over the last decade has provided new impetus to support the examination of skill learning from a 'situated' perspective. Specifically, Chow, Davids, Button, Shuttleworth, Renshaw & Araújo (2007) highlighted how a Nonlinear Pedagogical approach can explain and provide practical implications for researchers and practitioners to better understand the complexities that are inherent in dynamic learning situations. Nonlinear pedagogy describes pertinent concepts relating to perception-action, movement variability and self-organization processes that support an embodied approach to comprehend how skill learning occurs in physical education.

In this chapter, insights about the emerging ideas that support a Nonlinear Pedagogical approach are shared. Further to that, recommendations on practice are discussed and implications for its value to physical education especially in Eastern societies are provided.

2. An embodied and nonlinear approach to understanding learning

The acquisition of knowledge is imperative in the process of learning and the Cartesian view of separating cognition and body may be a reductionist approach that requires re-examination. Clark (1997, 1999, 2001), Port and van Gelder (1995) and Varela, Thompson and Rosch (1995) have emphasized the need to understand the development of cognition from a situated and embodied perspective. Learning takes place when the learner is in the context of the learning environment and the acquisition of knowledge occurs as a consequence of the interactions between the learner and the environment. Below, we explore an embodied approach to cognition and the implications for motor learning within a nonlinear pedagogical framework.

2.1. *Embodied approach: a nonlinear perspective*

Arguments against a fragmented approach to studying the brain and behavior have received increased attention over the last decade. Davids, Button & Bennett (2008) proposed a post modern approach emphasizing concepts of pattern formation and processes of coordination between components of a complex system to develop understanding of brain, mind and behavior. Such an approach is required to replace the popular trend of examining brain areas in isolation, leading to perceiving the brain and behavior from a reductionist point of view (Edelman, 1992; Kelso, 1995).

Further arguments have surfaced in cognitive science for cognition to be examined from an embodied approach. The mind, body and the environment are to be seen as equal partners in the construction of robust and flexible behaviors (Clark, 1997). Clark (1997, 2001) further emphasized the incorporation of the role of evolution in our understanding of how the human neural machinery developed in a coordinative manner to opportunistically exploit sources of order and coherence already in the environment and body. It may not be adequate to view the brain as a computer-like device, storing specific symbolic codes and mapping input from the environment with a detailed programmed output although such an arrangement could be seen as optimal. The use of the computer analogy that reduces knowledge and the mind to disembodied and socially inactive data processing (Davis & Sunara, 1997; Light & Fawns, 2001) cannot explain the complex workings of human thoughts. However, the processes of evolution has help shaped the human system in highly variable ways and Davids et al. (2008) propose that the biological nervous systems should be seen as complex, 'open' systems whose micro-components are continually modifying and adapting their structural organization in response to a range of constraints. The role of the environment should have a larger role to play and it is not necessary for the organism to plan and use all the resources from within the organism to perform a task. Strong arguments have also been made to see the environment as offering information in the form of material content, patterns and invariant properties which allows learners to construct meaningful relations (Barab, Cherkes-Julkowski, Swenson, Garrett, Shaw & Young, 1999). Further implications from such a dynamic perspective augment suggestions that the control of behavior is an emergent property of a self-organizing, distributed system embracing brain, body and aspects of the world (Clark, 1997).

Key dynamical systems concepts emanating from the work of dynamicists (see Kelso, 1995; Thelen & Smith, 1994) have also provided a plausible theoretical framework to explore cognition and adaptive behavior. Moreover, since dynamical approach focuses on the evolution of a system over time, it is appropriate for examining interactions between components in a system (Clark, 1999), which is the essence of a learning model. Dynamical systems theory concepts like self-organization, state space, phase transitions, order and control parameters, attractor states, perturbation and bifurcations are some of the cornerstones in a nonlinear framework of research relating to motor learning and control (see Handford, Davids, Bennett & Button, 1997; Newell, Liu & Mayer-Kress, 2001), as well as systemic interactions and behaviors observed in many biological, physical and even social systems (see Kelso, 1995). But, how does an embodied approach to cognition within a dynamical systems perspective help our understanding of movement generation and control?

2.2. *Embodied cognition and control of movements: perception-action coupling*

In many sport situations, real time adjustments of actions have to be provided by the performer in response to the task requirements. These real time adjustments can be considered a kind of coordination between the inner worlds (brain and body) and the outer worlds (environment) (Clark, 1999). Gibson (1979) purported that perceiving is a psychomatic act, not of the mind or body but by the observer. The individual will need to perceive to move and similarly, move to perceive. Information from the environment, in the form of huge arrays of light energy provides important information for the performer to determine affordances of actions, which are opportunities for actions. Gibson (1979) further suggests that information from the environment is not stored as it is always available and perception is more than explicit knowledge since optical information that is present cannot be explicitly described in words. Gibson's concept of *perception-action coupling* (or information-movement coupling), which emanates from ecological psychology, lends support to online control of action which emphasizes the availability of information in the surroundings that allows the performer to continuously use for movement control and vice versa, movement for information. Online control of action enables the performer to use the information for action-happening in real time and emphasizes the importance of understanding online cognition in the context of the performing situation. Work by Milner and Goodale (1995) on the presence of two visual pathways (dorsal and ventral) lends support to the idea of an embodied online cognition through the function of the dorsal visual pathway (which specializes in fluent motor interaction, in the here and now, with the target physically present) available to the performer. Van der Kamp, Oudejans and Savelsbergh (2003) furthered some of these ideas and suggested that visual control of goal-directed movements for the dorsal visual pathway (i.e., vision for action) is fast, short-lived and implicit. Moreover, the use of information to guide movement is instantaneous or online and one which the performer is not aware of.

What about the role of explicit information delivered through verbal or visual instructions in an embodied cognition framework? Offline cognition in the form of knowledge for movements and actions needs to be similarly embedded, relating to the context of body, mind and environment. Knowledge or memorial representation of an object or event in the brain can be conceived as a spatiotemporal firing pattern of neurons in the cortex (Calvin, 1996). Edelman (1992) further argued in his work on Theory of Neuronal Group Selection (TNGS) that thoughts, emotions, ideas, beliefs, images and actions are merely the neural traffic constantly being produced between billions of neurons in the CNS. Connections between neuronal groups can be possibly strengthened when a functional behavior, such as an idea or action occurs. Similarly, the neural network patterns connected with less successful behaviors are unlikely to be selected. From a Neo-Darwinism perspective, more functional connections will be selected over time as the individual executes appropriate movements and behaviors successfully, embodying the mind and the brain and this is likely to be facilitated by the strengthening of neural pathways connecting different parts of the brain by a chemical neurotransmitter acting as a 'value system' (Edelman, 1992).

In relation to offline cognition, it may be possible to associate Clark's (1997) proposed concept of action-oriented 'representations', which simultaneously describe aspects of the world and 'prescribe' possible actions, for a less online approach to cognition and movement control. Action-oriented 'representation should not be seen as strictly coded programs for detail action but be seen as 'representation' that uses information from the interaction with the environment to guide the completion of a goal directed movement. For example, an action-oriented 'representation' could provide the intention to pick up a ball on the ground but as the performer moves towards the ball, information from the environment is available to guide the action towards completion, using online perception-action couplings. Although classical cognitive science refers to 'representation' as the basic building blocks, dynamical models usually reconceived such 'representations' as dynamical entities (e.g., system states, or trajectories shaped by attractor landscapes) (van Gelder, 1999). This 'dynamical entities' or 'intention for action' could be in the form of neural synapses and connections as proposed by Edelman's (1992) TNGS concept. In relation to visual control systems, van der Kamp et al. (2003) proposed that the acquisition of information from the environment or the self through the ventral pathway (i.e., vision for perception) is a slow, long and mainly explicit process. There are further suggestions that vision for perception also allows performers to identify goal for action or to decide about the appropriate action. Empirical work from Gentilucci, Chieffi, Daprati, Saetti and Toni (1996) have also supported how vision for perception can be used to control goal directed movements in situation where there is a time delay between the detection of information and the initiation of movement. Similarly, vision for perception was also involved in movement control when it was accompanied by explicit verbalization (Rossetti, 1998). Thus, it is plausible to further suggest that offline cognition for movement through intentional selection of actions can be seen as the capacity to consciously use the perceptual arrays of information in the environment (from verbal or visual instructions) to identify goals and 'plan' actions and the action emerges as a result of the interactions of the neuromuscular properties of the performer, the goals of the task and the environmental context.

As pointed out by Thelen and Smith (1994), action and cognition may not be explained by reference to genetic blue prints or programs because they are emergent out of the intentions of multiple forces spanning brain, body and world. Solutions to movements are decentralized and dependent on the interaction with the environment. An ecological model predicated on the principles of self-organization brings meaning to learning by contextualizing the learning situation to real world settings which is imperative for encouraging learner-teacher interaction (Barab et al., 1999). Thus, a framework that endorses an embodied approach, capturing the interactions between the performer, the task and the environment, would provide the theoretical foundations to understand motor learning from a nonlinear perspective.

2.3. *Variability as an inherent phenomenon for control and change*

Noise in the human movement system is often seen as 'noise' and something that is undesirable in the control of human movement (Broadbent, 1958). However, in the motor learning literature, there is increasing support for 'noise' in the human movement system to be considered as functional (Davids, Bennett & Newell, 2006). Particularly, movement variability that is inherent in all motion can be considered as playing a critical role to allow adaptability and flexibility in the control of human movement (Riley & Turvey, 2002). For example, an investigation on expert stone knappers in India by Biryukova and Bril (2008) demonstrated how these stone knappers were able to manipulate multiple segments of their body in the knapping action with compensatory joint actions to produce functional trajectories to the hammering action.

Increasing evidence has also been available empirically to suggest that movement variability is a pertinent phenomenon for change between movement behaviors during learning. Chow, Davids, Button and Rein (2008) reported successful novice participants in a soccer kicking task demonstrated increased kicking pattern variability prior to the acquisition of a new kicking pattern during an intervention phase which included 570 practice trials. It seems that the presence of movement variability in the kicking patterns was an important learning phase where participants could explore and discover ways to refine and alter their kicking patterns to achieve more success in performance. Even in small-sided game play, Araújo, Davids, Bennett, Button and Chapman (2004) also found that, in a 1 v 1 basketball dribbling situation, attackers who demonstrated greater movement/ dribbling variability while approaching a defender, had greater success in beating the defender and progressed towards the basket. In this regard, the increase in movement variability was a key attribute for success in destabilizing the attacker-defender relationship from a situation when the defender had the advantage to a new situation when the attacker gained an edge in the 1 v 1 situation.

The functional role of movement variability was appropriately suggested by Hamill and colleagues (2006) to be not all good but it is also not all the time bad. So, in any learning situation, movement variability should be an expected observation and it is not necessary paramount for it to be eliminated. The incorporation of using movement variability as a channel to help encourage exploration and search for functional movement solutions within an embodied approach should also be an important cornerstone for a nonlinear basis to skill learning.

3. Foundations for a nonlinear basis to skill learning

3.1. *An embodied approach to the interactions of constraints*

The role of constraints in setting up boundaries for learners to search within a perceptual motor workspace is a key feature of a nonlinear basis for skill acquisition. Newell (1986) first proposed a constraint model with performer, task and environmental constraints as the key constraints in a learning context. Briefly, performer constraints include physical and structural characteristics of the performer. Task constraints related to goal of the task, rules of the activity and equipment used in these learning activities. Environmental constraints incorporate the physical and social aspects of the environment.

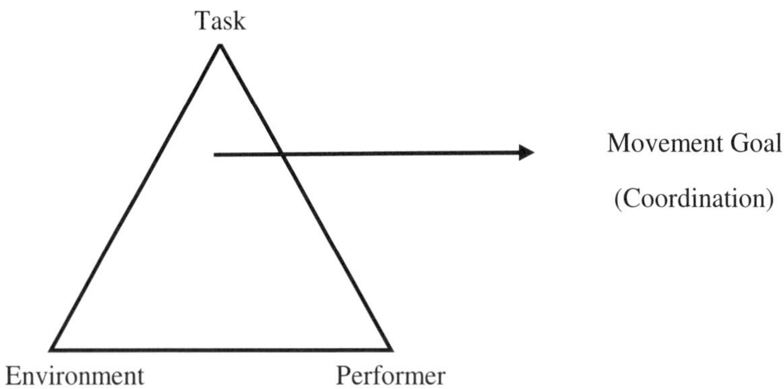

Figure 1: Schematic diagram of constraints model (Adapted from Newell, 1986).

The constraints model provides strong theoretical foundations for explaining the emergence of behavior in motor learning and motor development (see Figure 1). The different categories of constraints present in learning and teaching situations sets boundaries from which learners can develop specific goal-directed behaviors in various task contexts. Newell's (1986) constraints model provides an excellent conceptualization to guide nonlinear pedagogical practice because it adequately captures the rich range of diverse constraints in skills learning and participation in games present in physical education and sports. Such a dynamical perspective views learning new behaviors, not as acquiring rules of action encoded in the Central Nervous System (CNS), but acquiring new relationships to the laws of nature that underlie the action system of the learner and the association to environmental properties (Shaw & Alley, 1985). Thus, the emergence of movement coordination in learners occurs within an embodied framework where the performer, task and the environment plays significant roles in shaping the development of movement outcomes.

Thelen and Smith's (1994) work on infant treadmill stepping provides a classic example on the application of a constraints-led model based on dynamical systems theory in examining emergence of behavior (stepping movements in infants) as a consequence of manipulating tasks constraints in different experimental environments. Stepping movements were observed for infants at seven months old, who under normal circumstances did not demonstrate the ability to step, as compared to when they were held in an upright position and placed on a moving treadmill. The observation of infant stepping in Thelen and Smith's (1994) work demonstrated how a target behavior (stepping) emerges when the key physical attributes of the infants, muscles, joint and tendons, interacts with the appropriate task context (provision of treadmill). The presence of infant stepping thus depends on complex interactions between neural states, the biomechanics of the legs and the specific environmental parameters (Thelen & Smith, 1994).

Chow, Davids, Button and Koh (2008) recently investigated the impact of presenting specific task constraints on the acquisition of a soccer kicking task among novice male participants. For the task, participants were required to kick a ball over a height barrier (1.6m to 1.7m high) and to targets located at specific distances (10m to 14m). In the absence of explicit instructions on kicking, only the task outcome, in the form of a video clip depicting the ball flight to the target, was shown. In the study, participants developed their own individualised kicking patterns to achieve the task outcome by the end of the 4 weeks practice phase. It was clear in Chow et al. (2008) that participants searched for functional movement solutions based on the interactions among the key constraints of performer, task and the environment.

Other motor learning studies on bimanual finger coordination (Zanone & Kelso, 1992), ski learning using a ski simulator (Vereijken, van Emmerik, Whiting & Newell, 1992; Vereijken, Whiting & Beek, 1992), cascade juggling (Beek, 1989), cricket bowling (Renshaw, 2004), volleyball serve (Davids, Bennett, Handford & Jones, 1999), soccer kicking (Anderson & Sidaway, 1994) and ball bouncing (Broderick & Newell, 1999) have also demonstrated the interactive influences of the various performer, task and environmental constraints in performing situations.

3.2. *Advocating a nonlinear pedagogical approach*

From the basis of the ideas relating to an embodied and constraints-led perspective, Chow et al. (2007) proposed a Nonlinear Pedagogical approach to help researchers and practitioners understand the dynamic and interactive nature of game skill acquisition. Key considerations of such an approach are highlighted below.

3.3. *Allow for explorative learning: search within the perceptual motor workspace*

Nonlinear pedagogy recommends an explorative and discovery type of learning where the search for movement solutions are bounded by the constraints in the learning context. Building on the ideas shared in the earlier sections, the acquisition of goal-directed behaviors is heavily dependent on how performer, task and environmental constraints act on each other. The role of the teacher in a physical education setting is to function as a facilitator. Appropriate manipulation of constraints, especially task constraints, can effectively channel learners to acquire functional movement solutions that meet the task goal. For example, in badminton, when the dimensions of the playing area are manipulated such that it becomes long and narrow, the short and long play of badminton will be accentuated. Similarly, when the playing area is short and wide, net play will be encouraged. It is through the expert manipulation of constraints by teachers or coaches with the relevant knowledge of the game that learners can search within a smaller pool of possible solutions in the specific learning context without explicit instructions to do so.

Key pedagogical principles espoused in the physical education pedagogy literature such as 'modification by exaggeration' (see Rink, 2001) is one teaching approach that can be supported by the ideas in Nonlinear Pedagogy. Exaggerating certain task constraints such as instructions, equipment or playing area can accentuate the self-organization of specific behaviors (like the earlier badminton example).

3.4. *Allow implicit and less conscious type of learning*

The ideas shared earlier on an embodied cognition with learning being implicit can be further explored. It is possible to move away from having overly prescriptive instructions or learning activities. Ideas of implicit learning have been actively pursued by Masters and colleagues (e.g., Liao & Masters, 2001; Maxwell, Masters & Eve, 2000; Masters, 1992). The idea of implicit learning is to allow learners to acquire key features of the movement skill without using conscious analytic strategies (Berry & Dienes, 1993). The key advantages of such implicit learning as suggested by Masters (1992) is that learners presented with implicit learning are less likely to be affected under high anxiety situations when the skill needs to be performed because there are no explicit knowledge that can be reinvested under such stressful situations. Specifically, learners with implicit learning will not have access to explicit knowledge and therefore, less likely to be affected in making cognitive decisions about the movement.

Some of the methods used to elicit an implicit learning context included the use of analogy for instructions pertaining to the movement. In a recent table-tennis study, Masters, Poolton, Maxwell and Raab (2008) used the analogy having the table-tennis bat move up the slope of a mountain to help learners learn the forehand drive without explicit knowledge about the movement itself. It was found that analogy learners were just as good as explicit learners. More importantly, analogy learners were able to process multiple streams of information in the learning setting that mimics the performance of expert players. From a practical perspective, it may be effective to use analogies to direct learners in their search for suitable movement solutions.

Other similar research studies have also reported that instructions which help learners focus their attention on outcome of movement could also be useful. Wulf (2007) has over the last decade purported an 'External' focus of attention to be more effective than 'Internal' focus of attention. Specifically, attention focused on effects or outcomes of a movement is termed an external focus of attention, while attention focused on movement of body parts is considered an internal focus of attention (Wulf, 2007). For example, instructions such as, 'Focus on the ball flight over the defender' constitutes an external focus while instructions like, 'Focus on bending your knees' is an example of internal focus of attention instructions. Studies conducted over the last decade have overwhelmingly reported the advantage of external focus of attention over an internal focus of attention (e.g., Totsika & Wulf, 2003 in learning to ride a pedalo; Wulf, Lauterback & Toole, 1999 in practicing golf pitch shots; Wulf & McNevin, 2003 in balancing on a stabliometer; Wulf, McConnel, Gärtner & Schwarz, 2002 in learning sports skills like soccer kicks and volleyball serves; Wulf, Zachry, Granados & Dufek, 2007 in a maximal jump-and-reach task).

The effectiveness of external focus of attention instructions stems from the suggestion that actions are best planned and controlled by their intended effects (Wulf & Prinz, 2001). Wulf (2007) further explained that conscious attempts to control movement tend to interfere with automatic control processes. From a Nonlinear pedagogical perspective, the use of external focus of attention instructions does not disrupt the self-organization processes of the movement dynamics as athletes explore the task (Chow et al., 2007).

3.5. *Allow for movement variability*

The earlier discussion on the functional role of variability provides the theoretical and empirical basis for practical implications to organise practices where variability can be encouraged. Practices should be variable to challenge learners to transit from one preferred movement pattern to new functional movement solutions. However, it should be noted that high variability in practice may frustrate the learners although there are benefits to transfer of learning (Davids et al., 2008). The challenge is for practitioners to keep the learners motivated during such practices.

Most recently, Schöllhorn, Mayer-Kress, Newell and Michelbrink (2009) discussed ideas relating to how variability can be incorporated into skill practices. It was suggested that different practice conditions of variability can account for different amount of learning. Ideas like variable practice, where different variation of the same skill can be presented (e.g., shooting to the right, left or centre of goal in soccer) can result in higher contextual interference (i.e., interference that occurs as a consequence of performing various tasks or skills within the context of practice (Battig, 1979)). Similarly, random practices as compared to block practices can also create greater contextual interference. Notably, higher interference could have a beneficial learning effect during retention and transfer contexts (Brady, 1998). Schöllhorn et al. (2009) also emphasized that children or novice learners should be exposed to practice schedules with lower contextual interference while adults or skilled learners be presented with practice schedules with higher contextual interference. This differential approach to infusing contextual interference to learners at different learning stages highlights the need to adjust the amount of variability during practices even though there are suggestions that such variability can be functional.

4. Implications of nonlinear pedagogy in the East

While explorative and discovery type of learning has become increasingly popular in western societies, it is less prevalent in the east. There is a tendency for most Asian societies to adopt more traditional and top-down approach of teaching and learning. In such approaches, the teacher provides prescriptive instructions with explicit information about the skill requirement and learners have minimal involvement in terms of discovering the dynamics of the movement. Such traditional practices do stem largely from the cultural and societal norms present in the east.

However, with increasing development and adaptation of western type pedagogical approaches in the east, there are greater opportunities for practitioners in Asian countries to explore discovery-type pedagogy models. As so far espoused in this chapter, a nonlinear pedagogical approach can provide the framework for a facilitative based teaching perspective. For example in Singapore, the Ministry of Education has undertaken the Games Concepts Approach (GCA) as the key vehicle to teach game skills in Singapore Schools (Ministry of Education, 2006). The GCA approach is similar in concept to the Teaching Games for Understanding (TGfU) (see Bunker & Thorpe, 1986;

Hopper, Butler & Storey, in press; Rink, 2001 for more discussion) approach commonly used in many western countries such as Canada, America, Australia and the United Kingdom. Such an approach uses modified games where tactical concepts are exaggerated to help learners explore and understand the tactics required to play these games. Questioning and eliciting answers about the tactical knowledge taught in the modified games are emphasized. Many of the modified games use ideas relating to manipulating task constraints to accentuate the tactical knowledge to be shared. However, the theoretical principles underlying the perceived effectiveness of the GCA or TGfU are not clear although there have been previous discussions (see Chow et al., 2007). More recently, nonlinear pedagogy has been purported to support the processes that underpin such game teaching approaches (Chow et al., 2007).

Certainly, the adaptation of pedagogical approaches emanating from nonlinear pedagogy has tremendous potential for an Asian context. Nevertheless, such adaptation does take time and is dependent on the willingness of key educational institutes in these Asian countries to embrace facilitative-type of pedagogical approaches.

5. Conclusion

This chapter provided valuable insights to the development in motor learning that can augment the pedagogical practices in physical education. Specifically, a nonlinear pedagogical approach based on the tenets of nonlinear dynamics has pertinent framework for an explorative-based teaching and learning perspective.

Key theoretical concepts relating to an embodied learning, perception-action coupling and functional role of movement variability were also shared to clarify the theoretical underpinnings of a nonlinear pedagogical approach. Some practical implications for nonlinear pedagogy and its role in the changing Asian educational context were also discussed. Nevertheless, more synergetic transfer of knowledge between motor learning and physical education pedagogy should be emplaced to help the development of our understanding about teaching and learning.

References

1. Anderson, D. I., & Sidaway, B. (1994). Coordination changes associated with practice of a soccer kick. *Research Quarterly for Exercise and Sport, 65*(2), 93-99.
2. Araújo, D., Davids, K., Bennett, S., Button, C., & Chapman, G. (2004). Emergence of sport skills under constraint. In A. M. Williams & N. J.

Hodges (Eds.), *Skill Acquisition in Sport: Research, Theory and Practice* (pp. 409-433). London: Routledge, Taylor & Francis.

3. Barab, S. A., Cherkes-Julkowski, M., Swenson, R., Garrett, S., Shaw, R. E., & Young, M (1999). Principles of self-organizations: Learning as participation in autocatakinetic systems. *The Journal of the Learning Sciences, 8*(3&4), 349-390.
4. Battig, W. F. (1979). The flexibility of human memory. In L. S. Cermak & F. I. M. Craik (Eds.), *Levels of processing in human memory* (pp. 23-44). Hillsdale, NJ: Erlbaum.
5. Beek, P. J. (1989). Timing and phase locking in cascade juggling. *Ecological Psychology, 3*, 55-96.
6. Berry, D. C., & Dienes, Z. (1993). *Implicit learning: Theoretical and empirical issues.* Hillsdale, NJ: Erlbaum.
7. Biryukova, L., & Bril, B. (2008). Organization of goal-directed action at a high level of motor skill: The case of stone knapping in India. *Motor Control, 12,* 181-209.
8. Brady, F. (1998). A theoretical and empirical review of the contextual interference effect and the learning of motor skills. *Quest, 50*, 266-293.
9. Broadbent, N. A. (1958). *Perception and communication.* London: Pergamon Press.
10. Broderick, M. P., & Newell, K. M. (1999). Coordination patterns in ball bouncing as a function of skill. *Journal of Motor Behavior, 31*(2), 165-188.
11. Bunker, D., & Thorpe, R. (1982). A model for the teaching of games in the secondary schools. *The Bulletin of Physical Education*, 5-8.
12. Calvin, W. H. (1996). *The Cerebral Code: Thinking a Thought in the Mosaics of the Mind.* Cambridge, MA: M.I.T. Press.
13. Chow, J. Y., Davids, K., Button, C., & Koh, M. (2008). Coordination changes in a discrete multi-articular action as a function of practice. *Acta Psychologica, 127,* 163-176.
14. Chow, J. Y., Davids, K., Button, C., & Rein, R. (2008). Dynamics of movement patterning in learning a discrete multi-articular action. *Motor Control, 12,* 219-240.
15. Chow, J. Y., Davids, K., Button, C., Shuttleworth, R., Renshaw, I., & Araújo, D. (2007). The role of nonlinear pedagogy in physical education. *Review of Educational Research, 77,* 251-278.
16. Clark, A. (1997). *Being there: Putting brain, body and world together again*. Cambridge MA: MIT Press.

17. Clark, A. (1999). An embodied cognitive science? *Trends in Cognitive Sciences, 3*(9), 345-351.
18. Clark, A. (2001). *Mindware. An introduction to the philosophy of cognitive science.* New York: Oxford University Press.
19. Davids, K., Bennett, S., Handford, C., & Jones, B. (1999). Acquiring coordination in self-paced, extrinsic timing tasks: A constraints-led perspective. *International Journal of Sport Psychology, 30,* 437-461.
20. Davids, K., Bennett, S., & Newell, K. (2006). *Movement system variability.* Champaign, IL: Human Kinetics.
21. Davids, K., Button, C., & Bennett, S. J. (2008). *Coordination and control of movement in sport: An ecological approach.* Champaign, IL: Human Kinetics.
22. Davis, B., & Sunara, J. (1997). Cognition, complexity and teacher education. *Harvard Educational review, 67*(1), 105-125.
23. Edelman, G. M. (1992). *Bright air, brilliant fire. On matter of mind.* New York: Basic Books.
24. Gentilucci, M., Chieffi, S., Daprati, E., Saetti, M. C., Toni, I. (1996). Visual illusion and action. *Neuropsychologia, 34*, 369-376.
25. Gibson, J. J. (1979). *An ecological approach to visual perception.* Boston, MA: Houghton-Mifflin.
26. Hamill, J., Haddad, J. M., Heiderscheit, B. C., Emmerik, R. E. A., & Li, L. (2006). Clinical relevance of variability in coordination. In K. Davids, S. Bennett, & K. M. Newell (Eds.), *Movement system variability* (pp. 153-165). Champaign, IL: Human Kinetics.
27. Handford, C., Davids, K., Bennett, S., & Button, C. (1997). Skill acquisition in sport: some applications of an evolving practice ecology. *Journal of Sports Sciences, 15,* 621-640.
28. Hoffman, S. J. (1990). Relevance, application, and the development of an unlikely theory. *Quest*, 42, 143-160.
29. Hopper, T., Butler, J., & Storey, B. (Eds.). (2009). *TGfU...Simply Good Pedagogy: Understanding a Complex Challenge*. Ottawa: Physical Health Education Association (Canada).
30. Kelso, J. S. (1995). *Dynamic patterns: the self-organization of brain and behaviour.* Cambridge, MA: MIT.
31. Kirk, D., & MacPhail, A. (2002). Teaching games for understanding and situated learning: Rethinking the Bunker-Thorpe model. *Journal of Teaching in Physical Education, 21,* 177-192.

32. Liao, C. M., & Masters, R. S. W. (2001). Analogy learning. A means to implicit learning. *Journal of Sports Sciences, 19*, 307-319.
33. Light, R., & Fawns, R. (2001). The thinking body: Constructivist approaches to games teaching in physical education. *Melbourne Studies in Education, 42*(2), 69-87.
34. Locke, L. F. (1990). Why motor learning is ignored: A case of ducks, naughty theories, and unrequited love. *Quest*, 42, 134-142.
35. Masters, R. S. W. (1992). Knowledge, knerves and know-how: the role of explicit versus implicit knowledge in the breakdown of a complex motor skill under pressure. *British Journal of Psychology, 83,* 343-358.
36. Masters, R. S. W., Poolton, J. M., Maxwell, J. P., & Raab, M. (2008). Implicit motor learning and complex decision making in time-constrained environments. *Journal of Motor Behavior, 40*(1), 71-79.
37. Maxwell, J. P., Masters, R. S. W., & Eves, F. (2000). From novice to no know-how: a longitudinal study of implicit motor learning. *Journal of Sport Sciences, 18,* 111-120.
38. McMorris, T. (1998). Teaching Games for Understanding: Its contribution to the knowledge of skill acquisition from a motor learning perspective. *European Journal of Physical Education, 3,* 65-74.
39. Milner, A. D., & Goodale, M. A. (1995). *The visual brain in action.* Oxford: Oxford University Press.
40. Ministry of Education (2006). *Physical Education syllabus.* Curriculum Planning and Development Division. Ministry of Education, Singapore.
41. Newell, K. M. (1986). Constraints on the development of coordination. In M. G. Wade & H. T. A. Whiting (Eds.), *Motor development in children. Aspects of coordination and control* (pp. 341-360). Dordrecht, Netherlands: Martinus Nijhoff.
42. Newell, K. M., Liu, Y. T., & Mayer-Kress, G. (2001). Time scales in motor learning and development. *Psychological Review, 108*(1), 57-82.
43. Port, R. F., & van Gelder, T. (1995). *Mind as motion: Explorations in the dynamics of cognition*. Cambridge, MA: MIT Press.
44. Renshaw, I. (2004, April). *Informational Constraints on Cricket Batting.* Communication to 31st Australasian Experimental Psychology Conference, Dunedin, New Zealand.
45. Renshaw, I., Chow, J. Y., Davids, K., & Hammond, J. (in press). A constraints-led perspective to understanding skill acquisition and game play:

A basis for integration of motor learning theory and physical education praxis? *Physical Education and Sport Pedagogy.*

46. Riley, M. A., & Turvey, M. T. (2002). Variability and determinism in motor behavior. *Journal of Motor Behavior, 34*(2), 99-125.
47. Rink, J. E. (2001). Investigating the assumptions of pedagogy. *Journal of Teaching in Physical Education, 20*, 112-128.
48. Rossetti, Y. (1998). Implicit perception in action: Short-lived motor representation of space. *Consciousness and Cognition, 7*, 520-558.
49. Rovegno, I. (2006). Situated perspectives on learning, in *The Handbook of Physical Education*. D. Kirk, D. Macdonald and M. O'Sullivan (Eds). London: Sage.
50. Rovegno, I., & Kirk, D. (1995). Articulations and silences in socially critical work on physical education: Toward a broader agenda. *Quest, 47,* 447-474.
51. Rovegno, I., Nevett, M., & Babiarz, M. (2001). Learning and teaching invasion-game tactics in 4th Grade: Introduction and theoretical perspectives. *Journal of Teaching in Physical Education*, 20, 341-351.
52. Rossetti, Y. (1998). Implicit perception in action: Short-lived motor representation of space. *Consciousness and Cognition, 7*, 520-558.
53. Schöllhorn, W. I., Mayer-Kress, G. M., Newell, K. M., & Michelbrink, M. (2009). Time scales of adaptive behavior and motor learning in the presence of stochastic perturbations. *Human Movement Science.*
54. Shaw, R. E., & Alley, J. R. (1985). How to draw learning curves: Their use and justification. In T. D. Johnston & A. T. Pietrewicz (Eds.), *Issues in the ecological study of learning*. Hillsdale, NJ: Erlbaum.
55. Thelen, E., & Smith, L. B. (1994). *A dynamics systems approach to the development of cognition and action.* London: MIT Press.
56. Totsika, V., & Wulf, G. (2003). The influence of external and internal foci of attention on transfer to novel situations and skills. *Research Quarterly for Exercise and Sport, 74*, 220-225.
57. van der Kamp, J., Oudejans, R., & Savelsbergh, G. (2003). The development and learning of the visual control of movement: An ecological perspective. *Infant Behavior & Development, 26,* 495-515.
58. van Gelder, T. J. (1999) Dynamic approaches to cognition. In R. Wilson & F. Keil (Eds.), *The MIT Encyclopedia of Cognitive Sciences* (pp.244-246). Cambridge MA: MIT Press.
59. Varela, F. J., Thompson, E., & Rosch, E. (1995). *The embodied mind. Cognitive science and human experience.* London: MIT Press.

60. Vereijken, B., van Emmerik, R. E. A., Whiting, H. T. A., & Newell, K. M. (1992). Freezing degrees of freedom in skill acquisition. *Journal of Motor Behavior, 24*(1), 133-142.
61. Vereijken, B., Whiting, H. T. A., & Beek W. J. (1992). A dynamical systems approach to skill acquisition. *Quarterly Journal of Experimental Psychology, 45A*, 323-344.
62. Wulf, G. (2007). *Attention and motor skill learning*. Champaign, IL: Human Kinetics.
63. Wulf, G., Lauterbach, B., & Toole, T. (1999). Learning advantages of an external focus of attention in golf. *Research Quarterly for Exercise and Sport, 70*, 120-126.
64. Wulf, G., McConnel, N., Gärtner, M, & Schwarz, A. (2002). Feedback and attentional focus: Enhancing the learning of sport skills through external-focus feedback. *Journal of Motor Behavior, 34,* 171-182.
65. Wulf, G., & McNevin, N. H. (2003). Simply distracting learners is not enough: More evidence for the learning benefits of an external focus of attention. *European Journal of Sport Science, 3*(5), 1-13.
66. Wulf, G., & Prinz, W. (2001). Directing attention to movement effects enhances learning: A review. *Psychonomic Bulletin & Review, 8*(4), 648-660.
67. Wulf, G., Zachry, T., Granados, C., & Dufek, J. S. (2007). Increases in jump-and-reach height through an external focus of attention. *International Journal of Sports Science and Coaching, 2*(3), 275-284.
68. Zanone, P. G., & Kelso, J. A. S. (1992). Evolution of behavioral attractors with learning: Nonequilibrium phase transitions. *Journal of Experimental Psychology: Human Perception and Performance, 18,* 403-421.

EXERCISE IN CHILDHOOD FOR A LIFE-LONG BONE HEALTH

YOSHIHISA UMEMURA
School of Health and Sport Sciences, Chukyo University, Japan

TAKERU KATO
Faculty of Health Science, Suzuka University of Medical Science, Japan

Exercise improves bone development especially in young children, because it provides mechanical stress to bones. Exercise increases bone mass and bone size, both of which are thought as important factors for persevering bone strength against bending and torsion stresses. In young adults or aged women, the positive effects of previous sport activities during youth, especially before adolescence, on bone size are retained, according to research using magnetic resonance imaging (MRI). Thus, exercise in childhood is very important for a life-long bone health. These results are also demonstrated in animal studies where high-impact, low-repetition and low-frequency mechanical stress was effective for bone development. The details of two studies are presented.

Study 1: Effect of previous sport activity on the preservation of bone

1.1. *Introduction*

Weight-bearing exercise during childhood is shown to increase peak bone mass and may have long-lasting benefits on bone health in later life. New bone tissue is formed where mechanical stimuli are the most pronounced. Dual energy x-ray absorptiometry (DXA)-measured bone mineral content (BMC) and areal bone mineral density (aBMD) has provided useful data on bone status. Because of the two-dimensional planar nature of DXA measurements, however, the scan provides limited information about bone structure and geometry such as size and shape.

We investigated whether childhood sports participation, particularly weight-bearing sports, has any preservational effect on DXA-measured BMC and aBMD and on bone geometric characteristics of the femur, such as femoral mid-diaphyseal cross-sectional area, periosteal (outer), endosteal (inner) perimeters and second moment of area in the planes of least and maximum resistance to bending in premenopausal young and postmenopausal middle-aged women.

Geometric parameters provided by magnetic resonance imaging (MRI) were used to evaluate the preservational effects of exercise during childhood.

1.2. *Method*

Subjects comprised 43 premenopausal healthy young women (mean age, 21.2±0.6 years; range, 20-23 years) and 46 postmenopausal women (mean age, 60.2±5.6 years; range, 52-73 years). Subjects completed a questionnaire regarding current and past (at elementary school, i.e., 6-12 years old, at junior high school, i.e., 13-15 years old, at high school, i.e., 16-18 years old) physical activity, smoking habit, and background information including any history of bone disease, medication use and bone fracture.

Forty-three pre-menopausal young women were classified into three groups according to starting age of previous sport participation, (i) commencing from elementary school group, (ii) commencing from junior high school to college group and (iii) low-impact non-weight-bearing sports swimming or no sports participation, or no sports group. Forty-six postmenopausal middle-aged women were classified into two groups according to previous sport participation at junior high school and high school; weight-bearing sports, including high-impact weight-bearing activities such as athletic sprinting, handball, softball, volleyball and basketball; and low-impact non-weight-bearing sports such as swimming or no participation. No subjects commenced regular sports activity during elementary school in postmenopausal middle-aged women.

1.3. *DXA and MRI measurements*

BMC and aBMD were assessed using DXA (DCS-3000; ALOKA, Tokyo, Japan) of the left proximal femur. The femoral neck region was selected for analysis. Muscle cross-sectional area and bone cortical area of the left femur were measured using a 1.0-T system (Magnex αII, SMI-50C; Shimazu, Tokyo, Japan). Scans of femoral mid-diaphyseal cross-sectional area, periosteal perimeter and endosteal perimeter were obtained at the midpoint between the femoral head and the upper edge of the patella.

1.4. *Analysis*

Mean physiological characteristics and calcium intake were compared among the three groups, classified by starting age of sports participation using a one-way analysis of covariance (ANOVA) (Table 1). Analysis of covariance (ANCOVA) was used to compare significant differences in DXA (Figure 1) and MRI-determined (Figure 2) parameters between groups without the effects of height and weight for premenopausal young women and age and weight for postmenopausal middle-aged women. SPSS version 15.0J was used for the all statistical analysis. The significance level was set at 0.05, and all comparisons were two-tailed.

1.5. *Results*

No significant differences in age, height, weight, body-mass index (BMI), daily dietary calcium intake were seen in both premenopausal young women among the three groups and postmenopausal middle-aged women between the two groups, respectively (Table 1).

Periosteal perimeter, bone cross-sectional area and maximum second moment of area were significantly greater in the junior high-college group than the no sports group. Minimum second moment of area was significantly grater in the elementary school group than the no sports group in premenopausal young women. In postmenopausal middle-aged women, periosteal perimeter, bone cross-sectional area, maximum and minimum moment of area were significantly greater in weight-bearing sports group than no sports group. Conversely, no significant difference was seen in endosteal perimeter among the three groups. In addition, no significant difference in muscle cross-sectional area of the mid-thigh was seen both in premenopausal young women and postmenopausal middle-aged women.

1.6. *Discussion*

One significant finding was that postmenopausal middle-aged women with participation in weight-bearing sports during junior high to high school (at 12-18 years old) displayed significantly greater BMC in femoral neck regions, and also showed significantly greater femoral mid-diaphyseal bone cross-sectional area, periosteal perimeter and maximum and least second moment of area than the non-weight-bearing sports group. Since none of these subjects were currently participating in regular weight-bearing sports (36 subjects were currently participating in regular swimming exercise, with a mean history of swimming was 6.0±5.0 years, while the remaining 10 subjects were not participating in any regular training), the present results suggest that weight-bearing sports activity in adolescence can affect bone structure, and that cortical bone expands toward the outside due to weight-bearing exercise during junior high and high school. The present findings support the idea that weight-bearing exercise in youth affects bone, and geometric advantages may be preserved even after 40 years.

We also found that although pre-menopausal young women did not differ in DXA-measured projected 2-dimensional bone area, BMC or aBMD between elementary school and junior high-college groups, the elementary school group showed significantly greater MRI-determined cross-sectional bone geometric parameters such as femoral mid-diaphyseal bone cross-sectional area, periosteal perimeter and maximum second moment of area than the junior high-college group. These findings suggest that weight-bearing sports activities before and during early puberty exert greater effects on bone geometry and structure, rather than DXA-measured BMC and aBMD. In the elementary school group, mean staring age of sports participation was 9.2±1.5 years. This result may support the

Table 1. Physiological characteristics of the subjects and calcium intake

	Premenopausal young women			Postmenopausal middle-aged women	
	Elementary school (n=18)	Junior- high school (n=18)	No sports (n=7)	Weight-bearing sports (n=16)	Non sports (n=30)
Age (yr)	21.3 ± 0.6	21.1 ± 0.2	21.6 ±1.0	59.9±5.3	60.4±5.9
Height (cm)	158.0 ± 5.6	158.1 ± 5.5	159.9 ± 4.6	156.8±4.0	154.8±4.5
Weight (kg)	48.6 ± 6.8	49.3 ± 6.1	49.8 ± 6.5	54.4±12.9	52.9±8.3
BMI	19.4 ± 1.7	19.8 ± 2.1	19.5± 2.5	22.1±4.7	22.0±3.0
Calcium (mg)	511.0 ± 395.2	406.6 ± 173.6	552.0 ± 574.6	703.3±280.8	704.6±245.5

Values are means±SD.

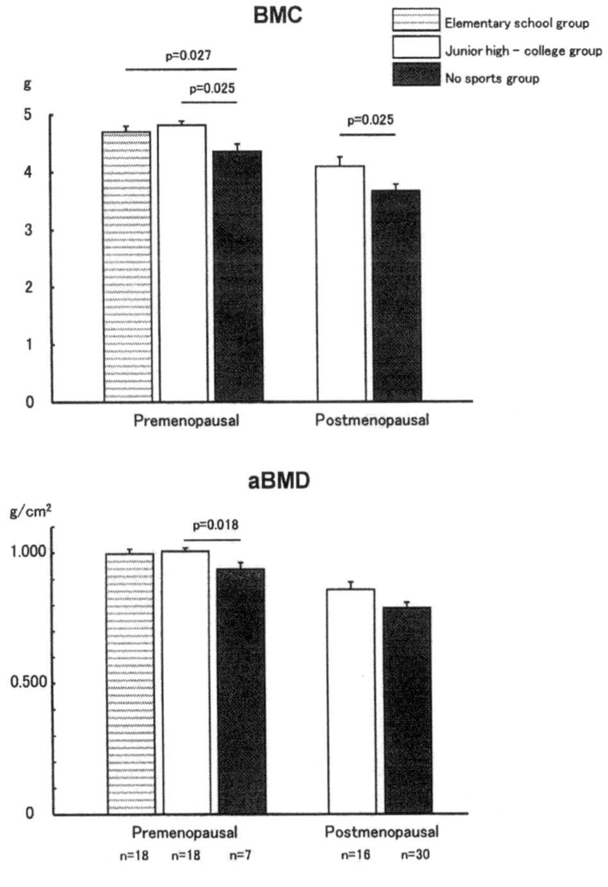

Figure 1. DXA-measured BMC and aBMD at femoral neck (n=89).
Values are means±SEM and adjusted for covariate values of height=158.3cm and weight=49.1kg (premenopausal), age =60.2 years and weight=53.4kg (postmenopausal).

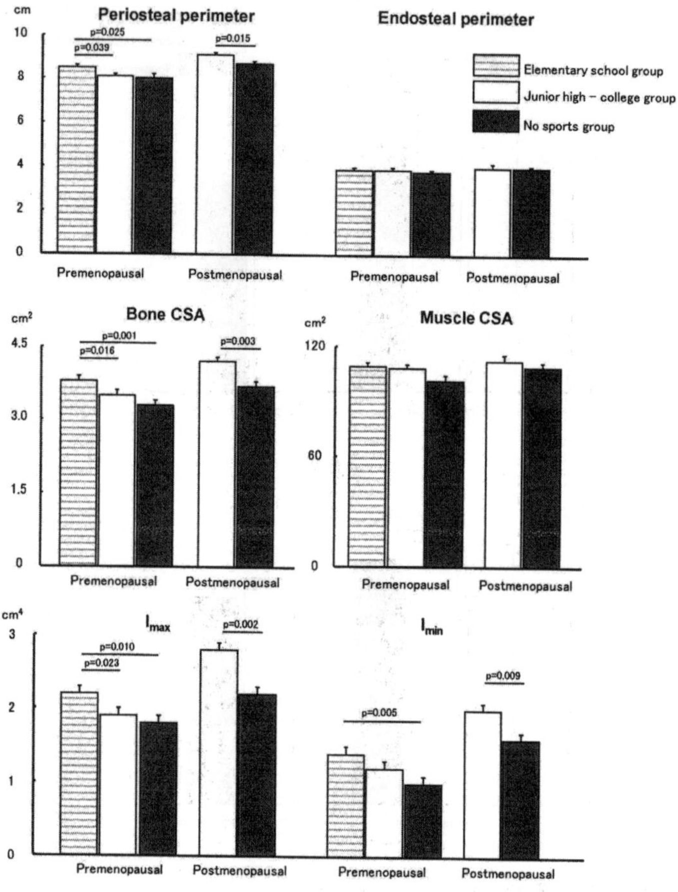

Figure 2. MRI-determined periosteal and endosteal perimeters, maximum and minimum second moment of area, and bone and muscle cross-sectional area (CSA). Values are means±SEM and adjusted for covariate values of height=158.3cm and weight=49.1kg(premenopausal),age =60.2 years and weight=53.4kg (postmenopausal). Imax & Imin indicate maximum & minimum second moment of area.

idea that cortical bone expands more effectively toward the outside from the neutral axis of the long bone due to regular weight-bearing exercise before and in early puberty period (elementary school, 6–12 years old) than after puberty (junior high-college, ≥13 years old), and these benefits were effectively preserved in young adult women.

We found a significantly greater BMC at the total proximal femur in elementary school group, and at femoral neck in junior high-college group than no sports group. Weight-bearing exercise had a systematic, positive effect on the loaded axial and appendicular bones, indicating that high-impact weight-bearing exercise programs are specifically effective as site stimuli, especially for the proximal femoral region (Kato, 2006). And this type of weight-bearing exercise is more advantageous than other types of exercise in that it has preservational effects on bone (Honda, 2008; Singh, 2002; Umemura, 2008a). The postmenopausal middle-aged women with participation in weight-bearing sports during junior high to high school (at 12-18 years old) displayed significantly greater BMC in femoral neck regions, and also showed significantly greater femoral mid-diaphyseal bone cross-sectional area, periosteal perimeter and maximum and minimum second moment of area than the non-weight-bearing sports group (Kato, 2009).

Adolescent weight-bearing exercise exerts preservational effects on femoral mid-diaphyseal size and shape. Weight-bearing exercise in youth affects bone, and that these effects may be preserved as geometric and structural advantages even after 40 years.

2. Study 2: An effective exercise protocol for bone development

2.1. *Introduction*

High dynamic mechanical stress is an effective stimulator of bone formation or remodeling (Turner, 1998). Thus, high-impact exercises which generate great and dynamic ground reaction forces are considered as an appropriate exercise mode for bone development. We used laboratory animals to study an effective exercise protocol for bone development in detail, because rigid controlled studies were needed. Jump exercise in rats is regarded as a high-impact exercise, because high ground reaction forces are imposed on the rat's lower limb at the take-off during each jump. In this animal model, we examined daily repetition number (Umemura, 1997) and daily or weekly frequency (Umemura, 2008b) for an effective osteogenic response. Additionally, we examined whether the interval time between each jump affected the osteogenic response (Umemura 2002).

2.2. *Method*

In the daily repetition number study, we used five-week-old female Fischer 344 rats. They were assigned to five jump groups or a control group (each, n=10).

The five jump groups comprised of 5-, 10-, 20-, 40- and 100-jump groups according to the number of daily jumps. In daily exercise, the rats were jumped continually in one bout.

In the daily frequency study, we used eleven-week-old female Wistar rats. They were assigned two jump groups or a control group (each, n=10). The two jump groups comprised of daily 1- and 2-bout groups according to the number of daily exercise bout. One exercise bout consisted of ten continual jumps. In the weekly frequency study, we used eleven-week-old female Wistar rats. They were assigned to four jump groups (each, n=10) or a control group (n=8). The four jump groups comprised of weekly 1-, 3-, 5- and 7-bout groups according to the number of weekly exercise bout. One exercise bout consisted of ten continual jumps, and each exercise bout was conducted on alternate days. The weekly 7-bout group exercised one bout everyday.

In the interval study, we used five-week-old female Fisher 344 rats. They were assigned two jump groups or a control group (each, n=10). The two jump groups comprised of 3s- and 30s-interval groups. The rats in the 3s-interval group jumped 20 times everyday with 3 seconds interval for each bout and the rats in the 30s-interval group jumped with a 30 seconds interval.

In all the jump studies, each rat was placed at the bottom of a handmade box and jumped from the floor to catch up the top of the box. The jump exercise was initiated by electric stimulation. After 8 weeks of training, the rats were sacrificed, and their tibia was dissected for bone analysis. The bone strength was measured with a tree-point bending test apparatus (RX1600, I. Techno, Tokyo), the fat-free dry weight was measured after chloroform-methanol immersion and drying, and the bone periosteal perimeter was obtained at the mid-shaft.

2.3. *Results*

In the all studies, there were no significant differences among groups in final body weight and tibial length. This result meant that the jump exercise did not affect longitudinal growth. In the daily repetition number study, the 5-jump group had significantly heavier and stronger bone with greater perimeter (b $p>.05$) than the control group. Although the 100-jump group had the heaviest, strongest and greatest perimeter bone among the groups, the differences between the exercise groups were diminished. This result indicated that a large number of loading was not always necessary for bone development.

In the daily frequency study, there were no significant differences in bone weight, strength and cross-sectional size between the daily 1- and 2-bout groups, although there were significant differences between the two exercise groups and the control group. This result indicated that daily two exercise bouts were not necessary for bone development. In the weekly frequency study, the weekly 1-bout group had significantly stronger and greater perimeter bone than the control group. Although the weekly 7-jump group had the heaviest, strongest and greatest perimeter bone among the groups, the differences between the exercise groups were somewhat diminished. This result indicated that a weekly single loading had positive potential, although loading every day did have the greatest effect.

In the interval study, the 30s-interval group had significantly heavier bone weight per body weight than the 3s-interval group, although the differences among two exercise groups in the other variables did not reach significance. This result indicated that some loading interval enhanced the osteogenic response.

2.4. *Discussion*

Our result that daily low-repetition loading had potential to evoke the osteogenic response contrasted with a previous study by Rubin (1984), in which artificial bending loads was imposed on rooster's ulna. Turner (1998) discussed that a long continual loading decreased mechano-sensitivity of the bone, and returns were diminished. Moreover he pointed out that the relation between daily loading number and bone mass gained was fitted by a logarithmic curve. Thus, a large number of continual loading is not always necessary for bone development.

Robling (2001) pointed out the decreased mechano-sensitivity by a continual loading would return within a several hours. Furthermore he showed that osteogenic response is enhanced if daily loading was separated into multiple bouts, with his animal model in which the ulnas of the rats were longitudinally compressed under anesthesia. Our results were not consistent with his studies and indicated that the decreased mechano-sensitivity by a continual loading did not return within a several hours, because two loading bouts daily, did not enhance the effects. Moreover our weekly frequency study suggested that the decreased mechano-sensitivity did not return entirely within a day. In high-impact loading like jumping, frequent exercise is not always necessary for bone development.

Results showed that decreased mechano-sensitivity did not return within a day in jump exercise, and it might return to some extent only within 30 seconds. Therefore, the 30s-interval jumping enhanced the effect on bone compared to 3s-interval jumping. This result was supported by Srinivasan (2007) who reported that inserting a 10-s interval between each load cycle amplifies osteogenic response. In high-impact loading, the long interval between each loading also enhances the effect.

2.5. *Conclusion*

High-impact exercise in youth increases bone mass and size, and these effects are retained over a long life period. For women, high-impact exercise before adolescence is very important to increase the cross-sectional area of bone, which makes it resistant to bone fracture later in life. In the high-impact exercise protocol, a large number of loading or a high-frequency loading bout is not always necessary for bone development. School-based exercise for bone development should be encouraged for a life-long bone health.

References

1. Honda A, Sogo N, Nagasawa S, Kato T & Umemura Y. (2008). Bones benefits gained by jump-training are preserved after detraining in young and adult rats. *J Appl Physiol*, 105: 849-853.
2. Kato T, Terashima T, Yamashita T, Hatanaka H, Honda A & Umemura Y. (2006). Effect of low-repetition jump training on bone mineral density in young women. *J Appl Physiol*, 100: 839-834.
3. Kato T, Yamashita T, Mizutani S, Honda A, Matumoto M & Umemura Y. (2009). Adolescent exercise associated with long-term superior measures of bone geometry: A cross-sectional DXA and MRI study. *Br J Sports Med*, 43: 932-935.
4. Robling AG, Burr DB & Turner CH. (2001). Recovery periods restore mechanosensitivity to dynamically loaded bone. *J Exp Biol,* 204: 3389-3399.
5. Robling AG, Hinant FM, Burr DB, & Turner CH. (2002). Improved bone structure and strength after long-term mechanical loading is greatest if loading is separated into short bouts. *J Bone Miner Res,* 17: 1545-1554.
6. Rubin CT & Lanyon LE. (1984). Regulation of bone formation by applied dynamic loads. *Bone Joint Surg Am,* 66: 397-402.
7. Singh R, Umemura Y, Honda A & Nagasawa S. (2002). Maintenance of bone mass and mechanical properties after short-term cessation of high impact exercise in rats. *Int J Sports Med,* 23: 77-81.
8. Srinivasan S, Ausk BJ, Poliachik SL, Warner SE, Richardson TS & Gross TS. (2007). Rest-inserted loading rapidly amplifies the response of bone to small increases in strain and load cycles. *J Appl Physiol,* 102: 1945-52.
9. Turner CH. (1998). Three rules for bone adaptation to mechanical stimuli. *Bone,* 23: 399-407.
10. Umemura Y, Ishiko T, Yamauchi T, Kurono M & Mashiko S. (1997). Five jumps per day increase bone mass and breaking force in rats. *J Bone Miner Res,* 12: 1480-1485.
11. Umemura Y, Sogo N and Honda A. (2002). Effects of intervals between jumps or bouts on osteogenic response to loading. *J Appl Physiol,* 93: 1345-1348.
12. Umemura Y, Nagasawa S, Sogo N & Honda A. (2008a). Effects of jump training on bone are preserved after detraining regardless of estrogen secretion state in rats. *J Appl Physiol,* 104: 1116-1120.
13. Umemura Y, Nagasawa S, Honda A & Singh R. (2008b). High-impact exercise frequency per week or day for osteogenic response in rats. *J Bone Miner Metab,* 26: 456-460.

MEASUREMENT OF BLOOD LACTATE DURING SPORTS

KAORU KITAGAWA

Exercise and Sports Physiology, Chukyo University, Japan

The measurement of blood lactate in sporting activities provides useful information to athletes, coaches and sports scientists for individualizing training programs and also for evaluating the effectiveness of the training programs. The chapter provides an overview of the how blood lactate measurements are conducted and applied in soccer, synchronized swimming, alpine skiing and in swimming in a sports science laboratory in Japan.

1. Introduction

The energy required for muscular contraction is released by the breakdown of adenosine triphosphate (ATP) to adenosine diphosphate (ADP) and inorganic phosphate (Pi). As the stores of ATP in skeletal muscle are very small, the energy of ATP resynthesis comes from three different series of chemical reactions. Exercise intensity determines the ratio of contribution in the cellular energy supply process, such as alactic energy processes, lactic energy processes and aerobic energy processes. High intensity and short duration activities—such as sprinting, weight lifting, and fast breaks in basketball or soccer—require immediate and a rapid energy supply (Zumerchik, 1995). In such high intensity activity, which often lasts less than 10 seconds, energy is supplied to the working muscles solely from the high-energy phosphate molecules that are present in the muscle cells. So, this energy source is depleted after about 7 seconds of such high intensity activity. In a 100 m sprint, for example, the available store of muscle ATP runs out before the finish line.

For prolonged strenuous exercise, the main cellular energy supply is from lactic energy processes. The main process for ATP synthesis during strenuous exercise is the anaerobic process of glycolysis, which uses glucose and stored glycogen as fuel and produces lactic acid. This process is the fast anaerobic breakdown of glucose for energy, but only provides limited amount of molecules of ATP along with a product called lactic acid and too much of this causes muscle fatigue.

Aerobic energy processes provide ATPs especially at low intensity exercise such as slow jogging and walking. Oxygen consumption reflects the energy demands during relatively low intensity exercise (less than 50 % of maximal oxygen uptake), but does not reflect energy demands during high intensity exercise.

There is heightened interest among athletes and coaches in using the lactic energy processes, as a basis for developing training programs. Wilmore et al. (2008) suggest that there is, however, no gold-standard method for determining an athlete's anaerobic capacity. Several methods are available; but the respective validity of each method is not strong, and at best each offers only a crude estimate of anaerobic capacity. An early attempt to estimate anaerobic capacity is blood lactate measurement after exhaustive exercise. In spite of controversy involving the quantitative estimate of the anaerobic energy production, it is generally agreed that increased blood lactate concentration is indicative of the contribution of lactic energy processes during exhaustive exercise. The maximal EPOC (excess post-exercise oxygen consumption) and the maximal oxygen deficit methods are also suggested as a means of estimating anaerobic capacity. Despite the limitations in each of these methods, sports scientists continue to use these methods as indirect indicators of anaerobic capacity.

At the Laboratory for Exercise Physiology and Biomechanics in Chukyo University, Japan, research has focused on the anaerobic capacity of elite to semi-elite athletes during games, such as soccer players, synchronized swimmers, alpine ski racers and competitive swimmers, in order to individualise sport-specific training program for athletes, by means of blood lactate measurements. This chapter provides an overview of research involving blood lactate measurements in competitive sports.

2. Blood lactate concentration during sports

Blood lactate sampling is usually conducted during pre-exercise rest, bicycling, intermittent rest and post-exercise recovery periods. Whilst it is easy for blood sampling to be done under laboratory conditions, most sports scientists favour blood lactate sampling of athletes during game conditions to fine-tune the training program. In this regard, we investigated a variety of athletes' blood lactate concentration during different types of sports under game conditions.

2.1. *Soccer*

Ekblom (1986) explained that soccer is a sport that can be categorized as a high intensity, and intermittent non-continuous exercise. Players cover approximately 10 km on the pitch per game. A greater percentage of the game is performed at maximal speed. Blood lactate concentration among players at half time and after a regular game ranged from 3.6 to 12.8 mM. Most studies on soccer, however, including those involving female players (Davies, et al., 1993) did not measure blood lactate concentration during the game, but only measured the blood lactate concentration at half time and after game.

One study from our laboratory investigated the change of blood lactate concentration to determine the exercise intensity of the game, using a percentage of maximal lactate during a soccer game (Miyagi et al., 1995). Four well-trained adult soccer players, consisting of center forwarder (CF), offensive mid-fielder (OM), defensive mid-fielder (DM) and stopper (ST) were subjects in the study. The physical characteristics of the subjects are shown in Table 1.

Table 1 Physical characteristics and body composition of the subjects (Miyagi et al., 1995)

Subject	Height	Weight	Fat	Fat	LBW	40s cycling	$\dot{V}O_2max$
	(cm)	(kg)	(%)	(kg)	(kg)	(watt/kg)	(ml/kg/min)
CF	178.7	71.78	8.0	5.74	66.04	6.2	62.1
OM	166.5	61.43	8.5	5.22	56.21	7.0	64.9
DM	173.0	66.49	7.8	5.19	61.30	6.9	67.0
ST	175.5	69.18	9.1	6.30	62.88	6.2	57.6
mean	173.4	67.22	8.4	5.61	61.61	6.6	62.9
SD	5.2	4.42	0.6	0.52	4.10	0.4	4.1

CF: Center forwarder, OM: Offensive mid-fielder, DM: Diffensive mid-fielder,
ST: Stopper,
LBW: Lean body weight

Body composition was estimated by densitometry using an underwater weighing method and a pulmonary residual volume measurement (Kitagawa et al., 1978). Percentage of body fat was calculated by the equation of Brožek et al. (1963). Maximal oxygen uptake was measured by a treadmill exhaustive running test. Peak blood lactate concentration was computed from five blood lactate measurements after a 40-second maximal pedaling exercise using a electrically braked bicycle ergometer (POWER MAX-V: Combi Wellness Corp., Japan) in the laboratory. Blood lactate concentrations were analyzed by an enzymatic membrane method (1500 Sports: YSI Corp., Tokyo, Japan). Table 2 shows individual and mean values, of which mean peak lactate concentration was 11.7 ± 0.6 mM.

Finger stick blood lactate concentration of the players during the game was measured at the 15th, 30th and 45th minute of each half, and at 5th and 10th minute of the half time. While blood sampling during the game, other players substituted for the subjects. The game for this study was a practice game but a very serious one because of soon coming final game. Temperature and humidity during the game were 27.1 °C and 62 %RH.

Table 2 Changes of blood lactate concentration after 40-second maximal effort cycling (Miyagi et al., 1995)

Subject	1 min (mM)	3 min (mM)	5 min (mM)	7 min (mM)	9 min (mM)	Peak LA (mM)
CF	10.0	10.60	11.5	10.4	10.0	11.5
OM	8.9	10.90	12.1	10.8	11.0	12.1
DM	8.8	9.80	10.3	11.0	10.2	11.0
ST	9.7	10.90	12.3	11.0	9.4	12.3
Mean	9.4	10.55	11.6	10.8	10.2	11.7
SD	0.6	0.52	0.9	0.3	0.7	0.6

La: blood lactate

Table 3 shows the lactate concentration and percentage of peak lactate concentration of each subject and averaged values. Mean values of lactate concentration and percentage of peak lactate concentration during the game according to positions were 5.8 mM and 50.1 % for CF, 5.6 mM and 46.6 % for OM, 5.2 mM and 46.8 % for DM, and 4.4 mM and 35.9 % for ST. Mean peak lactate concentration of the subjects was 11.7 ± 0.6mM shown in Table 2. Lactate concentration and percentage of peak lactate concentration during the game were 5.2 ± 1.0 mM and 44.9 ± 9.1 % on average, respectively. But there were significant differences in lactate concentration and percentage of peak lactate concentration between the two halves: 5.7 ± 0.9 mM and 49.0± 8.2 %, and 4.8 ± 0.9 mM and 40.7 ± 8.3 % in the second half.

Table 3 Changes of blood lactate concentration and percentage of peak blood lactate concentration during the game (Miyagi et al., 1995)

Subject	First half					
	15 min		30 min		45 min	
	La (mM)	%peakLa (%)	La (mM)	%peakLa (%)	La (mM)	%peakLa (%)
CF	5.7	49.6	7.4	64.3	5.6	48.7
OM	6.2	51.2	6.9	57.0	5.5	45.5
DM	5.7	51.8	6.3	57.3	4.4	40.0
ST	5.1	41.5	5.7	46.3	4.3	35.0
mean	5.7	48.5	6.6	56.2	5.0	42.3
SD	0.4	4.8	0.7	7.4	0.7	6.0
	Second half					
	15 min		30 min		45 min	
	La (mM)	%peakLa (%)	La (mM)	%peakLa (%)	La (mM)	%peakLa (%)
CF	5.5	47.8	5.9	51.3	4.5	39.1
OM	6.2	51.2	4.9	40.5	4.1	33.9
DM	5.5	50.0	4.7	42.7	4.3	39.1
ST	4.3	35.0	4.0	32.5	3.1	25.2
mean	5.4	46.0	4.9	41.8	4.0	34.3
SD	0.8	7.5	0.8	7.7	0.6	6.6

La: blood lactate concentration

% peakLa: percentage of peak blood lactate concentration

In order to verify the removal rate of lactate during half time, the removal rate was calculated by the equation described below; {(lactate at 45th minute of first half − lactate at rest) − (lactate at 5th or 10th minute during half time − lactate at rest)}/ (lactate at 45th minute of first half − lactate at rest). Table 4 shows that lactate concentration and lactate removal rate of the players during the half time were 2.9 ± 0.4 mM and 30.7 ± 6.3 % at the 5th minute, and 1.9 ± 0.3 mM and 54.9 ± 6.7 % at the 10th minute. Table 4 also shows that there were no players who regained the resting level in 10th minute of the half time.

Table 4 Blood lactate concentration and blood lactate removal rate in the half-time (Miyagi et al., 1995)

Subject	Rest	Half-time			
		5th min		10th min	
	La (mM)	La (mM)	Removal rate (%)	La (mM)	Removal rate (%)
CF	0.8	3.1	35.4	2.0	58.3
OM	0.9	3.3	28.3	2.1	54.3
DM	0.9	2.7	22.9	1.9	45.7
ST	0.7	2.3	36.1	1.4	61.1
mean	0.8	2.9	30.7	1.9	54.9
SD	0.1	0.4	6.3	0.3	6.7

La: blood lactate, Removal rate: see the text.

These results indicate that most players play at above 4 mM level of lactate concentration during the game, and anaerobic metabolism plays an important role in well trained adult soccer players. Therefore soccer player and coach must pay sufficient attention on anaerobic exercise training, and also use the half-time period to actively rest players so that the overall blood lactate concentration is reduced. This will also spare the muscle glycogen for the latter parts of the game, in the second half.

2.2. *Synchronized swimming*

Synchronized swimmers conduct complex and precise maneuvers while floating, and sometimes undergo prolonged apneic conditions in water. In particular, swimmers must execute physical maneuvers of a high intensity many times during any competition. In addition to these dynamic movements, gracefulnesses as well as shapeliness in action are also important factors for artistic evaluation.

Our laboratory investigated the physiological loads on synchronized swimmers during the team technical and free routines by measuring blood lactate concentrations and percentage of peak blood lactate concentration (Yamamura et al., 2000). The components in the study were classified into six skill elements by videotape; deck movement, stroke figure, underwater movement, body boost, rocket and lift. Four trained college female synchronized swimmers aged 19.6 ± 1.4 years were subjects in the study. All were the finalists in the 1995 Japan

Synchronized Swimming Open Championships. The physical characteristics of the subjects are shown in Table 5.

Table 5 Physical characteristics of the subjects (Yamamura et al., 2000)

Height (cm)	Weight (kg)	Fat (%)	LBW (kg)	$\dot{V}O_2max$ (ml/kg/min)	Peak La (mM)
162.5±7.8	53.4±5.2	17.2±2.6	44.2±3.4	51.6±1.5	10.2±1.1

Values are mean and SD (n=4). LBW: lean body weight

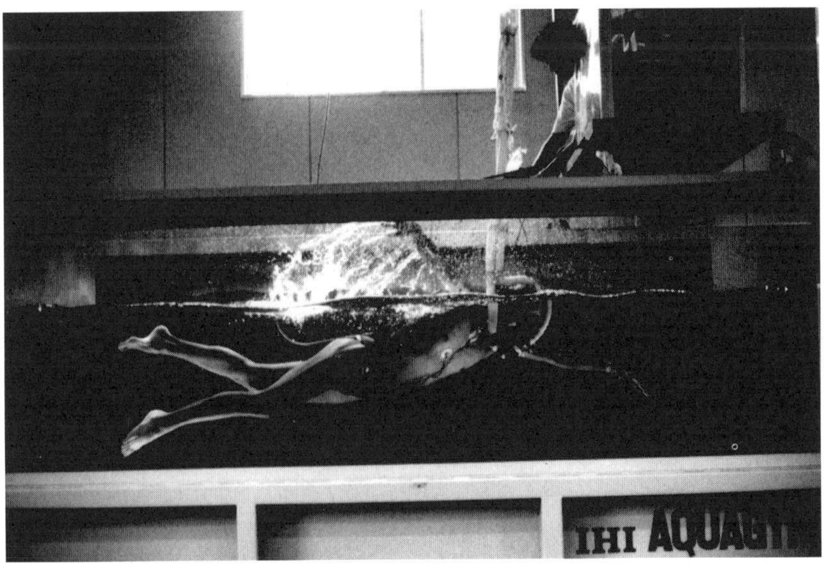

Figure 1 Swimming flume (AQUAGYM: IHI Corp., Tokyo, Japan)

Body composition was measured by densitometry using an underwater weighing method and a pulmonary residual volume measurement. The equation of Brožek et al (1963) was used to calculate the percentage of body fat. Maximal oxygen uptake was measured by exhaustive swimming test in the swimming flume (AQUAGYM: IHI Corp., Tokyo, Japan) shown in Figure 1.

Peak blood lactate concentration was measured after maximal exertion in a100-m freestyle swim. Blood samples were taken from the fingertips at 3, 5, 7 and 9 minutes after exercise. The highest concentration value was selected as the value presenting peak blood lactate concentration. Blood lactate concentrations were analyzed by an enzymatic membrane method (1500 Sports: YSI Corp., Tokyo, Japan). The blood lactate concentration was measured in the first and middle periods and after the team technical and free routine as shown in Figure 2.

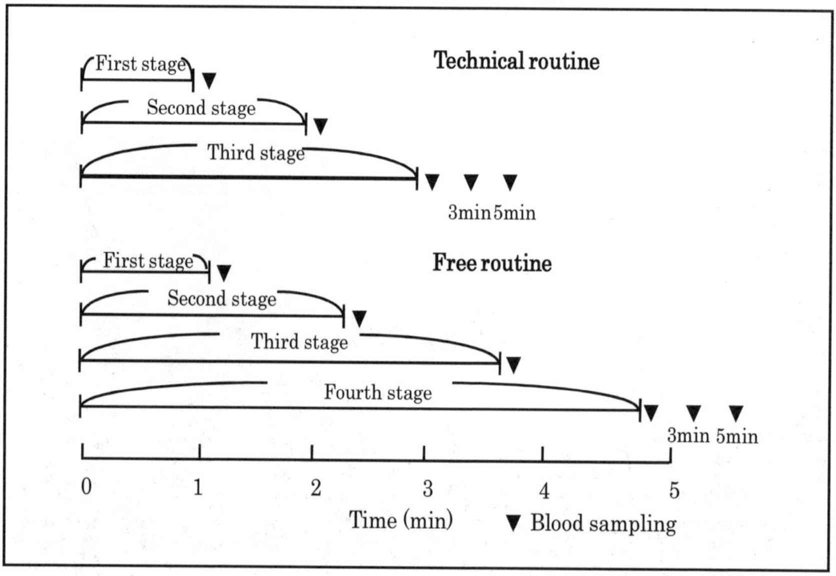

Figure 2 Blood sampling time in the team technical and free routines (Yamamura et al., 2000)

Each stage was performed from start to finish. A resting period of more than 45 minutes was allowed between the second and the third stages of the team technical routine, and between the third and the fourth stages of the team free routine. The resting period among the other stages was more than 30 minutes. Blood samples were taken immediately, then at 3 and 5 minutes after the final stages; the highest blood lactate concentration value was selected as the value of the final stage of the team technical and free routines. At each of the other stages blood was taken immediately after.

Averaged values of blood lactate concentration and the percentage of peak blood lactate concentration after team technical and free routine were 4.7 ± 1.1

mM, 46.2 ± 11.0 % and 4.3 ± 1.1 mM, 42.8 ± 11.5 %, respectively shown in Table 6.

Table 6 Lactate concentration and percentage of peak blood lactate concentration during the team technical and free routines (Yamamura et al., 2000)

	1st stage	2nd stage	3rd stage	4th stage
Technical routine				
La (mM)	2.9±0.3	3.9±0.8	4.7±1.1[a]	
%peak La (%)	28.6±5.3	38.6±7.1	46.2±11.0[a]	
Free routine				
La (mM)	3.1±0.4	2.6±0.7	3.7±1.0	4.3±1.1[b]
%peak La (%)	30.7±7.8	26.2±9.7	36.8±15.3	42.8±11.5

Values are mean and SD (n = 4).

La: blood lactate concentration, %peak La: percentage of peak blood lactate concentration

[a]: first stage vs. third stage($p < 0.05$), [b]: second stage vs. third stage ($p < 0.05$)

The blood lactate concentration and percentage of peak blood lactate concentration after the technical routine were significantly higher than those in the first period, and the blood lactate concentration after the team routine was significantly higher than in the middle period. The blood lactate concentration of synchronized swimmers during team technical and free routines in the study tended to increase with the performance time. Thus, in the first period for the technical routine and the middle period for the free routine, the predominant sources of energy may be phosphocreatine stores and aerobic metabolism. On the other hand, in the final period, glycolysis may also play an important role in relation to the energy requirements of the routines.

2.3. *Energy source contribution in alpine skiing*

Åstrand et al. (2003) reported that one of the first studies on elite alpine skiing was carried out by Agnevik et al. They measured various physiological variables such as heart rate, oxygen uptake and blood lactate concentration both in the laboratory and during regular international competitions. Peak lactate concentrations after the races were about 14 mM for the special slalom racers and about 15 mM for thc giant slalom racers. After that study, Veicsteinas et al.

(1984) measured the energy source contribution in special slalom and giant slalom skiing by means of the Douglas Bag method. This method, however, has an intrinsic disadvantage in field studies. The Douglas Bag bothered skiing and racers could not ski with the bag as freely as without the bag.

Our laboratory investigated the energy source contribution in giant slalom (GSL) and slalom (SL) skiing (Yamamoto et al., 1999). The subjects were five Japanese male varsity alpine ski racers, ranked in the semi-elite class in Japan. Their SAJ (Ski Association of Japan) points were 52.48~73.71 for GSL skiers and 20.96~110.41 for SL skiers. Their physical characteristics were shown in Table 7.

Body composition was estimated by densitometry using underwater weighing method and a pulmonary residual volume measurement. Percentage of body fat was calculated by the equation of Brožek et al (1963). Their physical fitness characteristics were shown in Table 8.

Table 7 Physical characteristics of the subjects (Yamamoto et al., 1999)

Age (year)	Height (cm)	Weight (kg)	Fat (%)	LBW (kg)
20.7±1.5	173.2±4.3	70.22±4.6	9.2±2.2	63.69±3.4

Values are mean and SD (n = 5). LBW: lean body weight

Table 8 Physical fitness characteristics of the subjects (Yamamoto et al., 1999)

$\dot{V}O_2max$		HRmax	Alactic power		Lactic power		Peak La
(l/min)	(ml/kg/min)	(beats/min)	(W)	(W/kg)	(W)	(W/kg)	(mM)
3.94±0.19	55±4	204±4	1296±71.3	18.3±0.8	698.2±31.4	9.9±0.4	11.4±0.8

Maximal oxygen uptake was determined by a treadmill run test to exhaustion. Maximal alactic power and lactic power were measured by an electrically braked bicycle ergometer (POWER MAX-V: Combi Wellness Corp., Tokyo, Japan) in the laboratory. Aerobic and anaerobic metabolisms during and just after SL and GSL skiing were measured by oxygen uptake and blood lactate concentrations, respectively. Oxygen uptake was measured by the portable apparatus (Mac Quarto VM4-064: VINE Corp., Tokyo, Japan) and blood samples were taken at 3, 5 and 7 minutes after goal in. Ski courses were set under the regulations of SAJ affiliated to FIS (Fédération Internationale de Ski); the course profile of GSL was 800m long, 280m altitude with averaged 17 degree and profile of SL was 450m long, 130m altitude with averaged 15 degree. Their performance times were 53.2 seconds for GSL and 46.9 seconds for SL on average.

Lactate concentration and percentage of peak lactate concentration during skiing were 6.8 ± 1.0 mM and 60.9 ± 6.0 % for GSL, and 6.9 ± 0.5 mM and 62.6 ± 6.2 % for SL. Table 9 shows the aerobic and anaerobic energy sources in GSL, SL and 40 second maximal effort cycling on POWER MAX-V. Figure 3 also shows the energy contribution of the components in GSL, SL and cycling.

Table 9 Aerobic and anaerobic energy sources in giant slalom, slalom and 40 second maximal effort cycling (Yamamoto et al., 1999)

	ΔVO_2tot (l)	ΔVO_2ex (l)	ΔVO_2rec (l)	ΔVO_2La (l)
Giant slalom	6.17±0.64	1.77±0.33	3.21±0.45	1.19±0.15
Slalom	6.95±0.79	1.72±0.35	4.03±0.49	1.20±0.11
40s cycling	7.34±0.44	1.44±0.39	3.74±0.30	2.16±0.25

Values are mean and SD (n = 5).

ΔVO_2tot:total oxygen cost

ΔVO_2ex:liters of O_2 above resting consumed during exercise

ΔVO_2rec:liters of O_2 above resting consumed during recovery

ΔVO_2La:O_2 equivalent of the net accumulated lactate

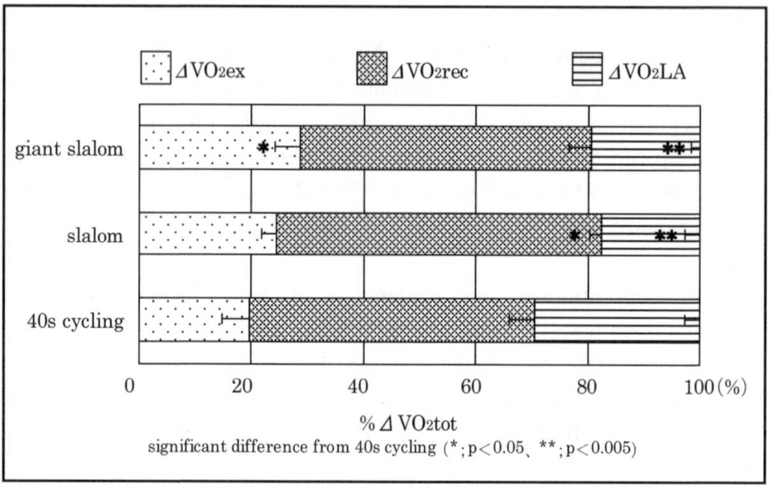

Figure 3 Energy contribution of the components in giant slalom, slalom and 40 second cycling by permission of *Jap. J. Biomech. Sports Exer.* with minor modification (Yamamoto et al., 1999)

The results showed that the body dimensions of the racers in this study were smaller, and that they had lower maximal oxygen uptake and anaerobic power than the elite world class racers in the previous studies. The contribution of the three energy systems was estimated by measuring oxygen uptake during SL and GSL skiing. Approximately 55 % of total energy came from the alactic energy system, 20 % from the lactic energy system and 25 % from the aerobic energy system. Compared to the elite world-class racers in the previous study, the results showed that racers in the study had less contribution to the lactic energy system, a higher oxygen expenditure and smaller lactate accumulation.

2.4. *Critical swimming velocity*

Critical swimming velocity (Vcri) is recognized to be the swimming speed corresponding to the maximal lactate steady state (MLSS), and it is expressed as the slope of a regression line between swimming distances and their sustained times. Vcri has been utilized as an index for determining training speed and evaluating endurance capacity in the field of competitive swimming. Vcri has its origin in critical power (Wcri), which was defined by Monod and Scherrer (1965) as the slope of the regression line based on the total work performed and the corresponding time until exhaustion, which can be theoretically maintained and continued without exhaustion. Wakayoshi et al. (1992) applied the concept of Wcri to the field of competitive swimming as Vcri, and showed that Vcri corresponds to MLSS.

2.4.1. *A simplified method for freestyle sprinter and distance swimmer*

In order to determine Vcri, the conventional practical test requires a swimmer to swim a distance of 200-m and 400-m twice. Our laboratory researched into a simpler method for the determination of Vcri (Takahashi et al., 2002). Eight sprinters (50-m and 100-m freestyle) and eight distance swimmers (400-m and 1500-m freestyle) performed 50-m, 100-m, 200-m, 300-m, 400-m and 1500-m at maximal effort in a 25m-swimming pool. The obtained Vcri were 1.409 ± 0.064m/sec for sprinters and 1.482 ± 0.026m/sec for distance swimmers. Then, so as to find the simpler method, the relationships between Vcri and swimming velocities at each swimming distance (V50m, V100m, V200m, V300m, V400m and V1500m) were investigated.

Both sprinters and distance swimmers showed significant relationships between Vcri and swimming velocities at distances over 200 m. From the viewpoint of the aerobic energy supply system to muscle, however, V300m was the most appropriate swimming velocity to estimate Vcri as an endurance index from the shortest swimming distance. In order to make sure that Vcri shows the maximal lactate steady state, the subjects were instructed to swim 2500m at the three constant velocities (98.5 %, 100 % and 101.5 % of Vcri). Blood samples were taken from the finger tips at intervals of each 500 m swim. As shown in Figure 4, 100 % of Vcri showed a higher steady state than 98.5 % of Vcri, but 101.5 % of Vcri did not demonstrate the steady state. Thus, we recognized that 100 % of Vcri was at the highest steady state level. Therefore one timed 300 m maximal effort swimming test is believed to be a simpler, more rational method to determine Vcri for both freestyle sprinters and distance swimmers.

2.4.2. *A simplified method for breaststroke swimmer*

The laboratory also determined whether the critical swimming velocity (Vcri) estimated by the swimming velocity for a distance of 300 m at maximal effort breaststroke reflects MLSS (Takahashi et al., 2009). The subjects were nine male and three female trained college swimmers with more than nine years experience as competitive swimmers; eight swimmers were specialized in the breaststroke and four in the individual medley. They swam 50 m, 300 m and 2000 m at maximal effort for determination of Vcri that averaged 1.167 ± 0.045m/sec. Since Vcri was equivalent to 90.5 % of the mean swimming velocity

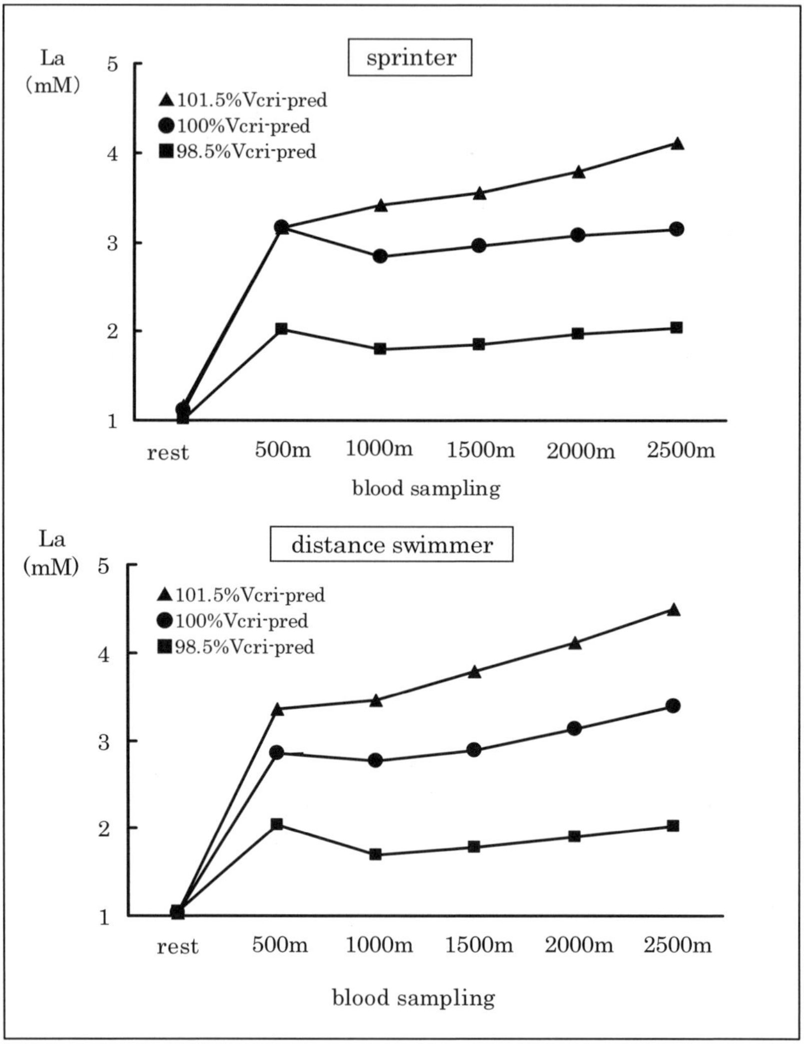

Figure 4 Changes of blood lactate concentration in 2,500m endurance swimming at three different velocities by permission of *Jap J Biomech Sports Exer* with minor modification (Takahashi et al., 2002)

over the distance of 300-m at maximal effort, the swimming velocity obtained by multiplying the swimming velocity for the distance of 300-m of each subject by 90.5 % was taken to be 100 % of the predicted critical swimming velocity (Vcri-pred). Then, in an MLSS test, the subjects were instructed to swim breaststroke 2000 m (5×400 m) at three constant velocities (98 %, 100 %, and 102 % of Vcri-pred), interrupted by four short rest periods from 30 to 45 seconds for blood sampling and heart rate measurement.

As a result, the blood lactate concentration at 100 % Vcri-pred showed a higher steady state than the slow velocity, but at high velocity did not show the steady state. Thus, the present results indicate that a one timed 300 m maximal effort swimming test is a simpler, more effective indicator of endurance capacity and to determine the training pace in breaststroke swimming without significantly interfering with the daily training regimen. In conclusion, we can accurately estimate the Vcri for breaststroke by a one-time 300-m maximal effort swimming test.

3. Conclusion

It is generally agreed that blood lactate accumulation in the blood indicates increased anaerobic glycolysis in the muscle as a result of high intensity exercise. Blood lactate accumulation during incremental exercise tests are used routinely to determine peak lactate concentration and the onset of blood lactate accumulation (OBLA) is a measurement which is commonly used to evaluate the effectiveness of a training program. These tests conducted in the laboratory do not provide complete answers about the anaerobic capacity of athletes, especially in real game-like situations in the field. The research team at Chukyo University demonstrated that field measurement of blood lactate concentration in various sporting contexts provided useful information to athletes and coaches alike which can be used to refine training programs that can bring out the best in each athlete.

References

1. Åstrand, P.-O., Rodahl, K., Dahl, H.A., and Stromme, S.B. (2003). *Textbook of Work Physiology* 4th ed. Human Kinetics, Champaign, IL, USA. pp 491-493.
2. Brožek, J., Grande, F., Anderson, J.T. and Keys, A. (1963). Densitometric analysis of body composition: Revision of some quantitative assumptions. *Annals of New York Academy of Science, 110*, 113-140.

3. Davis, J.A. and Brewer, J. (1993). Applied physiology of female soccer players. *Sports Medicine, 16*, 180-189.
4. Ekblom, B. (1986). Applied physiology of soccer. *Sports Medicine*, *3*, 50-60.
5. Kitagawa, K. and Miyashita, M. (1978). Muscle strength in relation to fat storage rate in young man. *European Journal of Applied Physiol*ogy, *38*, 189-196.
6. Miyagi, O., Shimazaki, T., Taki, H., Ishiko, T. and Kitagawa, K. (1995). Exercise intensity of soccer game using blood lactic acid of well trained adult soccer players. *Japanese Journal of Sports Science, 14*, 639-645.
7. Monod, H. and Scherrer, J. (1965). The work capacity of a synergic muscular group. *Ergonomics*, *8*, 329-337.
8. Takahashi, S., Wakayoshi, K., Nagasawa, S. and Kitagawa, K. (2002). A simplified method for determination of critical swimming velocity as a swimming fatigue threshold for sprinter and distance simmers. *Japanese Journal of Biomechanics, Sports and Exercise*, *6*, 110-115.
9. Takahashi, S., Wakayoshi, K., Hayashi, A., Sakaguchi, Y. and Kitagawa, K. (2009). A method for determining critical swimming velocity. *International Journal of Sports Medicine, 30*, 119-123.
10. Veicsteinas, A., Feretti, G., Margonato, G.R. and Tangliabue, D. (1984). Energy cost of energy sources for alpine skiing in top athletes. *Journal of Applied Physiology Respiration and Environmental Exercise Physiology, 56,* 1187-1190.
11. Wakayoshi, K., Ikuta, K., Yoshida, T., Udo, M., Moritani, T., Mutoh, Y. and Miyashita, M. (1992). Determination and validity of critical velocity as an index of swimming performance in the competitive swimmer. *European Journal of Applied Physiol*ogy, *64*, 153-157.
12. Wilmore, J.H., Costill, D.V. and Kenney, W.L. (2008). *Physiology of Sport and Exercise* 4th ed. Human Kinetics, Champaign, IL, USA. pp110.
13. Yamamoto, S., Matsui, N. and Kitagawa, K. (1999). Energy metabolism in giant and slalom skiing of Japanese alpine ski racers. *Japanese Journal of Biomechanics, Sports and Exercise, 3*, 95-102.
14. Yamamura, C., Matsui, N. and Kitagawa, K. (2000). Physiological loads in the team technical and free routines of synchronized swimmers. *Medicine and Science in Sports and Exercise, 32,* 1171-1174.
15. Zumerchik, J. (Ed). *Encyclopedia of Sports Science* Vol. 2. Simon and Schuster MacMillan, New York, USA, 1997. pp. 646-648.

ASSESSMENT OF BODY COMPOSITION

GOVINDASAMY BALASEKARAN

Physical Education and Sports Science, National Institute of Education, Nanyang Technological University, Singapore

NIDHI GUPTA

Physical Education and Sports Science, National Institute of Education, Nanyang Technological University, Singapore

VISVASURESH VICTOR GOVINDASWAMY

Texas A&M University, Texarkana, U.S.A.

Body composition is a term used to categorise the different components in the human body, which collectively make up an individual's body weight. The human body consists of a variety of components such as metabolically active tissue like fat-free mass or lean mass, which includes muscle, bone and organs and non- metabolically active tissue such as fat. With modernisation, health professionals and researchers are focusing on accurate measurements of body composition. An accurate evaluation of body composition is indispensable in identifying body fat and fat-free mass which are used to categorise individuals in exercise and clinical settings, and are used as scaling factors to normalize physiologic variables such as metabolic rate, physical activity, and physical fitness. There are different types of body composition assessment models and these are commonly divided into the two compartment model; fat mass and fat-free mass, which may be measured accurately by total body potassium, total body water and under water weighing techniques. The underwater weighing technique was considered as the gold standard in measurement of body composition until recent advancements in technology where new sophisticated methods have made this technique outdated. This chapter focuses on recent advancements in body composition assessment and discusses the limitations and advantages of the various techniques of body composition available.

1. Introduction

In the modern era, health professionals including scientists, health workers and researchers from different disciplines are focusing on body composition in assessment, physiology, psychology, nutrition etc. Information garnered from research and applied in clinical practice is an important factor in the classification and treatment of obesity via different intervention programmes that employ exercise, dieting and behaviour modification. Body composition helps to maintain proper work capacity, muscular strength, and the ability to perform daily tasks such as walking and lifting. Negative changes in body composition can lead to a decline in physical performance capabilities of an individual (Bemben et al., 1995).

Body composition analysis evolved from the single unit of body weight through the classical division of fat and fat free mass (FFM), known as the two compartment model and then to the three, four or more compartment models. The first model is a single compartment model that includes measurement of body weight. Although, weight alone does not give an accurate indication about body composition, it was popular in categorising level of obesity in adults. The two compartment model divides the body composition into two compartments; Fat mass (FM) and FFM (Jebb et al., 2000). This model is the basis of most classical body composition techniques such as total body water (TBW), total body potassium (TBK), and underwater weighing (UWW). Previously, hydrostatic weighing was the 'gold standard' or 'reference method' for measuring body composition and it was based on assumed constant densities of fat and FFM (Balasekaran, 2003). However, water, protein and mineral FFM fractions vary considerably according to age, ethnicity and sex. Furthermore, this method presented many technical problems especially the determination of residual lung volumes (Davies and Cole, 1995). Longitudinal studies also show that UWW does not reliably measure small changes in body composition (Institute of Medicine, U.S., Committee on Body Composition, Nutrition and Health of Military Women, Institute of Medicine, U.S., 1998). Additionally, it does not take hydration status into account and this leads to erroneous readings (Davies & Cole, 1995; Institute of Medicine, U.S., Committee on Body Composition, Nutrition and Health of Military Women, Institute of Medicine,

U.S., 1998). Hydrostatic weighing also does not take into account the variations in FFM among different ethnicities like African-American and Caucasian subjects (Clark, Kuta, & Sullivan, 1993; Visser et al., 1997).

The three compartment model divides the body into fat, water and protein and minerals (Siri, 1961). Firstly, TBW is measured and removed from its contributor, total body density (Db), so that, Db including protein, fat and minerals can be calculated (Wang et al., 2005). One of the best models to determine body composition is the four compartment model (Aleman-Mateo et al., 2007). This model consists of bone mineral density (BMD; Dual Energy X- Ray Absorptiometry; DXA) along with the three compartment model (TBW) to eliminate the errors related to individual differences in the bone (Wang et al., 2005). The body mass (BM) is- BM = FM + TBW + bone mass (Mo) + residuals (includes protein, soft tissues such as minerals and glycogen) (Wang et al., 2005)

For healthy, similar-weight categories, and ethnically-similar participants with similar age range, two, three and four compartment body composition models give accurate and similar measurements. But in cases of diseased and varied-weight categories or in varied subjects differing in age, sex, and race, four compartment model is the only method that provides accurate fat measurements (Heymsfield et al., 1993). Currently, the four compartment model is used as a reference method to measure body fat percent (fat%) and FFM estimation in homogenous and heterogeneous population (Institute of Medicine, U.S., Committee on Body Composition, Nutrition and Health of Military Women, Institute of Medicine, U.S., 1998; Aloia, Vaswani, & Flaster, 1996; 1997). Lohman (1992) supported the use of four compartment model for children owing to changes in FFM density due to a decrease in TBW and an increase in BMD during growth and development. Four compartment models require good techniques to measure components of body composition. It includes measurement of Db, BMD and TBW in the body. Traditionally Db is measured through hydrodensitometry but selections of methods for measuring body composition depends on accuracy, easiness and invasiveness. Descriptive methods (Body Mass Index; BMI, DXA, Skinfolds, and Bioelectric Impedance Analysis; BIA) are more preferable than mechanistic methods (dilution techniques, densitometry) because they are non-invasive, inexpensive and fast as compared to more elaborate mechanistic methods (Lichtenbelt et al., 2004). In hydrodensitometry, some children and older adults, specially overweight or obese children, face difficulty in performing some of the testing procedures (Heyward, & Wagner, 2004) and also the density of FFM keeps fluctuating due to changes in water, protein, and minerals components due to growth and maturation influences (Roemmich et al., 1997). An important recent advancement is the use of DXA (descriptive method) for the measurement of body composition. For absolute measurements of FM the measurement of BMD is essential. DXA, based on the three compartment model including FM, FFM and BMD, utilizes a simple technique for measuring BMD. DXA has been validated against the four compartment model and has been proven to be a gold standard for body fat, BMD and FFM estimation. However, DXA can be combined with variety of multi- compartment models for producing more qualitative results such as combination of DXA with TBW gives researchers more information on mineral, water, fat and the remaining fat free soft tissues which is predominantly proteins (Heymsfield et al., 1990). This combination model is preferred over four compartment model proposed by Heymsfield (1990) in which Invitro Neutron Activation analysis (ICNAA) is used to measure total body calcium as the estimate of mineral mass and nitrogen for protein measurement. However, glycogen amount is unmeasured by Invitro Neutron Activation four compartment model (Heymsfield, 1990).

Every component of body composition has its own importance. The absolute amount of fat, termed as FM that includes all extractable lipids and adipose tissues (Heyward & Vivian, 2004). Literature suggests that women have high fat percentage than men due to physiological reasons such as child-bearing (Science Daily, 2009). The preferred methods for identifying extra body fat are high BMI and high waist hip ratio (WHR) which indicates increased obesity and a risk for coronary heart disease (Park, Heymsfield, & Gallaghar, 2002). The types and the level of participation in physical activities influence body fat percentage (% BF). Individuals engaged in elite sports which is dynamic and utilises more muscle mass tend to have lower % BF (Balasekearan, 2003).

2. Bone mineral density (BMD)

BMD is an important factor in osteoporosis. Osteoporosis is a serious health hazard in many parts of the world. It causes softening, and weakening of the bone leading to an eventual loss of bone mass that may lead to increase in risk of fractures (Ondrak & Morgan, 2006). The main causes for such fractures are decreased bone mass and bone mineral content (Cummings et al., 1993). Women are more prone than men to such fractures especially during the post menopausal phase due to the depletion of the hormone estrogen to lower levels leading to the eventual reduction in BMD (Riggs, Khosla, & Melton, 1998). BMD at any time of the life span is dependent upon bone gained during the early years of growth and bone loss with advancing age. Studies on preventive strategies for loss of BMD show that performing physical activity in the growing years can reduce bone loss in later years of life (Karlsson, 2002). Some studies show that maximizing peak bone density to one's full genetic potential during early years of growth is a good way to prevent or delay the onset of osteoporosis (Heaney, 1991). Overweight individuals add more mechanical stress on their bone and may lead to increased BMD and prevent age-induced osteoporosis (Toth et al., 2005; Cobayashi, Lopes & Taddei, 2005), But some studies do not support this assertion (Chao et al. 2000).

Bone mass is related to muscle mass and FM and these variables are important predictors of bone mass. Visser et al (1998) observed positive correlations between total body BMD with muscle mass ($P = 0.007$) and body fat percentage ($r = 0.38$; $P = 0.0001$) among 504 women aged 72-93 years and among 285 older men, muscle mass was directly related to BMD ($P = 0.02$) but not FM ($r = 0.32$; $P = 0.32$). Cui et al (2007) also indicated that muscle mass is an important predictor in pre-menopausal women while, FM is the important predictor in post menopausal women in South Korea. In pre-menopausal women, muscle mass was the only variable correlated with BMD for all sites; Lumbar Spine (L1-L4; $r = 0.245$; $P = 0.007$), Femoral neck ($r = 0.372$; $P = 0.000$), Ward's triangle ($r = 0.335$; $P = 0.0001$), Trochanter ($r = 0.540$; $P = 0.000$), Distal Forearm ($r = 0.401$; $P = 0.000$), and Calcanus ($r = 0.314$; $P = 0.0001$). But in post menopausal women, FM was positively correlated with BMD at lumbar ($r = 0.153$; $P = 0.011$), distal forearm ($r = 0.157$; $P = 0.002$), and calcaneus sites ($r= 0.226$; $P = 0.0001$), and both muscle ($r = 0.341$; $P = 0.0001$) and FM ($r = 0.105$; $P = 0.042$) was associated to BMD at the hip. Douchi et al (2003) reported a positive correlation between muscle mass and BMD ($r = 0.545$, $P < 0.0001$). Sun et al (2003) observed that pre-menopausal women among African-American, Asian American, and European American and post menopausal European American women have a strong positive relation between total BMD and total appendicular muscle mass ($r = 0.925$; $P = 0.001$) but had a negative relation in post menopausal African American ($r = -0.013$; $P = 0.021$) and post menopausal Asian-American women ($r = -0.019$; $P = 0.087$).

3. Hydrodensitometry

Assessment of body composition is necessary to determine athletes' status of preparation as well as to profile the unique sports specific characteristics that differentiate athletes from one another. It is also necessary to determine the efficacy of physical training and nutritional and energy requirements (Wang et al., 1995). Body composition encompass many different components, ranging from body fat, water compartment, and cell mass to bone minerals.

Until recently, UWW or hydrodensitometry, was considered as a gold standard, and was used as a criterion measure for measuring body composition (Gulick, 1999; Sutton & Miller, 2006). This technique is based on measurement of body volume of human body. The term densitometry means the method which assesses body composition through the measurement of body density. This technique is based on Archimedes Principle that 'a body immersed in a fluid is acted on by a buoyancy force, which is evidenced by a loss of weight equal to weight of displaced fluid (DeTurk & Cahalin, 2004). The body volume is equal to loss of body weight in water, which is then corrected for the density of water (Dw) corresponding to temperature of water at the time of submersion (Heyward & Vivian, 2004). This formula is shown below.

$$BV = \frac{(Wa - Ww)}{Dw}$$

Wa and Ww are the weights of the subject in air and water respectively including residual air left in lungs after exhalation and flatus in gastrointestinal tract (GI tract) at the time of measurement. The GI gas volume is generally considered to be minimal, with constant value of 100 ml while the residual volume in the air is measured through indirect measurement derived from vital capacity which is considered to be fixed as 1.3 L for men and 1.0 L (Buskirk 1961). The preferable method for assessing residual gas in lungs is nitrogen washout procedure by Wilmore (Wilmore, 1969). With the correction for residual volume (RV) and flatus in GI tract, the calculation of body density becomes as follows:

$$Db = \frac{Wa}{\{[(Wa\text{-}Ww)/Dw]\text{-}(RV+100cc)\}}$$

The validity of hydrostatic weighing is limited in clinical settings because of the time and space required to perform this technique (Pollock & Jackson, 1984). The standard error of estimate of this technique is 2.7 %, primarily because of the variation in FFM density within specific populations (Lohman, 1981). It also requires expertise both on part of examiner and subject. It can be difficult for a novice as it is necessary to expel air as much as possible from lungs when subject's head is immersed in water. The limitations of hydro-densitometry method, gave rise to more feasible and practical technique which is based on measuring body volume, called as air displacement plethysmograph. This technique uses pressure - volume relationship to compute density and volume (Heyward, 2006). It is proven to be a better technique to avoid many of errors of hydro-densitometry. This technique is based on Boyle's law that is a quantity of air compressed under isothermal conditions will decrease its volume in proportion to the increasing pressure (Dempster & Aitkens, 1995)

The relation between pressure and volume is: $P1/P2 = (V2/V1)^r$, where r is the constant represent ratio of specific heat of gas at constant pressure and constant volume (Going, 2005; Sly, Lanteri, & Bates, 1990). Change of pressure and compression of air under isothermal condition is easier than in adiabatic conditions (Going, 2005). This difference leads to significant volume measurement error of 2.5%, which limits its use in a research setting where a higher level of accuracy is needed. The Bod Pod body composition equipment is based on the air displacement technique. The technique of body composition analysis is based on Poisson's law, which at appropriate conditions (that the subject be dry, and that the testing environments temperature remain stable; BOD POD body composition system, 2000) is more precise and accurate compared to other past methods including hydrostatic weighing (Fields, Higgins, & Hunter, 2004). The equipment includes two chambers: testing chamber of 450L where the subject is seated, and a reference chamber of 300L.

4. Bioelectric impedance analysis (BIA)

BIA was introduced for the measurement of body composition, (Hoffer, Meader, Simpson, 1969; Lukaski et al.,1986), which is based on the principle of impedance; a current is supplied to the body by two electrodes placed on the body and two detection electrodes are placed to detect the resistance and reactance in the body (Nyboer, 1959). In the human body, the bioelectric impedance method measures impedance of water (conductor) with the help of resistance, as in non-biological conductors, and reactance, caused by capacitant effect of cell membranes, tissue interfaces, and non-ionic tissues that retard a portion of electric current through multiple current pathways (Barnett & Bagno, 1936). The usual distance between the electrodes is the length of the conductor and the minimal allowed distance between the electrodes is 4-5 cm to avoid electric interference. The limb and trunk of the human body is not a uniform conductor (Chumlea & Sun, 2005). Limbs are usually made up of a high amount of muscles and offer a high electrical resistance due to the high amount of water in the muscles (Chumlea & Sun, 2005). The human trunk is composed of complex organs like lungs, heart, liver and kidneys and the majority of the commercial impedance analyzers may not be able to produce uniform current in the body (Chumlea & Sun, 2005).

Advanced technology has led to two types of impedance analyzers; the single frequency and multiple frequency analyzers. Single frequency analyzer uses frequency at 50 kHz approximately and is not sensitive to changes in body composition (Alvarez et al., 2007). Segmental BIA and multi-frequency BIA are sensitive to body composition changes and compute body composition regionally. It is based on the fact that 85 % of the total impedance is from the arms and the legs (Heitmann, 1994) but the legs and trunk contributed to only about 15-17 % approximately (Chumlea, Baumgartner, & Mitchell, 1990). Additionally, the volume assessed by segmental BIA is lower than the volume assessed by DXA (Bracco et al., 1996). In earlier days of impedance analysis, the measurements were taken in the supine position in order to counter-balance the effect of gravity on body fluid in the standing position.

Due to modern advancement in impedance analyzers (multi-frequency, segmental impedance analyzer), measurements can be taken in standing as well as in the supine position depending upon the model. In case of disproportionate size, shape and composition of limbs and trunk, measurements are affected (National Institute of Health, 1994). Measurements are also not accurate in case of obese subjects due to high proportion of body fat, tissue, water in FFM and also due to increase proportions of ICW and ECW (Sun et al., 2005). There are no reference norms for impedance values for data interpretation and these values are not accurate in clinical settings [wider limits of agreement between $\%BF_{DXA}$ and $\%BF_{BIA}$ (male: 6.7%; Female: 6.1%; unpublished data]. Additionally, accurate readings are not possible in cases of malnutrition in subjects due to the disturbance in the level of ICW in the body.

BIA is also not accurate in case of acute body weight changes due to dieting and glycogen changes in extreme weight loss. However, it is doubtful as to whether the validity and reliability of equations derived from impedance for prediction of body composition are better and whether BIA is better than anthropometry alone (Cohn, 1985; Diaz et al., 1989)

5. Computed tomography (CT) and magnetic resonance imaging (MRI)

Computed Tomography (CT) is an accurate technique to measure body composition and it measures skeletal muscle and adipose tissue. A basic system of CT consists of x-ray tube and a receiver. An attenuation of x-ray is detected by the receiver and is called a linear coefficient or CT number. Then an image is reconstructed with mathematical techniques based on two dimensional fourier analysis, a filtered back projection or combination of both methods (Heymsfield et al., 2004). These images have pixels and each pixel is assigned by a CT number which gives contrast to the image and each CT value reflects the composition of tissue (Heymsfield et al., 2004). Muscle and adipose tissue have high and low density than water and have 30 to 100 CT, -190 to -30 CT, respectively (Heyward & Vivian, 2004).

Magnetic Resonance Imaging (MRI) is different from CT in terms of the image acquired. This method is based on the interaction of hydrogen (proton) nuclei, which are abundant in biological tissue and have a non-zero magnetic field and thus, act as tiny magnets (Heymsfield et al., 2004). When a subject is placed inside the magnet, all the protons get arranged and aligned to the magnetic field. After this, a pulsed radio–frequency field is applied to the tissues causing a number of hydrogen protons to absorb energy (Heymsfield et al., 2004). When the radio frequency pulse is turned off, the protons gradually return to their original positions, and in the process release energy that is absorbed in the form of a radio frequency signal (Heymsfield et al., 2004). This signal helps to develop cross–sectional images. But, in case of noise caused by respiratory motion, it blurs the borders between tissues in the abdomen to a greater extent in Magnetic Resonance Imaging (MRI) than CT (Heymsfield et al., 2004). The MRI and CT methods are hard to get access to and are extremely expensive, and thus remain an obstacle for routine use for most laboratories.

6. Anthropometry

Anthropometry is an easy, relatively convenient, portable, inexpensive and non-invasive method to measure body composition. It can be used in large populations in clinical practice, rural and urban conditions. It is commonly assumed that all tissue, to be measured, is in a standard state. All the measurements of the breadth and length are measured at different sites of the body and are known as skeletal dimensions because measurements are taken between bony landmarks (Bellisari & Roche, 2005). But these measurements may be affected due to the amount of soft tissue on the measured site.

Skinfolds includes the double layer of skin and subcutaneous adipose tissue (SAT; adipocytes that contain triglycerides, and connective tissue that include blood vessels, nerves, and tissue fluids) underlying the subcutaneous tissue (Bellisari & Roche, 2005). Measurements are taken by pinching the double layer of skin in order to raise the fold including the subcutaneous tissue but not the muscles (Snetselaar, 1997). The skinfold calliper is applied 1 cm below and at right angle to the pinch of the subcutaneous fat. Usually the thickness of double layer of skin is 1.8 mm but becomes varied due to age and site to be measured (Bliznak, & Staple, 1975). Skinfold measurement is taken at different sites like triceps, biceps, subscapular, suprailiac, mid-axillary, among others, depending on the formula used and the purpose of the study.

Skinfold measurement is affected by the compressibility of SAT, age, gender, measurement site and sudden weight loss (Fanelli & Kock, 1987). Sometimes, pressure exerted by the calliper on the tissues may displace some amount of ECW, especially in the case of malnutrition where ECW content of SAT is increased (Martin, Ross, Drinkwater, & Clarys, 1985). Additionally, skinfold calliper may force some of adipose tissue to move to a less pressured area, especially among thick skinfolds of individuals (Roche, 1996). Such inter-site and inter-subject differences in skinfold compressibility reduce the utility of skinfold measurement.

Ultrasound is primarily used for the measurement of soft tissues in clinical practices but it can also measure tissue thickness such as SAT, muscle, and deep adipose tissue (DAT). It has gained popularity over anthropometry, especially in obese subjects. But due to its high cost, it is not the preferred method for measurement of body composition in population studies. It is shown to underestimate SAT volume at the upper arm and thigh. The validity of SAT and abdominal DAT is also uncertain (Bellisari, 1997).

7. Dual energy X-ray absorptiometry (DXA)

Recently some in-vivo techniques evolved into a modern technological innovation called DXA. Before 1990, the DPA (^{153}Gd dual-photon absorptiometry) was considered as an accurate and versatile method for measuring body composition (Gotfredsen et al., 1986). But its precision was less than optimal due to the decay of gadolinium source (Svendsen et al., 1991). So, DPA was further developed and this gave rise to DXA, which was with a stable x-ray generator instead of a decaying radioactive source. DXA was developed by

Mazess et al (1990) for bone mineral content and density measurement. Lukaski (1993) indicated in his report that X-rays at two discrete energy levels are collimated and directed into the body. Mazess et al (1990) reported that DXA used a constant potential x-ray source and a K-edge filter (cerium) to generate two main energy peaks (40 keV and 70 keV). Roubenoff et al (1993) claimed that the attenuation of soft tissue could be measured rather than assumed.

The DXA method requires the subject to lie supine on a padded table, and an x-ray beam is passed in a posterior-to-anterior direction through the bone and soft tissue of the subject upward to a detector. The ratio of x-ray beam attenuation at the lower energy relative to that at the higher energy is used to distinguish fat from the FFM (minus the bone component) (Lukaski, 2005). The increased photon flux improved the resolution and precision of the image and reduces scan time (Wagner & Heyvard, 1999). DXA has increased its validity in measuring regional and whole body soft tissue estimations (Lohman, 1996). It measures three components in the body as, FM, soft tissue lean mass and bone mineral content with precision error of 6.6 %, 1.9-3.1%, and 1.5 %, respectively (Haarbo et al., 1990; Mazess et al., 1990). Lukaski (1993) reported 99 % accuracy in measurement of bone mineral content and density with only 1 % error. The major advantages of this technique is, it takes short time (<10 mins) for measurement, precision is quite good (1-2 % variance), and dose of radiation is minimal (< 0.01 mSv, whole body) (Goran et al., 1996; Mazess et al., 1990). DXA is not affected by ethnicity, athletic status or musculoskeletal development (Aloia et al., 1999; Prior et al., 1997)

Recently, DXA is used as gold standard or criterion or reference method for assessing body composition in children, (Goran et al., 1996) young men and women (Mazess et al., 1990). Some investigators compared the two compartment model reference methods with four compartment models, and DXA was found to be the more accurate method than TBW, hydrodensitometry and TBK measurements (Friedl et al., 1992; Fuller et al., 1992; Prior et al., 1997). Lockner et al (2000) also supported the validity of DXA against UWW. Pritchard et al (1993) compared two densitometers, the Hologic QDR 1000W densitometer (QDR) and the Lunar DPX densitometer (DPX), with four traditional methods for the measurement of body fat: UWW, skinfold thickness measurements (SKF), bioelectrical impedance analysis (BIA) and deuterium oxide dilution (D_2O). The coefficient of variability (CV) was 1.8 % for percentage fat, 0.6 % for lean mass and 2.1 % for FM. In 10 repeated observations on three subjects, QDR_{CV} was greater than UWW_{CV} (CV fat % of QDR, 1.3 % (0.9-1.6 %) compared to 4.8 % (3.8-6.6 %) for CV fat % of UWW). The correlations between QDR and DPX with UWW for measuring percentage fat of 12 subjects are 0.916 ($P < 0.0001$) for QDR and 0.913 ($P < 0.00001$) for DPX. A limit of agreement estimate showed a between-method difference of +1.3 % (range -4 % to +7 %) for QDR compared with UWW. The DPX showed a between-method difference of +4.8 % (range +2 % to +9 %) compared to UWW. These two DXAs (Hologic QDR 1000W densitometer, QDR and the Lunar DPX densitometer, DPX) are highly correlated ($r = 0.986$, $P < 0.0001$). DXA also have high correlations with other body composition techniques (QDR: 0.824, $P < 0.001$; SKM; 0.972, $P < 0.0001$ for BIA; $r = 0.787$, $P < 0.002$ for D2O; for DPX: $r = 0.923$, $P < 0.00001$ for SKM; $r = 0.910$, $P < 0.00001$ for BIA; $r = 0.812$, $P < 0.001$ for D_2O). The CV and correction values indicated higher accuracy of QDR and DPX for measuring percentage fat than UWW. Predicted percentage fat measurements using QDR was 3 % lower than DPX, but both DXAs predicted percentage fat 1.3-4.8 % higher than UWW. The DXA also produced accurate results in regional measurement of bone mineral content (BMC), FM (FAT), lean mass (LEAN) and percentage fat (Pritchard et al., 1993).

Slosman et al (1992) validated DXA against body potassium –40 (K_{40}) on young adults. DXA is highly correlated with body potassium 40 (K_{40}) method in lean body mass (LBM) measurement ($LBM_{k\text{-}40} = 1.069$, LBM_{DXA}, $R^2 = 0.996$). Additionally, the authors assessed body composition by DXA on ten Acquired Immuno Deficiency Syndrome (AIDS) patients and ten Cystic Fibrosis patients. LBM on AIDS patients was slightly decreased, while, LBM and bone mineral body mass (BBM) were decreased in cystic fibrosis patients. The study showed DXA to be an accurate method for clinical practices in order to detect specific alterations of body composition. Maddalozzo et al (2002) reported high concurrent validity of DXA for assessing fat % in young women (19.4 +/- 1.4 years) with a BMI of 23.4 ± 2.3. Body fat % was estimated to be 24.3% (SE= 1.1) and 23.8% (SE = 0.8) using the Bod Pod and DXA techniques, respectively (Maddalozzo et al., 2002). Radley et al (2003) also observed high validity of DXA against air displacement plethysmography ($r = 0.84\text{-}0.95$, all $P<0.001$; SEE.= 3.42- 3.89 %). Jensen et al (1993) observed that DXA measurement of FM and FFM was significantly associated with bromide space technique measurement of extra cellular fluid volume but prediction of LBM measured by DXA, TBW and TBK were significantly different. Pietrobelli et al (1996) and Mazes et al (1990) reported the error of 0.8 % and 1.8 % for BMD and TBM, respectively, measured through DXA. The error for % BF in soft tissue, FM and lean tissue mass was 1.4 %, 1.0kg, and 0.8 kg respectively. The precision of DXA was also tested through measuring BMD of an isolated skeleton. The precision error was also determined by measuring the same skeleton 34 times with one DXA scanner, and by measuring another skeleton on 37 different scanners. The precision error for total BMD was less than 0.01 $g \cdot cm^{-2}$ in both cases.

Haarbo et al (1991) validated the use of DXA for measurement of body composition. The precision error (SD) for FM, fat %, lean tissue mass and total body BMD was 1.1 kg (6.4 %), 1.6 % (5.7 %), 1.4kg (3.1 %), and 0.03kg (1.2 %), respectively. The authors measured the accuracy using three materials such as dried bones, mixtures of water and alcohol, and mixture of ox muscle and lard. In the clinically range of values, there were only a small influence on DXA measurements of variation in amount and composition of soft tissue equivalents. The accuracy study in vivo compared components of body composition by DXA, dual photon absorptiometry, TBK and UWW in 25 healthy adult subjects. The results revealed good agreement fat % and lean body mass by DXA and three established measurement methods; mean differences were (-5.3 to -0.4 %) and (-0.7 to 2.5 kg) for fat % and lean body mass, respectively. The conclusion of the study revealed that DXA seems to be a method which measures body composition with precision and accuracy, and may be compatible with application of DXA in group research studies and probably also for clinical measurements of single subjects (Haarbo et al., 1991).

Levine et al (2000) compared CT and DXA, by measuring thigh muscle and FM to evaluate the random and systematic discrepancies between these two methods. Thigh skeletal muscle area measured by CT was fairly related ($r = 0.86$; $P < 0.0001$) to DXA measured FFM, in contrast to thigh FFM and fat measured by CT and DXA ($r^2 = 0.96$, $P < 0.0001$). The measured thigh fat by DXA was significantly lower than that measured by multislice-CT ($3{,}764 \pm 2{,}184\ cm^3 > 3{,}394 \pm 1{,}957g$; $P < 0.0001$). On the contrary, leg muscle mass measured by multislice-CT is less ($6\ 557 \pm 1\ 385\ g < 5\ 852 \pm 1\ 251g$; $P < 0.0001$) than that measured by DXA. Thus, appendicular soft tissue measured by CT and DXA are highly related. Glickman et al (2004) reported the validity of DXA in measuring abdominal adiposity against CT. 65 men and women aged 18-72 years participated in a series of studies. Bland-Altman analysis demonstrated good concordance between DXA and CT for abdominal total tissue mass with limits of agreement -1.56 to 2.54 kg and FM with limits of agreement -0.40 to 1.94 kg. DXA also showed excellent reliability among three different operators (vertebral L1–L4) to determine total fat and lean body mass ($r = 0.94$, 0.97, and 0.89, respectively). In conclusion, the DXA L1 - L4 region of interest compared with CT proved to be both reliable and accurate method to determine abdominal obesity.

Madsen et al (1997) investigated the reproducibility of total and regional body composition measurements performed on DXA. A group of 58 women aged 21-81 (52.4±17.8 yrs) years was scanned twice with repositioning to determine intra-observer reproducibility of measurements of BMD ($g{\bullet}cm^{-2}$), bone mineral content (BMC, g), lean mass (LM, kg) and FM (FM, kg) of the total body and of the major sub-regions of the body. In addition, the ability of the DXA machine to detect changes in LM and FM (simulated by placing 11.1 and 22.3 kg porcine lard on the body of 11 subjects) was examined. Coefficients of variations were as follow: (BMD, BMC, LM, FM) [corrected]: 1.4 %, 1.1 %, 1.4 %, 1.7 % (total body), 2.2 %, 2.1 % (head), 2.8 %, 2.8 %, 2.0 %, 2.2 % (trunk), 3.6 %, 3.9 %, 4.0 %, 4.9 % (arms), 2.7 %, 1.3 %, 2.6 %, 2.8 % (legs). Fat % of exogenous lard was 81.3 % (SD 3.5) as assessed by the absorptiometer which corresponded well with the result of chemical analysis (82.8 %). Estimated % fat of exogenous lard was not influenced by initial body mass or percentage body fat. The 11.1 kg lard were placed on the body and the expected mean values were 99.9 ± 0.3 kg for body mass, 100.5 ±2.1 kg for LM, 99.5 ±3.5 kg for FM and 103.2±2.2 $g{\bullet}cm^{-2}$ for BMD. With 22.3 kg lard on the body, the observed mean values were 99.4 ± 0.2 kg for body mass, 100.5 ±1.7 kg for LM, 98.1 ±2.0 kg for FM and 105.5±1.8 $g{\bullet}cm^{-2}$ for BMD. BMD was overestimated by 3.2 % (103.2 $g{\bullet}cm^{-2}$ > 1.01 $g{\bullet}cm^{-2}$; $P < 0.005$) when 11.1kg lard was added while BMD and BMC increased significantly ($P < 0.005$) when 22.3 kg lard was added on the body. Thus, added lard on the body may affect the measurement of BMD and BMC. Otherwise, results indicated that DXA measured BMD, BMC, LM, and FM of the total body accurately.

Chan et al (1992) studied the performance of the DXA method in evaluating bone mineral, fat, and lean soft tissue mass. DXA method produced accurate results in measuring known small amounts of lean tissues, calcium, and lard mass and evaluating bones of small animals and their fat, and muscle mass. It is sensitive to detect changes up to 40 mg for calcium, 180 mg for fat, and 270mg for lean tissue mass.

High correlation ($r = 0.998$) is also observed between single-photon absorptiometry method and DXA in measuring bone mineral content of radius bone of 32 children. Among old children, a difference is observed between the two methods. 14 newborn infants of age 28-41 weeks were scanned for their total-body, lumbar, and radial bone. The total-body bone mineral and FM increased with increasing age (from 28 weeks to 41 weeks) and weight. Total-body calcium of these infants is also related to length of lumbar and radial bone and their respective densities. Specifically, the density of the lumbar bone was related with birth weight, gestational age, length, BMI, body fat, and radial bone density. The ratio of lumbar bone density and total-body calcium among males is higher than that among females and DXA may be used in paediatrics with high accuracy, sensitivity, and precision.

8. Conclusion

In summary, sophisticated equipment such as the DXA can analyse body composition according to its constituents, which includes fat mass by body sections, fat-free mass and even bone density (Balasekaran and Loh, 2009). DXA is primarily developed for diagnosis of osteoporosis. Initially, it was used to measure lumbar spine, femoral neck, and forearm etc. but it was rapidly adopted for use in different clinical and exercise settings. As a result, DXA is also used to measure total skeleton and regional soft tissue measurement. Nowadays, DXA can measure three important components, FM, lean mass, and bone mineral mass, from a single whole body scan with high accuracy and precision with a low scanning time. The comprehensive view of body composition by DXA makes it more attractive to use in clinical practices and exercise settings such as in the prevention of cardiovascular and metabolic diseases, clinical management of different chronic diseases, and monitoring of the impact of treatment regimens on body tissues (Carlina, Diessel, & Genant 2003).

References

1. Adolph, E., & Dill, D. (1938). Observations on water metabolism in the desert. *American Journal of Physiology*, 123: 369–378.
2. Aleman-Mateo, H., Huerta, R.H., Esparza-Romero, J., Mendez, R. O., Urquidez, R., & Valencia, M.E. (2007). Body composition by the four-compartment model: validity of the BOD POD for assessing body fat in Mexican elderly. *European Journal of Clinical Nutrition, 61(7):* 830-836.
3. Aloia, J.F., Vaswani, A., Ma, R., & Flaster, E. (1996). Body composition in normal black women: the four compartment model. *Journal of Clinical Endocrinology & Metabolism,* 81: 2363–2369.
4. Aloia, J.F., Vaswani, A., Ma, R., & Flaster, E. (1997). Comparison of body composition in black and white premenopausal women. *The Journal of Laboratory and Clinical Medicine,* 129(3): 294-299.
5. Aloia, J.F., Vaswani, A., Mikhail, M., & Flaster, E.R. (1999). Body composition by dual-energy x-ray absoptiometry in black compared with white females. *Osteoporosis International*, 10: 114-119.

6. Balasekaran, G. (2003). Body composition in Track and Field: Measurement and application. *International Athletic Association Federation Bulletin*, 1.
7. Balasekaran, G., & Loh, M. K. (2009). School Physical Education Programmes: Health & Fitness Issues and Challenges. In N. Aplin (Ed.), *An Eye on the Youth Olympic Games 2010: Perspectives on PE and Sport Science in Singapore*. Singapore: McGraw-Hill. pp. 55- 72.
8. Barnett, A. & Bagno, S. (1936). The physiological mechanism involved in the clinical measure of phase angle. *American Journal of Physiology*, 114: 366-382.
9. Beddoe, A.H., Streat, S.J., & Hill, G. L. (1985). Hydration of fat free body in protein-depleted patients. *American Journal of Physiology*, 249: E227-E233.
10. Bellisari, A. & Roche, A.F. (2005). Anthropometry and Ultrasound. In S. Heymsfield, T.G. Lohman, & Z. Wang (Eds), *Human Body Composition* (2nd Ed.). Champaign, Illinois: Human Kinetics. pp. 129-127.
11. Bellisari, A. (1997). Validation of ultrasonic measurements of subcutaneous adipose tissue using magnetic resonance imaging. *American Journal of Human Biology*, 9: 123-124.
12. Bemben, M.G., Massey, B.H., Bemben, D.A., Boileau, R.A., & Misner, J.E. (1995). Age- Related Patterns in body composition for men aged 20-79 yr. *Medicine and Science in Sports and Exercise*, 27(2): 264-269.
13. Bliznak, I. & Staple, T.W. (1975). Roentgenographic measurement of skin thickness in normal individual, *Radiology*, 118: 55-60.
14. BOD POD body composition system. (2000). *Operator's manual.* Concord, CA: Life Measurement, Inc.
15. Bracco, D., Thiebaud, D., Chiolero, R.L., Landry, M., Burckhardt, P., & Schutz, Y. (1996). Segmental body composition assessed by bioelectric impedance analysis and DXA in humans. *Journal of Applied Physiology*, 81(6): 2580-2587.
16. Brooks GA. (2000). *Exercise physiology: human bioenergetics and its applications* (3rd ed.). Mountain View, CA: Mayfield.
17. Buskirk, E.R. (1961). Underwater weighing and body density: A review of procedures. In J. Bronzek & A. Henschel (Eds), *Techniques for Measuring Body Composition*. Washington, DC: National Academy of Sciences, National Research Council. pp. 90-105.
18. Carlina, V., A., Diessel E., & Genant H.K. (2003). Clinical applications of Body composition measurements using DXA. *Journal of Clinical Densitometry*. 6(2): 75-86.
19. Chan, G.M. (1992). Performance of Dual X ray Absorptiometry in evaluating bone, lean body mass, and fat in pediatric subjects. *Journal of Bone & Mineral Research*, 7(4): 369-74.

20. Chao, D. Espeland, M.A., Farmer, D., Thomas, D., Lenchik, C.L., Applegate, W., & Ettinger, W. (2000). Effect of voluntary weight loss on bone mineral density in older overweight women. *Journal of the American Geriatrics Society*, 48: 753-759.
21. Chumlea, W.C., Baumgartner, R. N. & Mitchell, C.O. (1990). The use of segmental bioelectric impedance in estimating body composition. In S. Yasumura (Ed), *Advances in In Vivo Body Composition Studies*. New York: Plenum. pp. 375-385.
22. Chumlea, W.C., & Sun, S.S. (2005). Bioelectrial Impedance Analysis. In A.F. Roche, S.B. Heymsfield & T.G. Lohman (Eds), *Human Body Composition*. Champaign, IL: Human Kinetics. pp. 79-87.
23. Clark, R.R., Kuta, J.M., & Sullivan, J.C. (1993). Prediction of percent body fat in adult males using dual energy x ray absorptiometry, skinfolds, and hydrostatic weighing. *Medicine and Science in Sports and Exercise*, 25(4): 528-535.
24. Cobayashi, F., Lopes, L.A., & Taddei. J.A.A.C. (2005). Bone mineral density in overweight and obese adolescents. *Journal of Pediatrics*, 81(4): 337-342.
25. Cohn, S.H. (1985). How valid are bioelectric impedance measurements in body composition studies? American Journal of Clinical Nutrition, 42: 889-90.
26. Cui, L.H., Shin, M.H., Kweon, S.S., Park, K.S., Lee, Y.H., Chung, E.K., et al. (2007). Relative contribution of body composition to bone mineral density at different sites in men and women of South Korea. *Journal of Bone and Mineral Metabolism*, 25: 165-171.
27. Cummings, S.R., Black, D.M., Nevitt, M.C., Browner, W., Cauley, J. Ensrud, K., et al. (1993). Bone density at various sites for prediction of hip fractures. *Lancet,* 341: 72-75.
28. Davies, P.S.W., & Cole, T.J. (1995). *Body composition techniques in health and disease*. Spain: Cambridge University Press.
29. Dempster, P., & Aitkens, S. A. (1995). New air displacement method for the determination of human body composition. *Medicine & Science in Sports & Exercise*, 27: 1692-1697
30. DeTurk, W., & Cahalin, L.P. (2004). *Cardiovascular and pulmonary physical therapy*. Columbus, OH: McGraw-Hill Professional.
31. Diaz, E.O, Villar, J., Immink, M., & Gonzales, T. (1989). Bioimpedance or anthropometry? European Journal of Clinical Nutrition, 43: 129-137.
32. Douchi, T., Kuwhata, R., Matsuo, T., Uto, H., Oki, T., & Nagata, Y. (2003). Relative contribution of lean and fat mass component to bone mineral density in males. Journal of Bone and Mineral *Metabolism*, 21 (1): 17-21.

33. Fields, D.A., Higgins, P.B., & Hunter, G.R. (2004). Assessment of body composition by air displacement plethysmography: influence of body temperature and moisture. *Dynamic Medicine*, 3: 1-7.
34. Friedl, K E., DeLuca, J. P., Marchitelli, L. J., & Vogel, J. A. (1992). Reliabiliry of body fat estimations from a four-compartment model by using density, body water and bone mineral measurements. *American Journal of Clinical Nutrition*, 55: 764-770.
35. Fuller, N.J., Jebb, S.A., Laskey, M.A., Coward, W.A., & Elia, M. (1992). Four component model for the assessment of body composition in humans: Comparison with alternative methods, and evaluation of the density and hydration of fat-free mass. *Clinical Science*, 84: 687-693.
36. Glickman SG., Marn CS., Supiano MA., & Dengel, D.R. (2004). Validity and reliability of Dual X Ray Absorptiometry for the assessment of abdominal Adiposity. *Journal of Applied Physiology*, 97(2): 509-514.
37. Going, S.B., Massett, M.P., Mathew, C.H., Bare, L.A., Root, P.A., Williams, D.P., et al. (1993). Detection of small changes in body composition by dual energy x-ray Absorptiometry. *American journal of Clinical Nutrition*, 57: 845-850.
38. Going. S.B. (2005). Hydrodensitometry and air displacement plethysmography. In S. Heymsfield, T.G. Lohman, & Z. Wang (Eds), *Human Body Composition* (2nd ed). Champaign, IL: Human Kinetics. pp. 17-33.
39. Goran, M.I., Driscoll, P., Johnson, R., Nagy, T.R., & Gary, H. (1996). Cross- calibration of body composition techniques against dual – energy x-ray absorptiometry in young children. *American Journal of Clinical Nutrition*, 63: 299-305.
40. Gotfredsen, A., Jensen, J., Borg, J., & Christiansen, C. (1986). Measurement of lean body mass and total body fat using dual photon absorptiometry. *Metabolism*, 35: 88-93.
41. Gulick, D.T. (1999). *Body composition assessment. Journal of Aquatic Physical Therapy*, 7(1): 19-21.
42. Guyton, A.C., Taylor, A.E., & Granger, H.J. (1975). *Circulatory Physiology II: Dynamics and Control of Body Fluids*. Philadelphia: W.B. Saunders.
43. Haarbo J., Gotfredsen A., Hassager C., & Christiansen C. (1991). Validation of body composition by dual energy x-ray absorptiometry (DXA). *Clinical Physiology*, 11(4): 331-341.
44. Heaney, R.P. (1991). Lifelong calcium intake and prevention of bone fragility in the aged. *Calcified Tissue International*, 49(suppl): S42-S45.
45. Heitman, B L. (1994). Impedance: a valid method in assessment of body composition? European Journal of Clinical Nutrition, 48: 228-240.

46. Heymsfield, S.B., Wang, Z., Baumgartner, R.N., Dilmanian, F.A., Ma, R., & Yasumura, S. (1993). Body composition and aging: a study by in vivo neutron activation analysis. *Journal of Nutrition*, 123(suppl 2): 432-437.
47. Heymsfield, S.B., Baumgartner, R.N., Allison, D.B., Shen, W., Wang, Z., & Ross, R. (2004). Evaluation of total and regional adiposity. In G.A. Bray, & C. Bouhard (Eds), Handbook of obesity: Etiology and pathophysiology (2nd ed). London, UK: Informa Healthcare. pp, 33-80.
48. Heymsfield, S.B., Lichtman, S., Baumgartner, R.N., Wang, J., Kamen, Y., Aliprantis, A., et al. (1990). Body composition of humans: Comparison of two improved four compartment models that differ in expense, technical complexity and radiation exposure. *American Journal of Clinical Nutrition*, 52: 52-58.
49. Heyward, V.H (2006). *Advanced fitness assessment and exercise prescription* (5th ed.). Champaign, IL: Human Kinetics.
50. Heyward, V., & Vivian, H. (2004). *Applied body composition assessment* (2nd ed). Champaign, IL: Human Kinetics.
51. Hoffer, E.C., Meader, C.K., & Simpson, D.C. (1969). Correlation of whole-body impedance with total body water. *Journal of Applied Physiology*, 27: 531-534.
52. Institute of Medicine (U.S.), Committee on Body Composition, Nutrition and Health of Military Women, Institute of Medicine (U.S). (1998). *Assessing readiness in military women: The relation of body composition, nutrition and health.* Washington, DC: National Academic Press.
53. Institute of Medicine (U.S.). Panel on Dietary Reference Intakes for Electrolytes and Water. (2005). *DRI, dietary reference intakes for water, potassium, sodium, chloride and sulphate.* Washington, DC: The National Academies Press.
54. Jebb, S.A., Cole, T.J., Doman, D., Murgatroyd, P.R., & Prentice, A.M. (2000). Evaluation of the novel Tanita body fat analyser to measure body composition by comparison with a four compartment model. *British Journal of Nutrition*, 83: 115-122.
55. Jensen, M.D., Kanaley, J.A., Roust, L.R., O'Brien, P.C., Braun, J.S., Dunn, W.L., & Wahner, H.W. (1993). Assessment of Body Composition with use of Dual Energy X ray absorptionmetry: Evaluation and Comparison with other methods. *Mayo Clinic Proceedings*, 68(9): 867-873.
56. Karlsson, M. (2002). Does exercise reduce the burden of fractures? A review. *Acta Orthopaedica Scandinavica*, 73: 691-705.
57. Kernbach-Wighton, G. (2009). Diagnostic problems with functional causes of death: Analytical approaches and procedures. *Legal Medicine*, 11: S31-S35.

58. Levine, J.A., Abboud, L., Barry, M., Reed, J.E., Sheedy, P.F., & Jensen, M.D. (2000). Measuring leg muscle and fat mass in humans: comparison of CT and Dual Energy X ray Absorptiometry. *Journal of Applied Physiology*, 88(2): 452-426.
59. Lichtenbelt, W.D.V.M., Hartgens, F., Vollaard, N.B.J., Ebbling, S., & Kuipers, H. (2004). Body composition changes in body builders: A method comparison. Medicine & Science in Sports & Exercise, 3: 490-497.
60. Lockner, D.W., Heyward, V.H., Baumgartner, R.N., & Jenkins, K.A. (2000). Comparison of air displacement Plethsmography, Hydrodensitometry, and Dual X ray Absorptiometry for assessing body composition of Children 10 to 18 years of age. *Annals of New York Academy Science*, 904: 72-78.
61. Lohman T.G. (1992). *Advances in body composition assessment*: Current issues in exercise science series (Monograph No. 3). Champaign, IL: Human Kinetics.
62. Lohman TG. (1981). Skinfolds and body density and their relation to body fatness: a review. *Human Biology*. 53: 181-225.
63. Lohman, T.G. (1996). Dual-energy X-ray absorptiometry. In A.F. Roche, S.B. Heymsfield & T.G. Lohman (Eds), *Human Body Composition*. Champaign, IL: Human Kinetics. pp. 63-78.
64. Lukaski H.C. (2005). Assessing muscle mass. In A.F. Roche, S.B. Heymsfield & T.G. Lohman (Eds), *Human Body Composition*. Champaign, IL: Human Kinetics. pp. 203-217.
65. Lukaski, H.C. (1993). Soft tissue composition and bone mineral status: Evaluation by dual energy x ray absorptiometry. Symposium: Aging and body composition: Technological advances and physiological interrelationships. *Journal of Nutrition*. 123: 438-443.
66. Lukaski, H.C., Bolonchuk, W.W., Hall, C.B., & Siders, W.A. (1986). Validation of tetrapolar bioelectrical impedance method to assess human body composition. *Journal of Applied Physiology*, 60: 1327-1332.
67. Maddalozzo, G.F., Cardinal, B.J., & Show, C.A. (2002). Concurrent validity of the BOD POD and dual energy X-ray absorptiometry techniques for assessing body composition in young women. *Journal of American Dietetic Association*, 102(11): 1677-1679.
68. Madsen O.R., Jensen J.E., & Sorensen O.H. (1997). Validation of dual X-ray absorptiometry: Measurement of bone mass and soft tissue composition. *European Journal of Applied Physiology and Occupational Physiology*, 75(6): 554-558.
69. Mazess, R.B., Burden, H.S., Bisek, J.P., & Hanson, J. (1990). Dual-energy x-ray absorptiometry for total-body and regional bone-mineral and soft

tissue composition. American Journal of Clinical Nutrition, 51: 1106-1112.

70. Modelsky, C.M., Cureton, K.J., Lewis, B.M., Prior, B.M., Sloniger, M.A., & Rowe D.A. (1996). Density of fat free mass and estimates of body composition in male weight trainers. *Journal of Applied Physiology*, 80: 2085-2096.
71. Nyboer, J. (1959). *Bioelectric impedance plethysmography*. Spring-field, IL: Charles Thomas.
72. Olsson, K.E., & Saltin, B. (1970). Variation in total body water with muscle glycogen changes in man. *Acta Physiologica Scandinavica*, 80(1): 11-18.
73. Ondrak, K.S., & Morgan, D.W. (2006). Factors influencing Bone mineral Density and Content in young girls. *Pediatric Exercise Science*, 17: 101-112.
74. Park, Y.W., Heymsfield, S.B. & Gallaghar, D. (2002). Is dual energy X-ray Absorptiometry regional estimates associated with visceral adipose tissue mass? *International Journal of Obesity*, 26: 978-983.
75. Penn I.W., Wang Z.M., K.M, Allison, D. B., Burastro, S.E., & Heysmfield, S.B. (1994). Body composition and two compartment model assumptions in male long distance runners. *Medicines and Science in Sport and Exercise*, 26: 392-397.
76. Pietrobelli, A., Formica, C., Wang, Z., & Heymsfield, S.B. (1996). Dual-energy x- ray absorptiometry body composition model: Review of physical concepts. *American Journal of Physiology*, 271: E941-E951.
77. Pollock, M.L., & Jackson, A.S. (1984). Research progress in validation of clinical methods of assessing body composition. *Medicine & Science in Sports & Exercise*, 16: 606-613.
78. Prior, B.M., Cureton, K.J., Modlesky, C.M., Evans, E.M., Sloniger, M.A., Saunders, M., et al. (1997). In vivo validation of whole body composition estimates from dual-energy x-ray absorptiometry. *Journal of Applied Physiology*, 83: 623-630.
79. Pritchard, J.E., Nowson, C.A., Strauss, B.J., Carlson, J.S., Kaymakci, B., & Wark, J.D. (1993). Evaluation of dual energy x-ray absorptiometry as a method of measurement of body fat. *European Journal of Clinical Nutrition*, 47(3): 216-28.
80. Radley, D., Gately, P.J., Cooke, C.B., Carroll, S., Oldroyd, B., & Truscott, J.G. (2003). Estimates of percentage body fat in young adolescents: a comparison of Dual Energy X-ray Absorptiometry and Air Displacement Plethysmography. *European Journal of Clinical Nutrition*, 57(11): 1402-1410.
81. Riggs, B.L., Khosla S., & Melton L.J. (1998). A Unitary Model for evolutional osteoporosis: Estrogen deficiency causes both type I and type

II osteoporosis in post menopausal women and contributes to bone loss in aging men. *Journal of Bone and Mineral Research*, 13: 763-773.

82. Roche, A.F. (1996). Anthorpometry and Ultrasound. In A.F. Roche, S.B. Heymsfield, & T.G. Lohman (Eds), *Human Body Composition*. Champaign, IL: Human Kinetics.
83. Roemmich J.N., Clark P.A., Weltman, A., & Rogol, A.D. (1997). Alterations in growth and body composition during puberty. Comparing multi-compartment body composition models. *Journal of Applied Physiology*, 83: 927-935.
84. Roubenoff, R., Kehayias, J.J., Dawson-Hughes, B., & Heymsfield, S.B. (1993). Use of dual-energy x-ray absorptiometry in body composition studies: Not yet a "gold standard." *American Journal of Clinical Nutrition*, 58: 589-591.
85. Salamone, LM., Fuerst, T., Visser, M., Kern, M., Lang, M., & Dockrell, M., et al., (2000). Measurement of Fat mass using DXA: A validation study in elderly adults. Journal of applied Physiology, 89(1): 345-352.
86. Sawka, M.N., Montain, & S.J., Latzka, W.A. (2001). Hydration effects on the thermoregulation and performance in the heat. *Comparative Biochemistry & Physiology - Part A*: 128: 679-690.
87. Sawka, M.N., & Pandolf, K.B. (1990). Effects of body water loss on physiological function and exercise performance. In C.V. Gisolfi D.R. Lamb (Eds), *Fluid homeostasis during exercise*. Carmel (IN): Benchmark Press. pp. 1-38.
88. Sawka, M.N. (1988). Body fluid responses and hypo-hydration during exercise heat stress. In K.B. Pandolf, M.N. Sawka, & R.R., Gonzalez (Eds), *Human performance physiology and environmental medicine at terrestrial extremes*. United States: Benchmark Press. pp. 227-266.
89. Schoeller, D.A. (2005). Hydrometry. In S. Heymsfield, T.G. Lohman, & Z. Wang (Eds), *Human Body Composition* (2nd ed.). Champaign, Illinois: Human Kinetics. pp. 35-49.
90. Siri, W.E. (1961). Body composition from fluid spaces and density: analysis of methods. In J. Brozek, & A. Henschel (Eds), *Techniques for Measuring Body Composition*. Washington, DC: National Academy of Science and National Research Council. pp. 223-244.
91. Slosman, D.O., Casez, J.P., Pichard, C., Rochat, T., Fery, F., Rizzoli, R., et al., (1992). Assessment of whole body composition with Dual Energy X- ray Absorptiometry. *Radiology*, 185: 593-598.
92. Sly, P.D., Lanteri, C., & Bates, J.H.T. (1990). Effect of the thermodynamics of an infant plethysmograph on the measurement of thoracic gas volume. *Pediatric Pulmonology*, 8: 203-208.
93. Snetselaar, L.G. (1997). *Nutrition councelling skills for medical nutrition therapy*. Sudbury, MA: Jones & Barlett Publishers.

94. Sun, G., French, C. R., Martin, G.R., Younghusband, B., Green, R.C., Gang Xie, Y., et al (2005) Comparison of multifrequency bioelectrical impedance analysis with dual-energy X-ray absorptiometry for assessment of percentage body fat in a large, healthy population. *American Journal of Clinical Nutrition*, 81: 74-78.
95. Sutton, R. A., & Miller, C. (2006). Comparison of Some Secondary Body Composition Algorithm. *College Student Journal*, 40(4): 791-801.
96. Svendsen, O.L., Haarbo, J. Heitmann, B.L., Gotfredsen, A., & Christiansen, C. (1991). Measurement of body fat in elderly subjects by dual energy X-ray absorptiometry, bioelectric impedance, and anthropometry, *American Journal of Clinical Nutrition*, 53: 1117-1123.
97. Toth, E., Ferenc, V., Meszaros, S., Csupor, E., & Horvath, C. (2005). Effects of body mass index on bone mineral density in men. *Orvosi Hetilap*, 10; 146(28): 1489-1493.
98. Visser, M., Kiel, D.P., Langlois, J., Hanna, M.T., Felson, D.T., Wilson, P.W.F. & Harris, T.B. (1998). Muscle mass and fat mass in relation to bone mineral density in very old men and women: the Framingham Heart Study. *Applied Radiation and Isotopes*, 49(5-6): 745-747.
99. Visser, M., Gallaghaer, D., Deurenberg, P., Wang, J., Pierson, R.N. & Heymsfield, S.B. (1997). Density of fat free body mass: Relationship with race, age, and level of body fatmass. *American Journal of Physiology*, 272: E781-E787.
100. Wagner, D.R., & Heyvard, V.H. (1999). Techniques of body composition assessment: A review of laboratory and field methods. *Research Quarterly for Exercise and Sport*, 70(2): 135-149.
101. Wang, Z. M., Heshka, S., Pierson Jr., R.N., & Heymsfield, S.B. (1995). Systematic organization of body-composition methodology: an overview with emphasis on component-based methods. *American Journal of Clinical Nutrition*, 61: 457-465.
102. Wang, Z., Shen, W., Withers, R.T., & Heymsfeld, S.B. (2005). Multicpmponent Molecular-Level models of body composition analysis. In S. Heymsfield, T.G. Lohman, & Z. Wang (Eds), *Human Body Composition* (2nd ed.). Champaign, Illinois: Human Kinetics. pp. 161-176.
103. Wardlaw, G.M., & Kessel, M.W. (2002). *Perspectives in nutrition* (5th ed). Boston, MA: McGraw-Hill.
104. Weinberg, A.D., & Minaker, K.L. (1995). American medical association CoSA. dehydration: evaluation and management in older adults. Journal of American Medical Association, 274: 1552-1556.
105. Wilmore, J. A. (1969). Simplified method for determination of residual lung volume. *Journal of Applied Pbysiology*, 27: 96-100.

REPEATED SHORT-TERM SPRINT PERFORMANCE OF ADULTS ON A NON-MOTORISED TREADMILL USING DIFFERENT WORK-TO-REST RATIOS

JAMIE MERVYN LIM

Tan Tock Seng Hospital, Singapore

MICHAEL CHIA

Physical Education and Sports Science, National Institute of Education, Nanyang Technological University, Singapore

Exercise duration, intra-session rest interval and exercise repetitions contribute to the recovery of power output from short-term high intensity intermittent exertions. There are inconsistent results in studies reported in the literature for the same work-to-rest ratio (WR). The aim of the study was to compare recovery capabilities of untrained male and female adults from short-term high intensity intermittent exercise using different WRs. Ten untrained male and ten untrained female subjects (mean age 25.4 ± 4.7 yrs, body mass 59.7 ± 11.0 kg) volunteered for the research. Three test sessions were organised. During each session, the subjects performed four 10-s maximal sprints on specially instrumented non motorised treadmill (NMT). The rest duration (60-s, 90-s and 120-s) between each sprint was randomly assigned, corresponding to a WR of 1:6, 1:9 and 1:12. Paired-sample T-tests were used to determine if there were significant differences ($p<.05$) in the composite fatigue index (CFI) between different WRs. Results showed that the WR of 1:6 registered the largest CFI_{pp} and CFI_{mp} after four sprints in both sexes. In male adults, there was a significant difference ($p<.05$) in peak power (PP) output and CFI_{pp}, for all three WRs. This indicated that optimal PP recovery was beyond either a WR of 1:9 or 90 s. Paired sample T-tests showed that mean power (MP) in sprints derived from the WR of 1:12 was not significantly different ($p>.05$) to that derived from a WR of 1:9. This demonstrated that a 90s recovery in male adults was sufficient to prevent a significant reduction in MP whilst sprinting on the NMT. For the female adults, the CFI_{pp} for WRs of 1:9 and 1:12 were not significantly different ($p >.05$), indicating that either at least a WR of 1:9 or a 90 s intra-session recovery was required to prevent a significant ($p<.05$) decrease in PP. There was also no significant difference ($p>.05$) in CFI_{mp} for the three WRs in female adults. The present study showed that male and female adults exhibited differences in recovery capabilities. Untrained female adults recovered faster than untrained male adults from short-term high intensity intermittent sprints of up to 10s.

1. Introduction

Exercise duration, intra-session rest interval and the number of exercise repetitions are factors that contribute to the recovery of power from short-term high intensity intermittent exertions. The literature highlighted variations in research methodologies used by various researchers. To date, these investigations have not arrived at a consensus on the ideal number of repetitions, ideal rest duration or the optimal work-to-rest ratio (WR) for sustained performance in intermittent exercises. This is not surprising since it is difficult to generalise these protocols to populations that are diverse in fitness status and sporting interests.

This situation is exacerbated by the fact that that inconsistencies exist from published results. Past research showed that even under the same WR, different results are obtained. For example, at a WR of 1:10, three studies (Blonc et al., 1998; Holmyard et al., 1988; Wootton & Williams, 1982) reported no significant ($p>.05$) decline in power while two studies (Thiriet et al., 1993; Weltman et al., 1977) reported a significant ($p<.05$) decline in power output. Data from the literature showed that most of the disagreement in results occurred within the WR range of 1:8 to 1:12. A study by Reilly et al. (1990) showed that after 10s of activity, a 30-s rest was sufficient to allow phosphocreatine (PCr) to be restored. Other studies showed that the initial power output was never restored under similar test conditions (Holmyard et al, 1988; Sahlin & Ren, 1989; Wootton & Williams, 1982). However, at very short and very long rest durations, results from studies are more consistent and is not investigated in the present study.

A sprint-duration of 10s was chosen in the present study to reflect the demands of sporting activities as far as possible. Drust et al (2000) attempted to simulate the physiological demands of a soccer game in the laboratory using a motorised treadmill with 10.5s sprints. Reilly (1997) reported that in competitive soccer, high intensity sprints 30-s intervals. The fatigue index is usually measured in studies on repeated sprints. Studies that report fatigue indices from high intensity sprints tend to measure the extent of power decline for each sprint (Hill & Smith, 1993; Spierer et al., 2004; Zajac et al., 1999). This method of measuring fatigue does not provide useful information for an intermittent sprint test.

Fatigue index is explained as the difference between the highest power output and the lowest power output expressed as a percentage. Introducing a precedent, a Composite Fatigue Index (CFI) was used. Instead of measuring fatigue within a single sprint, the CFI referred to the fatigue pattern after performing four 10 s sprints that were separated by recovery durations of 60 s, 90 s or 120 s. The calculation was based on the principle used in determining fatigue index, using the difference between the highest and lowest PP/MP over the multiple attempts.

$$CFI_{pp} = \frac{\begin{array}{c}\text{Difference between the highest and lowest}\\ \text{PP amongst the 4 sprints}^{*}\end{array}}{\text{Highest PP among the 4 sprints}} \times 100\%$$

$$CFI_{mp} = \frac{\begin{array}{c}\text{Difference between the highest and lowest}\\ \text{MP amongst the 4 sprints}^{*}\end{array}}{\text{Highest MP among the 4 sprints}} \times 100\%$$

Where,
$CFI_{pp:}$ peak power composite fatigue index,
$CFI_{mp:}$ mean power composite fatigue index

Current knowledge of recovery performance from short-term high intensity intermittent exercise is limited. The WR parameters used were different in the various studies. This made comparison between studies difficult. Moreover, fatigue was only reported for a single sprint and not for multiple sprints. Hence the objective of the study was to examine the short-term high intensity intermittent sprint performances under different WR between male and female adults.

2. Method

2.1. *Subject, test arrangement and equipment*

Institutional ethical approval for all procedures involving human subjects were granted by the National Institute of Education Physical Education and Sports Science Group and informed consent was obtained from all the subjects. Twenty subjects, male (n =10) and female (n =10) adults, were recruited, which gave a statistical power of more than 0.80, for PP and MP computations. Prior to testing, anthropometric measurements were taken. These included the age (yr), stature (cm), body mass (kg), lean muscle mass (kg) and lower limb muscle mass (kg). Age was calculated based on calendar age as at the month of the test. Stature was measured using the Harpendum Stadiometer, Holtain Limited, Britain. The body mass lean muscle mass and lower limb muscle mass of the participant were determined with a dual energy X-ray absorptiometry scan (Hologic QDR Series, Discovery W, Hologic Inc., MA, USA).

The subjects completed 3 test sessions on the non-motorised treadmill (NMT) on 3 separate days, over a 2-week period. On two pre-arranged days prior to the actual tests, the subjects were familiarised to the non-motorised treadmill (NMT) test. During the first familiarisation session, the subject started by walking on the treadmill, and then slowly progressing onto a brisk walk. Once the subject was comfortable with brisk walking, he/she was encouraged to jog and to gradually pick up speed. All the subjects eventually progressed to sprinting at a maximal effort on the NMT. The subjects were also encouraged to accelerate and decelerate repeatedly to simulate the initial acceleration during the test and thereafter, being able to decelerate from a maximal sprint in a controlled manner. This practice instilled confidence in the subjects. During the second familiarisation session, the subjects completed the entire test protocol as a trial. Each familiarisation session took about 45 min.

The NMT (SPRINT CLUB™ 2000, Médical Développement, Andrézieux-Boutheon, France) was set up according to instructions (Medical Development User Guide, 2002) provided by the manufacturers. A schematic representation is shown in Figure 1. The subject wore a hip belt, which was connected to a stress gauge force sensor on the treadmill via a rigid supporting tether bar. The joint between the bar and the stress gauge articulated to allow for vertical and side movements. The belt rested comfortably on the iliac crest. The height of the force sensor was adjusted such that in a standing position, the supporting tether bar was horizontal to the floor. The treadmill attachment end of the bar was a stress gauge force sensor that was capable of measuring the horizontal force exerted by the participant. As the subject ran, there would be an upward and downward displacement of the centre of mass. An optical encoder mounted at the axis of rotation of the supporting bar calculated this vertical displacement. The treadmill was set to the torque mode so that the resistance between the belt and the base of the treadmill was compensated. It therefore allowed the subject to drive the treadmill.

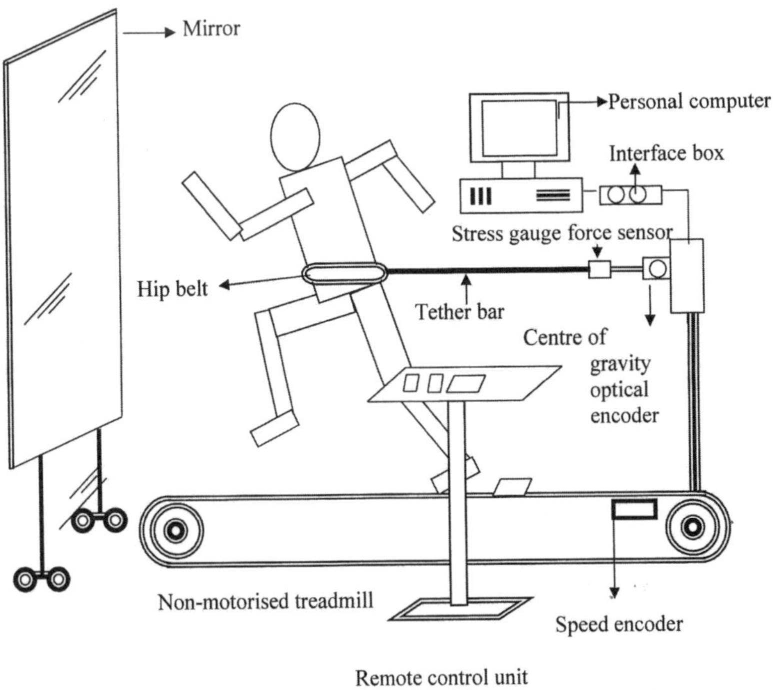

Figure 1: Schematic representation of the NMT test (Mukherjee & Chia, unpublished data, with permission)

Before each test, a standardised warm up protocol was performed consisting of 5 min of pedalling on the cycle ergometer at approximately 60 rpm and interspersed with four all out sprints each lasting 4 to 6 s. This was followed by general static stretching for 5 min. The NMT was initiated from a slow walking start. On the command "Go!", the subject sprinted as fast as he/she could on the treadmill for 10 s. Verbal encouragement was given by the investigator. At each session, the participant sprinted maximally on the NMT for 4 x 10 s. The intra-session recovery period between each sprint was randomly determined at the start of the session, either at 60-, 90- or 120-s. During the recovery period, the subject remained attached to the NMT via the waist harness. An active recovery was performed by walking on the NMT at a subject-selected pace.

2.2. *Power computations*

Power output on the NMT was determined electronically, based on the registered strain on the stress gauge force sensor. Both vertical and horizontal forces were measured. The following equations were used to calculate power (Medical Development User Guide, 2002).

Vertical power: P(v) = speed (v) x{mass x[9.81+acc(v)] + F(v)}

Where,

speed (v): vertical speed of the participant ($m.s^{-1}$),

mass : mass of the participant (kg),

9.81: earth's acceleration ($m.s^{-2}$),

acc (v): vertical acceleration of the participant ($m.s^{-2}$),

F(v): vertical resultant force (N),

F(v) = F(measured force) x sin *a*

Where *a* was the angle between the bar and horizontal.

Horizontal power: P(H) = F(h)xbelt speed

Where,

belt speed: speed of the belt generated by the participant ($m.s^{-1}$),

F (h): horizontal resultant force (N),

F (h) = F(measured) x cos *a*

Where *a* was the angle between the bar and horizontal

Total power output was the sum of the horizontal and vertical power.

2.3. *Statistical analysis*

All data were stored on computer and subsequently analysed using SPSS for Windows (Version 15.0). Descriptive statistics were generated for key dependent variables- PP, MP. Repeated measures ANOVA and post-hoc Tukey test were used to analyse differences in the CFI for the different WRs. The level of statistical significance was set at p<.05.

3. Results

3.1. *Subject measurements*

Descriptive statistics were computed for the subjects' characteristics and summarised in Table 1.

Table 1: Characteristics of the subjects

	Male adults (n = 10) (Mean ± SD)	Female adults (n = 10) (Mean ± SD)
Age (yr)	26.0 ± 4.4	24.7 ± 4.2
Stature (m)	1.71 ± 0.05*	1.62 ± 0.06*
Body mass (kg)	66.7 ± 10.6*	52.8 ± 6.1*
Lean muscle mass (LMM) (kg)	54.0 ± 5.9*	38.5 ± 3.6*
Lower limb muscle mass (LLMM) (kg)	18.7 ± 2.4*	12.8 ± 1.5*

* Significant difference between the sexes at p<.05. The computation of lean muscle mass and lower limb muscle mass excluded the mass of bone mineral content

3.2. *Power output*

Figures 1 and 2 provide illustrations of PP and MP achieved in the four sprints in male and female subjects under the different WRs. The decrease in peak power (PP) and mean power (MP) between subsequent sprints was greatest with the shortest rest duration (WR of 1:6) in male and female adults. Conversely, with a recovery of 120s, the decrease in PP was the least. In the test with a WR of 1:6, the largest decrease in PP and MP after four sprints was registered in male and female adults. Independent sample T-tests showed that there was a significant decrease (p<.05) in PP and MP after the repeated exercise, for both male and female adults, and also for all the three WRs. There was also a significant difference (p<.05) in PP for each sprint between male and female adults. The same was observed for MP.

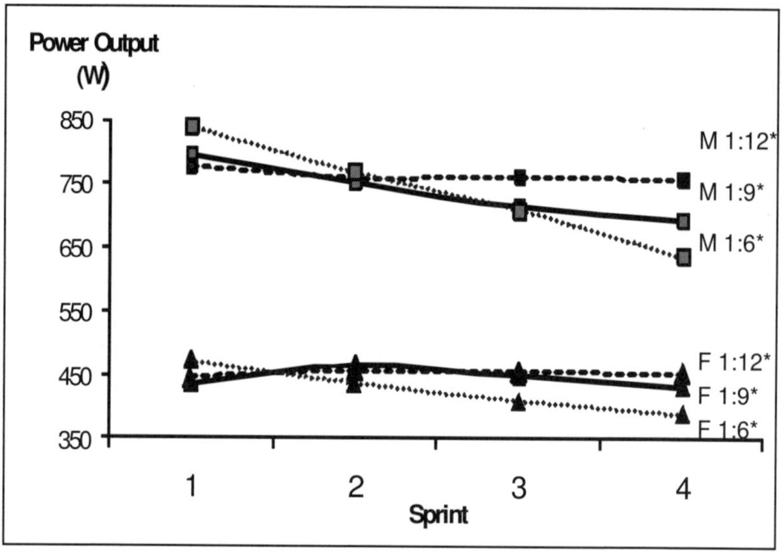

* Significant difference at p<.05 between highest and lowest PP output achieved in that particular series of 4 sprints. M=male adults (n=10), F=female adults (n=10). Peak power in each sprint was measured as the highest recorded power output (integrated over 1-s) in that specific 10s sprint.

Figure 1: PP between male and female adults for different WRs

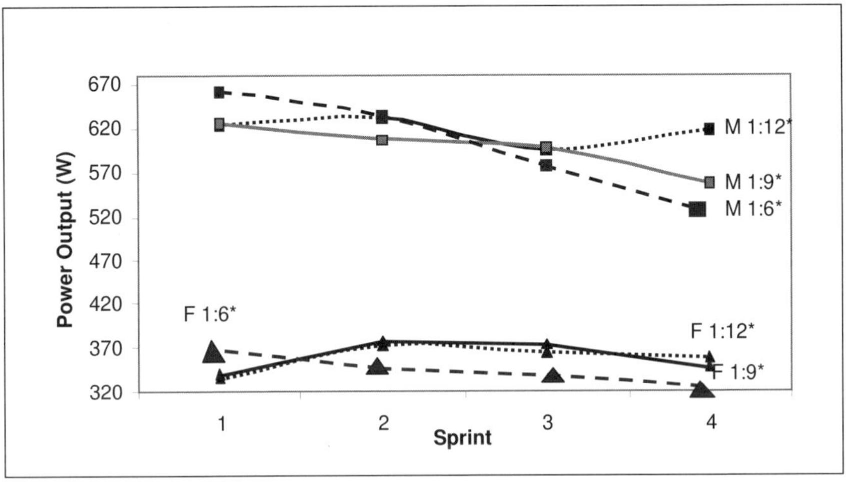

* Significant difference at p<.05 between highest and lowest MP output achieved in that particular series of 4 sprints. M=male adults (*n*=10), F=female adults (*n*=10). Mean power in each sprint was measured as the averaged power output recorded in that specific 10-s sprint.

Figure 2: MP between male and female adults for different WRs

3.3. *Composite Fatigue Index (CFI) for the different WRs*

CFI_{pp} and CFI_{mp} are the composite fatigue indices for PP and MP, respectively. They were calculated based on the percentage decline between the highest and the lowest PP or MP generated, amongst the four sprints. In the subject cohort, the highest PP output occurred within the first two sprints (e.g. For WR of 1:6, 15 cases in sprint 1 and 5 cases in sprint 2) whilst the lowest PP output occurred in the third or fourth sprint (e.g. WR of 1:6, 5 cases in sprint 3 and 15 cases in sprint 4). It is noteworthy that the highest PP and MP across the WRs were not significantly different (p<.016).

Pooled performance data showed that there was a significant difference ($p<.05$) in the extent of PP decline between a WR of 1:12 and a WR of 1:9, and between a WR of 1:9 and a WR of 1:6. The data sets showed that when the intra-session rest interval increased, PP declined less (Figure 3). Analysis of MP showed that the decline in MP was not significantly different between a WR of 1:12 and a WR of 1:9 ($p>.05$). It is indicative that when the WR was reduced to 1:9 or a 90-s intra-session recovery, the decline in MP was not significantly different as compared to the longer intra-session recovery time of 120 s. Mean power declined by 12.4 % with 90 s intra-session recovery and decreased by 9.5 % with 120 s recovery (Figure 4).

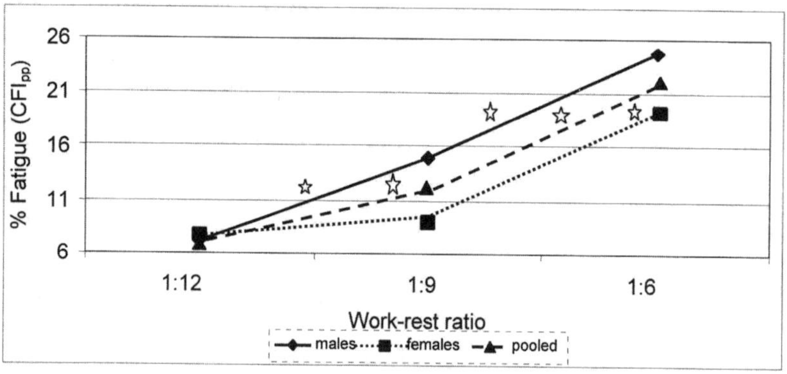

* Significant difference in CFI_{pp} (peak power composite fatigue index) at $p<.016$
CFI_{pp} was calculated based on the percentage decline between the highest and the lowest peak power generated, amongst the four sprints. Males adults (n=10) and females adults (n =10)

Figure 3: CFI_{pp} of male and female adults with different WRs

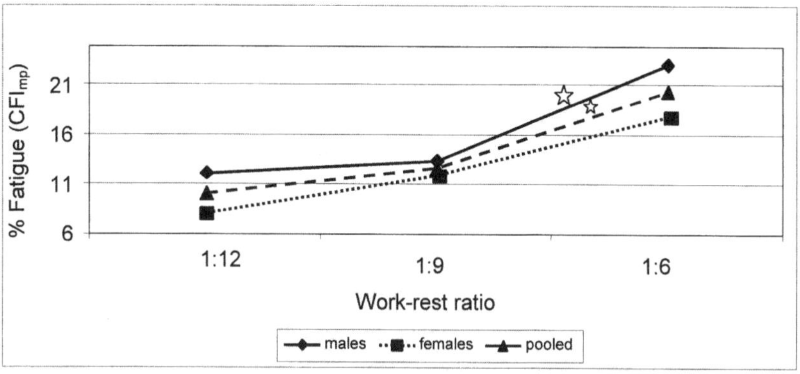

* Significant difference in CFI_{mp} (mean power composite fatigue index) at p<.05
CFI_{mp} was calculated based on the percentage decline between the highest and the lowest mean power generated, amongst the four sprints. Male adults (n=10) and female adults (n=10)

Figure 4: CFI_{mp} of male and female adults with different WRs

In male adults, there was a significant difference (p<.05) in CFI_{pp}, for all the three WRs (Figure 3). In terms of MP, the power generated from the WR of 1:12 sprints was not significantly different (p>.05) to that generated from the WR of 1:9, showing that a 90 s recovery after a 10 s sprint was sufficient to prevent a significant reduction in MP (Figure 4).

Peak power performance for female participants showed no significant decline, or no significant increase in CFI_{pp}, for a WR of 1:9 and a WR of 1:12 W (p>.05) indicating that there was no significant difference in the restoration of PP whether the intra session recovery time was 90 s or 120 s. PP did not decline further in four intermittent sprints when the intra session recovery period was reduced from 120 s to 90 s (Figure 2). Mean power decline was 17.4 % with a 60 s recovery. There was no significant difference in CFI_{mp} between the three WRs. The trend observed for male and female subjects in Figures 2 and 3 was an increasing CFI with the shortest rest duration (WR of 1:6).

4. Discussion

The aim of the study was to investigate performance of male and female subjects under the three different conditions of WRs (1:6; 1:9 and 1:12) for the maintenance of PP and MP over four 10 s sprints. The absence of equivalent research data in the extant literature, especially on untrained female adults make comparisons difficult. The majority of data on the recovery from short-term high intensity sprints are derived from male athletes. Two studies cited in the literature used a WR of 1:10. For example, Wootton and Williams (1982) reported a 3 % decrease in PP after the final bout of maximal sprint on a cycle exercise in 16 male athletes, with a 6-s sprint and 60-s rest over 5 bouts. Holmyard et al. (1988), reported on 10 Rugby Union backs over ten 6-s sprints. With a 60-s recovery period, they reported a 3 % and 4.2% decrease in PP and MP, respectively from the first to the last sprint.

The cited results were reported on trained athletes. In contrast, results of the current study showed that untrained male adults exhibited a decline of PP output, with CFI_{pp} (WR of 1:9) of 15 %, more than the 3-4 % decline demonstrated by trained male athletes (Holmyard et al, 1988; Wootton & Williams, 1982). The corresponding data for untrained female adults was a CFI_{pp}, of 9 %. No equivalent data are apparently available for comparison. This is indicative that more research attention should be devoted to this area. Bogdanis et al. (1998) reported that untrained male subjects were able to generate similar PP output after 2-min of recovery from a 10-s maximal cycle sprint. However, untrained participants in the current study reported a significant ($p<.05$) decrease in PP and MP after 2-min of recovery time, both in male and female adults. The recovery of PP up to the initial PP output was not observed, even after 120 s of recovery. Subject cohort differences may explain the difference between the present study and that of Bogdanis et al (1998). It is plausible that although both subject cohorts were described as untrained, the physical fitness status of the two subject cohorts were not determined.

The differences in the decrease in PP and MP, observed in the present study and that in the cited studies could be attributed to the training status of the subjects. Thoden (1991) reported that trained athletes relied less on non-oxidative sources and thus recovered faster during short-term high intensity intermittent exertions. Trained athletes have superior aerobic fitness and this supplemented anaerobic energy during the sprints and also provided aerobically-derived energy at a faster rate during the recovery period. This capability could be due to the increased concentration of aerobic enzymes, myoglobin and mitochondrial number, size and surface area (Holloszy & Coyle, 1984). Hamilton et al. (1991) explained that athletes consumed more oxygen immediately after exercise as compared to untrained subjects. Trained athletes are thus better able to restore adenonosine triphosphate (ATP) and phosphocreatine (PCr) quicker and to a fuller extent than untrained subjects and are hence more successful in maintaining PP in subsequent exercise bouts.

In another study, Hughes et al (2005) reported that in 10 X 6-s intermittent sprints, with rest periods of 25-, 40- and 55-s, there were significant ($p<.05$) differences in the recovery of untrained male adults. Force production was significantly lower in the 25-s recovery as compared to the 55-s recovery (71.2±5.9 N *vs* 76.4±6.8 N, $p<.05$) context. Results from the cited study were in agreement with the current investigations that either the WR was an important criterion for determining recovery, or that a rest interval of more than 90 s was necessary to ensure no further decline in PP for untrained male adults.

This conclusion is in agreement with the viewpoints articulated by others where the recovery of muscle function from intense exercise was a time dependent process and that recovery period played an important role in limiting fatigue (Ratel et al., 2003). This being the case, during high intensity intermittent exercises the fatigued muscles in adults is unlikely to regain full power restoration within the short intra-session recovery duration. Even though PCr is resynthesised during the recovery phase (McCully, 2002), intra-session rest intervals that are too short inevitably compromised subsequent muscle tension (DeLuca, 1984). Time must be allowed for the working muscles to replenish PCr, restore intramuscular pH, for the removal of metabolic end products and the return of impaired muscle membrane excitation to resting levels (Pincivero et al, 1998). Bogdanis et al. (1995) showed that PCr resynthesis after intense exercise has a half time of 56.6 s, therefore in a situation where the intra- session recovery period insufficient to allow full PCr resynthesis, the maintenance of PP is difficult.

One objective of the present study was to determine the WR needed to arrest a further decline in PP. Present results showed that the effects of time in power recovery between the sexes were different. Untrained male adults required a longer intra- session recovery time to arrest further power decline than untrained female adults.

5. Conclusion

Results from the present study showed that male and female adults exhibited differences in recovery capabilities. Female adults recovered faster than male adults from short-term high intensity intermittent sprints of up to 10 s.

References

1. Blonc, S., Casas, H., Duche, P., Beaune, B., & Bedu, M. (1998). Effect of recovery duration on the force-velocity relationship. *International journal of Sports Medicine, 19,* 272-276.
2. Bogdanis, G., Nevill, M., Boobis, L., Lakomy, H., & Nevill, A. (1995). Recovery of power output and muscle metabolites following 30s of maximal sprint cycling in man. *Journal of Physiology, 482,* 467-480.
3. DeLuca, C. (1984). Myoelectrical manifestations of localized muscular fatigue in humans. *CRC Critical Reviews in Biomedical Engineering, 11,* 251-279.
4. Drust, B., Reilly, T., & Cable, N. (2000). Physiological responses to laboratory-based soccer-specific intermittent and continuous exercise. *Journal of Sports Sciences, 18,* 885-892.
5. Hamilton, A., Nevill, M., Brooks, S., & Williams, C. (1991). Physiological responses to maximal intermittent exercise: Differences between endurance-trained runners and games players. *Journal of Sports Sciences, 9,* 371-382.
6. Holloszy, J., & Coyle, E. (1984). Adaptations of skeletal muscle to endurance exercise and their metabolic consequences. *Journal of Applied Physiology, 56,* 831-838.
7. Holmyard, D., Cheetham, M., Lakomy, H., & Williams, C. (1988). Effects of Recovery duration on performance during multiple treadmill sprints. In Reilly T, A. Lees, K. Davids & W. Murphy (Eds.), *Science and Football* (pp. 134-142). London: E & FN Spon.
8. Hughes, M., di Amaral, I., & Rose, G. (2005). The influence of recovery duration on blood lactate accumulation in repeated sprint activity. *Journal of Sports Sciences, 23,*130-131
9. Hill, D.W., & Smith, J.C. (1993). Gender difference in anaerobic capacity: role of aerobic contribution. *British Journal of Sports Medicine, 27,* 45-48.
10. McCully, K., Authier, B., Olive, J., & Clark, B. (2002). Muscle fatigue: The role of metabolism. *Canadian Journal of Applied Physiology, 27,* 70-82.
11. Mukherjee, S., & Chia, C. (2005). *Assessment of the capability to perform repeated high intensity running in youth professional soccer players.* Unpublished Thesis. National Institute of Education, Nanyang Technological University, Singapore.
12. Pincivero, D., Lephart, S., & Karunakara, R. (1998). Effects of intra-session rest interval on strength recovery and reliability during high intensity exercise. *Journal of Strength and Conditioning Research, 12,* 152-156
13. Ratel, S., Lazaar, N., Williams, C., Bedu, M., & Duche, P. (2003). Age differences in human skeletal muscle fatigue during high-intensity intermittent exercise. *Acta Pediatrica, 92,* 1248-1258.
14. Reilly, T. (1996). Energetics of high-intensity exercise (soccer) with particular reference to fatigue. *Journal of Sports Sciences, 15,* 257-263.

15. Reilly, T., Secher, N., Snell, P., & Williams, C. (1990). *Physiology of Sports*. London: E & FN Spon.
16. Sahlin, K., & Ren, J. (1989). Relationship of contraction capacity to metabolic changes during recovery from a fatiguing contraction. *Journal of Applied Physiology, 67,* 648-654.
17. Spierer, D., Goldsmith, R., Baran, D., Hryniewicz, K., & Katz, S. (2004). Effects of active vs passive recovery on work performed during serial supramaximal exercise tests. *International Journal of Sports Medicine, 25,* 109-114.
18. Tecmachine. (2002). *Sprint Club user's guide*. France: Medical development.
19. Thiriet, P., Gozal, D., Wouassi, D., Oumarou, T., Gelas, H., & Lacour, J. (1993). The effect of various recovery modalities on subsequent performance, in consecutive supramaximal exercise. *The Journal of Sports Medicine and Physical Fitness, 33,* 118-129.
20. Thoden, J. (1991). Testing aerobic power. In J. MacDougall, H. Wenger & H. Green (Eds.), *Physiological Testing of the High Performance Athlete* (pp. 107-174). Champaign, IL: Human Kinetics.
21. Weltman, A., Stamford, B., Moffatt, R., & Katch, V. (1977). Exercise, recovery, lactate removal and subsequent high intensity exercise performance. *Research Quarterly, 48,* 786-796.
22. Wootton, S., & Williams, C. (1982). The influence of recovery duration on repeated maximal sprints. In H. Knuttgen (Ed.), *Biochemistry of Exercise XIII* (pp. 269-273). Champaign, IL: Human Kinetics.
23. Zajac, A., Jarzabek, R., & Waskiewicz, Z. (1999). The diagnostic value of the 10- and 30-second Wingate test for competitive athletes. *Journal of strength and Conditioning Research, 13,* 16-19.

REPEATED HIGH-INTENSITY RUNNING PERFORMANCE IN SOCCER

SWARUP MUKHERJEE

Physical Education and Sports Science, National Institute of Education, Nanyang Technological University, Singapore

MICHAEL CHIA

Physical Education and Sports Science, National Institute of Education, Nanyang Technological University, Singapore

The overall activity pattern in soccer is of an intermittent high-intensity type and the capability to perform repeated high-intensity running is a discriminatory performance quality among soccer players at different standards of the game. Repeated high-intensity running derives energy from all three energy systems in different proportions depending upon the fitness level of the players and the physiological demands of the game in terms of duration, intensity and frequency of the high-intensity running efforts required during the game. Therefore, a measurement of repeated high-intensity running capability in soccer players provides a worthwhile index of their playing prowess. Both laboratory and field-based methods and protocols are used to assess this capability in soccer players. Some studies deal with high-intensity running and all-out sprint ability as separate entities while others combine them into one single category of high-intensity running. The majority of the laboratory-based test protocols are developed on the bicycle ergometer and relatively few use the motorized treadmill and the non-motorised treadmill. The field-based tests for the assessment of repeated sprint ability use different sprint distances and recovery intervals while intermittent high-intensity running ability are evaluated predominantly using the YoYo tests in soccer players. Long-term studies are required to determine the effect of age and environment on repeated high-intensity running capability in soccer players. Furthermore, it is desirable to conduct further studies determining the measures of repeated high-intensity running capability in the tests that can be objectively translated into measures of match performance.

1. Introduction

The game of soccer is extensively studied and it is well established that the exercise pattern in soccer is that of an intermittent high-intensity type and this nature of the game is independent of playing style and position (Bangsbo,

Norregaard & Thorsoe, 1991; Ekblom, 1986; Mohr, Krustrup & Bangsbo, 2003; Reilly & Thomas, 1976; Withers et al., 1982). A successful soccer player should therefore possess an outstanding capability to perform repeated high-intensity running. Moreover, the higher the level of soccer, the greater is the amount of high-intensity running performed by the players (Mohr et al., 2003).

Therefore, the most discriminatory fitness attribute between soccer players and teams of different standards is the overall intensity of activity during the game (Ekblom, 1986). While the total distance covered may vary from game to game for a player, the amount of high-intensity exercise appears to be a more constant measure of performance (Bangsbo, 1993). Hence, soccer at higher standards is characterised by the players' capability to perform high-intensity work repeatedly and this fitness attribute constitutes the most consistent, discriminatory, decisive and valid measure of performance in modern soccer. It is also evident during the soccer matches that the strategic execution of activities at high-intensity, with or without ball possession, often leads to decisive outcomes.

1.1. *Motion characteristics of soccer: with reference to repeated high-intensity running*

A soccer match requires more than a thousand discrete movements, with rapid and frequent alterations in pace and direction (Reilly & Thomas, 1976). Various elements of the game are presented in an acyclical manner with a change in the type or level of activity approximately every 4-6 s (Drust, Reilly & Rienzi, 1998; Reilly, 1997) reflecting the intermittent nature of the game. In competitive soccer, a player executes more than 75 high-intensity running efforts, including 18-20 all-out sprints (Bangsbo, 1993; Tumilty, 1993). This requires the players to perform a high-intensity effort every 30 s and an all-out sprint every 90 s. The average distance of these efforts is 15-20 m and in terms of duration, they last 2-5 s (Reilly, 1994; Reilly, Bangsbo & Franks, 2000). Moreover, the need for inter-positional play makes it imperative for the players in the team to be able to perform repeated high-intensity running independent of, and over and above the demands of their respective playing positions (Bangsbo et al., 1991).

The term 'high intensity running' can be based on the criteria of speed of running, on VO_2 as a percentage of VO_{2max} and on the HR as a percentage of HR_{max} (Table 1).

1.2. *Criteria for running intensity in soccer*

Criteria	Moderate intensity	High-intensity
Running speed	12-15 km·h^{-1}	> 15 km·h^{-1}
% VO_{2max}	65-80 %	> 80 %
% HR_{max}	80-90 %	> 80 %

Note: km·h^{-1} – kilometre per hour; % VO_{2max} – percentage of maximal oxygen uptake; % HR_{max} – percentage of maximal heart rate (Adapted from: Bangsbo, 1994b; Bangsbo, Norregaard & Thorsoe, 1991; Criswell et al., 1993, Nieman et al., 1993)

Different studies analysing motion characteristics of soccer document the percentage distance covered at high-intensity by the players (Table 2). The differences in the extent of high-intensity running shown in the cited studies during soccer matches is likely to be due to the differences in the motion-analysis methodology, and also to the differences in the motion descriptors used in respective studies. However, it is noteworthy that the amount of high-intensity running during soccer has greatly increased over the years.

Table 2 Percentage distance covered at high-intensity in soccer matches (Mean values)

Study	Team	Total distance covered (km)	% Distance covered at high-intensity
Reilly & Thomas, 1976	Professional	8.7	11.2
Withers et al., 1982	First team	11.5	18.8
Ekblom, 1986	1st– 4th Division	10.0	8.0
Van Gool et al., 1988	University	10.2	7.8
Bangsbo et al., 1991	Danish League	10.8	26
Mohr et al., 2003	Elite	10.8	22.3
	Professional	10.3	18.4
Krustrup et al., 2006	Fourth Division	9.7	16.4
Di Salvo et al., 2007	Professional	11.3	23.7
Rampinini et al., 2007	Professional	10.8	30.6

Note: km-kilometre, %-percentage

It is clear that the major discriminating performance attribute between the players of different quality is not the total distance covered during the game, but the percentage of the total distance covered at higher intensities and the absolute values of maximum speed play during the game. The elite players perform high-intensity running to a greater extent and also in terms of a greater number of high-intensity bouts than the lower-level players (Mohr et al., 2003). Mohr et al. reported that although the players of both elite-level and moderate-level covered greater distances at high-intensity as well as in sprints during the first half than in the second half of the game, the elite players performed 28 % more high-intensity running, and the distance covered in sprinting was reported to be 58 % more than that covered by moderate-level players. Further, the peak distance covered in high-intensity running in a particular 5 min period by top-level players was 27 % more than by the moderate-level players. It is noteworthy that even in younger age-group players (12-14 yr), the elite players are reported to perform greater higher-intensity activities compared to the non-elite players (Strøyer, Hansen & Klausen, 2004).

While the total distance covered may vary from game to game for any individual player, the amount of high-intensity exercise performed appears to be more constant (Bangsbo, 1993). High-speed running (cruising) and sprinting in combination represent the high-intensity activity during soccer play. Therefore the ratio of low-intensity to high-intensity exercise is approximately 2:1, if indicated by the distance covered (Reilly & Thomas, 1976) and when referred to a time base, the calculated ratio is about 7:1 (Reilly, 1997). As the nature of soccer is intermittent and acyclical, brief periods of repeated high-intensity running efforts are required throughout the game duration. A motion-analysis study on English FA Premier League soccer showed that about 40 % of recovery durations between subsequent high-intensity runs were less than 2 s (O'Donoghue, 2003). Another study by the same author on the repeated work-activity characteristics in elite soccer (O'Donoghue et al., 2005) reported that high-intensity work comprised of about 10.1% of the match time (~ 9 min) and the work-to-recovery ratio was reported to be 1:8.9 compared to 1:7 in a previous study by Reilly, 1997. Further, O'Donghue et al. stated that in soccer, a work period of any duration could be followed by a recovery interval of any length, thus highlighting the unpredictable nature of the game.

1.3. *Physiology of soccer- in relation to the performance of repeated high-intensity exercise*

The execution of technical and tactical skills in soccer is dependent on the player's physical and physiological capacities. Soccer is a sport which entails involvement of both aerobic and anaerobic energy systems (Bangsbo, 1994a; Reilly, 1997). More than 90 % of the game is fuelled by aerobic metabolism. The physiology of repeated high-intensity running however is a mixed bag, involving all the three energy systems (Dawson, Fitzsimons & Ward, 1993) that contribute in different proportions depending on the running intensity, sprint duration, number of repetitions, recovery interval and the fitness level of the players. Superimposed on the low-intensity activities are the repeated bouts of high-intensity running efforts, fuelled predominantly by the anaerobic energy systems (Reilly, 1997). The average work intensity in a game of soccer is around the lactate threshold or 70-75 % of VO_{2max} or 80-90 % of HR_{max} (Reilly, 1994).

A similar game intensity is reported even at the junior elite levels (Helgerud et al., 2001). However, it is impossible for the players to continuously sustain such a high work-intensity for an extended period of time as it will lead to increasing muscle and blood lactate accumulation. Hence, the actual duration spent at that intensity is about 20 min, as the players exercise either above (lactate accumulation) or below (lactate oxidation) this threshold (Helgerud et al., 2001). Therefore, the activity pattern in soccer involves alternate periods of high-intensity activity and lower-intensity periods of recovery.

1.4. *The phosphagen system in repeated high-intensity exercise*

The phosphagen system is the primary energy source for sprint starts and maximal efforts of short duration (Hirvonen et al., 1987; Serresse, et al., 1988). The intramuscular phosphocreatine (PCr) stores approximately amount to 80 $mmol \cdot kg^{-1} \cdot dm^{-1}$ (Bangsbo et al., 2001; Bogdanis, Nevill, Lakomy et al., 1995; Gaitanos et al., 1993). During maximal work, there is an exponential depletion of PCr at turnover rates of approximately 9 $mmol\ ATP \cdot kg^{-1} \cdot dm^{-1} \cdot s^{-1}$ (Hultman & Sjöholm, 1983). Approximately 50 % of the total anaerobic energy during a single short sprint of 5-6 s is provided by the degradation of PCr (Gaitanos et al., 1993). However, during repeated sprints, the extent of replenishment of the PCr stores during recovery determines the magnitude of its contribution in fuelling such activity.

The half-life for PCr recovery is about 20-60 s (Bogdanis, Nevill, Boobis et al., 1995; Harris et al., 1976) and in soccer, there might be a number of situations when the available recovery duration can be less than adequate for complete PCr recovery. Degradation of PCr and to a lesser extent the stored ATP provides a considerable amount of energy during the periods of high-intensity running in a match. While considerable extent of the phosphagen system replenishment occurs within 20-30 s, a full repletion may require more than 3-4 minutes (Dawson et al., 1993). Using a protocol of 10 × 6 s all-out sprints on the cycle ergometer, Gaitanos et al. (1993) reported that an interspersed recovery duration of 30 s could enable the PCr-based ATP resynthesis to contribute more than 50 % of ATP from the anaerobic sources.

Resynthesis of PCr during the periods of rest and low-intensity exercise probably causes the PCr concentration to alternate continuously as a result of the intermittent nature of the game (Bangsbo, 1994a). Although the net utilisation of ATP is quantitatively small during a soccer match, PCr has a very important function as an energy buffer, providing phosphate for resynthesis of ATP through the creatine kinase reaction during rapid increases in the exercise intensity (Bangsbo, 1994a).

1.5. *The anaerobic glycolytic system in repeated high-intensity exercise*

Immediately as a sprint is commenced, the glycolytic system also starts providing ATP (Hirvonen et al., 1987), and longer the sprint lasts, the greater is the proportion of energy supplied by the glycolytic system. The energy contribution from the glycolytic system becomes even more crucial during repeated sprint efforts with an insufficient recovery time in-between the successive efforts for an adequate replenishment of the phosphagen energy system.

As high-intensity sprints are repeatedly executed, the replenishment of the phosphagen system progressively decreases (Jansson et al., 1990; McCartney et al., 1986; Spriet et al., 1989) owing to the accumulation of H^+ ions interfering with the PCr replenishment. Hence, the performance of repeated high-intensity running efforts is likely to derive a substantial contribution from the glycolytic energy system. This is supported by the findings of BLa concentrations of 10-12 $mmol \cdot L^{-1}$ after RSA tests (Fitzsimmons et al., 1993). These values are close to the peak post-exercise BLa concentrations of 13-14 $mmol \cdot L^{-1}$ recorded after 30 s cycle sprints and 400 m track sprints (Dawson et al., 1993). Similar findings were observed in university soccer and rugby players (n=8) where after a repeated sprint exercise (6 × 6 s with 24 s between-sprint recovery) on a non-motorised treadmill, the peak BLa was found to be (Mean ± SD) 9.83 ± 0.86 $mmol \cdot L^{-1}$ (Mukherjee, 2008).

The percentage energy contribution from the glycolytic system in soccer however, is generally rated low, as most of the high intensity efforts last for less than 5 s (Barros, Valquer & Sant'Anna, 1999; O'Donoghue et al., 2005). Researchers often questioned the importance of glycolysis in team sports (Tumilty et al., 1988). Moreover, it is reported that the alterations in the metabolic environment during maximal intermittent work cause a gradual inhibition of glycolysis with repeated sprints (Bangsbo, 1996; Gaitanos et al., 1993). In participants performing 10 × 6 s maximal sprints with 30 s between-sprint recovery, Gaitanos et al. reported that glycolysis contributed to 44 % of the anaerobic ATP provision during the first sprint which reduced to 16 % by the tenth sprint. Furthermore, the glycolytic ATP provision was estimated to be nil by the tenth sprint in four of the participants.

Lactate samples obtained post-exercise or during formal breaks in the game show BLa concentrations in the range of 2-3 mmol·L^{-1} (Tumilty et al., 1988) whereas the samples obtained during actual play show much higher BLa concentrations of up to 8-12 mmol·L^{-1} (Ekblom, 1986; Smith et al., 1993). Therefore, the post-exercise samples or those collected during the scheduled breaks may not reflect the peak BLa levels during a game. Studies that estimated BLa during match play show a wide variation (Table 3).

Study	Sample source	Level of Play	First-half		Second-half	
			During	End	During	End
Ekblom, 1986	Not mentioned	1st division		9.5* (6.9-14.3)		7.2* (4.5-10.8)
		2nd division		8.0* (5.1-11.5)		6.6* (3.1-11.0)
		3rd division		5.5* (3.0-12.6)		4.2* (3.2-8.0)
		4th division		4.0* (1.9-6.3)		3.9* (1.0-8.5)
Rhode & Esperson, 1988	Finger tip	1st & 2nd division		5.1 ± 1.6**		3.9 ± 1.6**
Gerisch et al., 1988	Not mentioned	Top amateur league		5.6 ± 2.0**		4.7 ± 2.2**
		University match	6.8 ± 1.0**	5.9 ± 2.0*	5.1 ± 1.6**	4.9 ± 1.7**
Bangsbo et al., 1991	Finger tip	1st & 2nd division	4.9* (2.1-10.3)		3.7* (1.8-5.2)	4.4* (2.1-6.9)
Smith et al., 1993	Finger tip	College matches		5.2 ± 1.2**		
Bangsbo, 1992	Arm vein	League match	4.1* (2.9-6.0)	2.6* (2.0-3.6)	2.4* (1.6-3.9)	2.7* (1.6-4.6)
	Plasma	League match	6.6* (4.3-9.3)	3.9* (2.8-5.4)	4.0* (2.5-6.2)	3.9* (2.3-6.4)
Florida-James & Reilly, 1995	Finger tip	University soccer		4.4 ± 1.2**		4.5 ± 2.1**
Krustrup et al., 2006	Arm vein	4th Division	6.0 ± 0.4* (3.8-9.6)	4.1 ± 0.4* (1.3-6.0)	5.0 ± 0.4* (2.3-8.6)	3.9 ± 0.4* (2.1-5.9)

* Mean; ** Mean ± SD, within brackets- Range. (Adapted from Bangsbo, 1994a)

Although it is difficult to quantify the physiological contribution of the anaerobic lactacid energy system during a soccer match which is probably less than 10 % (Bangsbo, 1993), this system provides energy at very high rates during periods of intense exercise in a match, especially when there is a need to perform repeated bouts of high-intensity running with less than adequate recovery periods in between.

1.6. *The aerobic system in repeated high-intensity exercise*

The contribution of the aerobic system to maximal short duration sprint efforts is minor, but it plays a crucial role in replenishment of the intramuscular ATP, PCr and myoglobin stores during the recovery periods between sprints (Tesch et al., 1989). The aerobic energy system is also important for the breakdown and removal of lactate through various pathways (Åstrand et al., 1986). This provides strong support to the notion that improvements in aerobic fitness and thereby increasing the oxygen availability to the exercising muscles augments the performance of repeated high-intensity running efforts by enhancing the rate of phosphagen repletion and lactate removal.

Apor (1988) reported a rank-order correlation between the VO_{2max} and the league placement of Hungarian soccer teams. On similar lines, considerable difference was found in VO_{2max} in members of the top and the lowest placed teams of Norway (Wisloff et al., 1998). As further support to the importance of VO_{2max} in soccer, a study by Helgerud et al. (2001) showed that increasing the peak VO_2 by interval training in soccer players resulted in an increase in the total distance covered in the match by 20 %, an increase in the involvement with the ball by 23 % and an increase in the number of sprints executed by 100 %. Although the above studies support the notion that aerobic fitness may lead to enhanced repeated sprint performance capability, direct evidence as to how exactly endurance-training affects multiple-sprint performance is yet to be elucidated.

On the other hand, other studies report a low or non-significant correlation between the VO_{2max} and repeated high-intensity performance (Aziz et al., 2000; Wadley & Le Rossignol, 1998). Some researchers establish that there is a relationship between the peak VO_2 and the total distance covered in a match (Bangsbo, 1993; Krustrup et al., 2003). However, a non-significant correlation has been found between the maximal oxygen uptake and high-intensity running during a game (Krustrup et al., 2003, Mukherjee, 2008). Bangsbo (1993) found no difference in the VO_{2max} values between the top-level Danish players and non-regular players. A study on soccer by Wells et al. (2005) including amateur (n= 18) and professional (n=18) players found that both the groups despite having similar VO_{2max} (Mean ± SD: 57.1 ± 3.9 *vs* 58.1 ± 2.8 $ml \cdot kg^{-1} \cdot min^{-1}$) scored differently on the YoYo IRT level-2 (Mean ± SD: 716 ± 123 *vs* 840 ± 153 m).

A lack of consistency between VO_{2max} and the quality of soccer is suggestive that this physiological attribute does not necessarily determine quality performance in soccer. However, the consistent finding of values exceeding 60 $ml.kg^{-1}.min^{-1}$ in the elite soccer players is indicative of the existence of a threshold below which a player in unlikely to perform successfully in top-class soccer.

1.7. *Assessment of repeated high-intensity running in soccer: the methodological approaches*

Repeated high-intensity running in soccer include fast running (striding or cruising) at one end to all-out sprinting at the other extreme. Previous studies examined the capability to perform repeated high-intensity running by assessing repeated sprint ability (RSA) using different distance and rest interval (Aziz et al., 2004; Fitzsimmons, 1993), assessing intermittent high-intensity running capability (Krustrup et al., 2003, 2006; Wells et al., 2005) or evaluated the significance of aerobic fitness in performance of repeated high-intensity running (Bishop & Spencer, 2004; Castagna et al., 2006). Some studies however, due to the difficulties in accurately distinguishing between striding and sprinting have combined them into one single category of high-intensity running (Mayhew & Wenger, 1985; Van Gool et al., 1988).

1.8. *Field tests assessing repeated sprint running ability in soccer players*

The term 'repeated sprint ability' (RSA) was apparently introduced by Fitzsimmons et al. (1993) and this term represents the capability to repeatedly perform maximal sprint efforts (Dawson et al., 1993). RSA tests have the appeal of being more sports-specific than the 'single effort' performance tests of power and capacity of energy systems (Fitzsimons et al.). In an attempt to understand the various physiological mechanisms involved in RSA, a range of field tests have been developed. Most of these protocols, barring a few (Bangsbo, 1994b; Krustrup et al., 2003) are based on similar formats, with the sprint distances varying between 20-40 m, number of repetitions varying from 3-12 and the between-sprint recovery durations varying from 15-30 s (Table 4).

It is argued that a RSA test will challenge the energy systems in a manner which more closely replicates the game situation (Fitzsimmons et al., 1993). While some of the protocols are generally applicable to sports requiring repeated sprint ability (Baker & Davies, 2002; Baker, Ramsbottom & Hazeldine, 1993; Bishop et al., 2001; Dawson et al., 1993; Fitzsimmons et al.), others address the issue with specific reference to soccer (Balsom, Seger & Ekblom, 1992;

Bangsbo, 1994b; Krustrup et al., 2003; Rebelo et al., 1998; Tumilty et al., 1988; Wragg et al., 2000). A common approach of most of these studies is to measure the individual sprint time over the number of repetitions, to determine the peak speed, calculation of total and mean sprint time and the decrement in speed to estimate the fatigue index (FI).

Table 4 Field-based test protocols for repeated sprint ability (RSA)

Study	Sprint distance (m)	Repetitions	Recovery interval (s)
Tumility et al., (1988)	20	3 per set × 6 sets	20
Balsom, Seger &	40	15	60
Ekblom, (1992)	40	15	30
	15	40	30
Fitzsimmons et al., (1993)	40	6	24
Bangsbo (1994b)	34.2	7	25
Wadley & Le Rossignol (1998)	20	12	16-17
Rebelo et al., (1998)	30	7	25
Baker & Davies, (2002)	40 (20 × 2)	3	20
Newman et al., (2004)	20	12	20
Krustrup et al (2006)	30	5	25
Mukherjee (2008)	20	8	15
Pyne et al (2008)	30	6	20 s cycle

1.9. *Field tests assessing intermittent high-intensity running ability in soccer players*

While a range of RSA tests using different protocols and modes are used to assess the repeated all-out sprint running capability of players, apparently the only test protocol that is developed and widely studied to determine the intermittent high-intensity running capability in soccer players is the YoYo test. The YoYo test has an Intermittent Endurance Test (IET) and an Intermittent Recovery Test (IRT) version. (Bangsbo, 1994b; Bangsbo, 1996). In the YoYo IET, the players are required to perform repeated 2 × 20 m shuttle runs interspersed with an active recovery period of 5 s, during which the players jog (Figure 1). The YoYo IET evaluates a players' capability to repeatedly perform intense exercise over a prolonged period of time. The YoYo IET has two levels based on the starting speed. The YoYo IET level-1 has a starting speed of 8 km·h^{-1} and the level-2 has a starting speed of 11.5 km·h^{-1}.

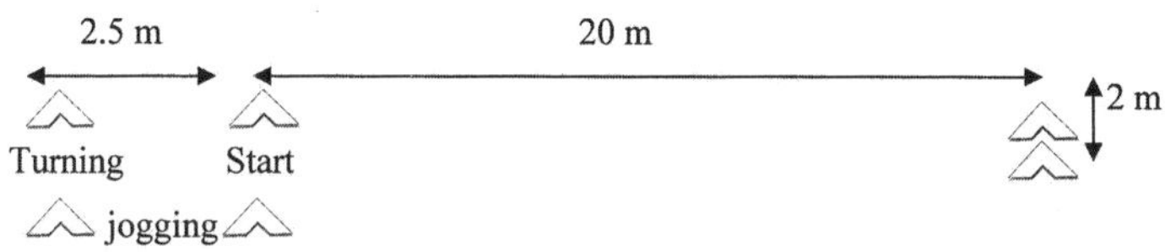

Figure 1: Schematic layout of the YoYo Intermittent Endurance Test (Adapted from Bangsbo, 1996)

The YoYo IRT evaluates a player's capability to recover from intense exercise. In this test the running speeds are higher than in the YoYo IET and there is a 10 s period of active recovery between each 2 × 20 m shuttle (Figure 2). It is particularly suitable for sports like soccer in which the capability to perform intense exercise after a short recovery period can be decisive for the outcome of the game (Krustrup et al., 2003). The YoYo IRT also has two levels. The test level-1 starts with a running speed of 10 km·h^{-1} and the test level-2 with a speed of 13 km·h^{-1} respectively.

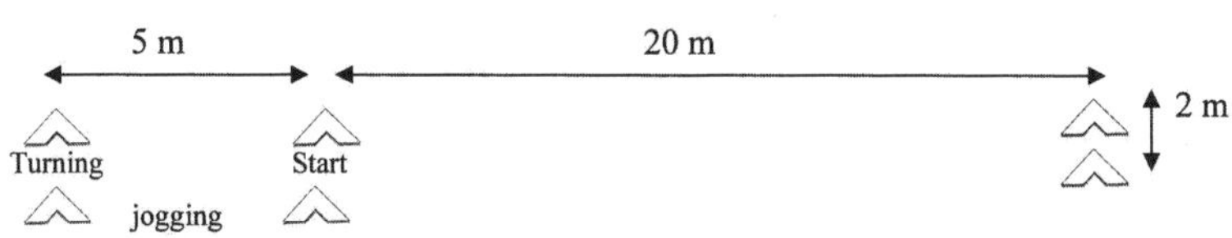

Figure 2: Schematic layout of the YoYo Intermittent Recovery Test. (Adapted from Bangsbo, 1996)

The YoYo IRT has a high reproducibility and a valid measure of physical performance in soccer (Krustrup et al., 2003). Moreover, the Yo-Yo IRT is suggested to be sensitive to changes in the performance level of adult elite (Krustrup et al., 2003; Krustrup et al., 2006) as well as youth elite soccer players (Mukherjee, 2008).

The performance on YoYo IRT level-1 is significantly correlated to the amount of high-intensity exercise performed during a soccer game by the players ($r = 0.71$, $p<0.05$, $n=37$; Krustrup et al., 2003) and soccer referees ($r = 0.75$, $p< 0.05$, $n=18$; Krustrup & Bangsbo, 2001). The test is sensitive allowing for a detailed analysis of differences between and the seasonal changes in the physical capacity of soccer players (Krustrup et al., 2003). The test can discriminate between the positional differences in the capability to perform high-intensity running, and between players of different levels (Krustrup et al., 2003; Krustrup, Mohr, Nybo et al., 2006; Mohr et al., 2003).

The YoYo IET (Aziz, Tan & Teh, 2005; Castagna et al., 2006; Rebelo et al., 1998) and YoYo IRT level-1 (Castagna et al., 2006; Dupont et al., 2008; Krustrup et al., 2003; Mohr et al., 2003) are well studied by different researchers. However, relatively fewer studies are focused on the YoYo IRT level-2 (Krustrup et al., 2006; Mukherjee, 2008; Wells et al., 2005). Since the YoYo IRT level-2 incorporates higher running speeds than the level-1 test, it is logical that the YoYo IRT level-2 is more suitable for the assessment of elite soccer players. The study by Wells et al. supports the use of Yo-Yo IRT level-2 as a measure of performance in soccer players. Further, with respect to stimulating the aerobic and the anaerobic energy systems, the YoYo IRT level-2 test may be more appropriate for the assessment of repeated high-intensity running capability in elite soccer players (Krustrup et al., 2006).

A recent study found that the performance in the YoYo IRT level 2 was significantly correlated (specify the range) with the amount of high-intensity work performed during professional soccer matches during different phases of a complete soccer season in youth professional soccer players (Mukherjee, 2008). Furthermore, the level 2 version is sensitive to the changes in the repeated high-intensity running performance through the season. It is recommended that the YoYo IRT level 2 is an appropriate tool to assess the capability to perform repeated high-intensity running in elite soccer players at both adult and youth levels, in particular in fitter players. Additional advantages of the YoYo tests are that they can be undertaken at low cost and in a short time with the possibility of testing multiple participants simultaneously.

1.10. *Laboratory tests assessing repeated high-intensity running in soccer players*

The activity pattern in soccer continuously varies through the game. Therefore, information derived from the simulated protocols and other field-based tests of performance may not reflect the true picture of match play that can be applied to every possible situation. Many researchers in sports and exercise science are discouraged in their attempts to study soccer by the lack of available experimental models (Reilly, 1990). Further, it might be problematic to attract the best players into laboratory tests due to motivational reasons (Kemi et al., 2003). As a consequence, few researchers have tried to develop soccer-specific laboratory-based protocols.

1.11. *Assessment of repeated high-intensity running capability on the motorised treadmill*

Apparently, there are few studies that use motorised treadmill-based test protocols to assess the capability to perform repeated high-intensity running capability in soccer players. A soccer-related protocol, constructed with a purpose of determining the VO_{2max} and the time to exhaustion (TTE), and to correlate these measures to the performance on a field test (YoYo IRT level-1) reported to be valid for assessing repeated high-intensity running in soccer players and to the high-intensity exercise performance during a game is reported by Krustrup et al. (2003). This protocol requires the participants to run on a motorised treadmill at the speeds of 10, 12, 14 and 16 $km{\cdot}h^{-1}$ in 6 min bouts, separated by 2 min rest periods followed by an incremental maximal test performed after 15 min of rest. Significant correlations are reported between the field test performance and the time to exhaustion and VO_{2max} on the treadmill test. However, neither the treadmill performance, nor the peak VO_2 are correlated to the high-intensity exercise performed during a game.

A recent study on youth professional soccer players used a motorised treadmill-based protocol (Figure 3) to specifically assess the capability to perform repeated high-intensity running (Mukherjee, 2008). This is schematically described in Figure 3.

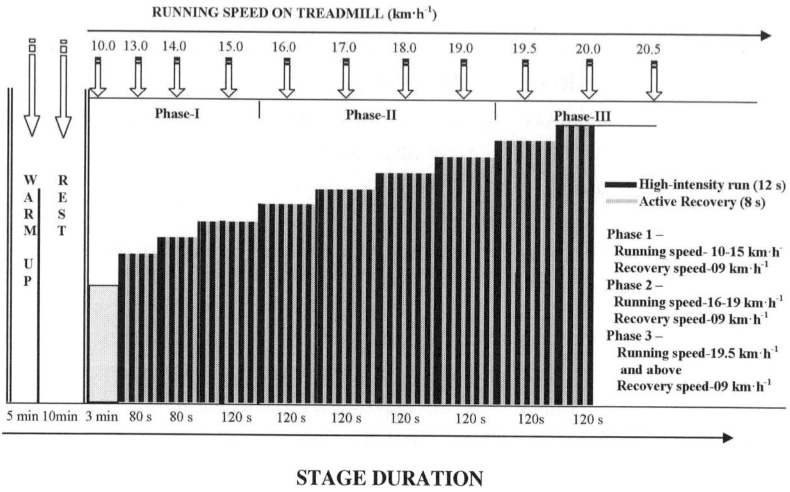

Figure 3: Schematic representation of laboratory test protocol for repeated high-intensity running capability in soccer players (Mukherjee, 2008)
Note: $km{\cdot}h^{-1}$ – kilometre per hour; min- minute; s- second

The test shows high reliability (ICC, 0.98; CV, 2.1 %; ratio Limits of Agreeement, 0.99 $^{\times}/\div$ 1.03) and the results of a longitudinal analysis of the measure of repeated high-intensity running in terms of distance covered (m) in the test showed a similar trend as the performance in the YoYo IRT L2. Further, the performance in this test showed a consistently significant correlation ($p < 0.05$) with the performance in the YoYo IRT L2 and with the high-intensity exercise performed during soccer games during different phases on the soccer season (Mukherjee, 2008). The criterion validity and sensitivity of this test with respect to the assessment of repeated high-intensity running capability in elite soccer players is therefore established. Moreover, the laboratory-based test provides the option of conducting different physiological measurements like oxygen uptake, HR and blood pressure monitoring and BLa estimation in a controlled testing environment, if warranted.

1.12. *Assessment of repeated high-intensity running capability on the non-motorised treadmill*

The development of a non-motorised running treadmill (NMT) has helped to overcome some of the practical shortcomings associated with laboratory-based intermittent exercise protocols. Apart from allowing maximal sprint running, the NMT also allows almost instantaneous alterations in the intensity of activity, similar to those observed during a soccer game. The non-motorised treadmill has the advantage of allowing sports-specific forms of locomotion with respect to sports with activity pattern like soccer. Despite these obvious advantages, few studies have been conducted on the NMT to assess repeated sprint running performance in soccer players (Drust et al., 2002; Holymard et al., 1988; Mukherjee, 2008).

The commonly measured performance indicators on the NMT are peak power, mean power, peak speed, force output and fatigue index. The NMT has been reported to be a reliable tool although the consensus is that the measures of speed and force have higher reliability than the measures of power output (Doherty, Hughes & Toms, 2007; Hughes et al., 2006; Tong et al., 2001). This is because the power output is not a directly measured parameter but calculated from the product of force and velocity and the trends in the power output data would represent observations intermediate between force and speed. Apparently the only study using NMT to assess RSA (6×6 s with 24 s recovery) in soccer players on a longitudinal basis, showed a significant change in the RSA of the players with the progress of the season (Mukherjee, 2008). However, non-significant correlations ($p > 0.05$) were observed between RSA test performance on the NMT and the amount of high-intensity exercise performed during soccer matches during the season.

1.13. *Assessment of repeated high-intensity running capability on the bicycle ergometer*

Bicycle ergometry is widely used for determining the RSA of athletes utilising different protocols (Table 5).

Table 5: Repeated sprint protocols on bicycle ergometer

Study	Sprint Duration	Number of Repetitions	Recovery Interval
Baker et al., 1993	30 s	1	Nil
Fitzsimmons et al., 1993	6 s	6	24 s
Dawson et al., 1993	6 s	6	24s
McMahon & Wenger, 1998	15 s	6	90 s (active)
Bishop et al., 2001	6 s	5	24 s
Baker & Davies, 2002	30 s	1	Nil
Bishop et al., 2003	6 s	5	24 s
Bishop & Spencer, 2004	6 s	5	24 s
Edge et al., 2006	6 s	5	24 s
Racinais et al., 2007	6 s	10	30 s

While the tabulated studies suggested different conclusions regarding reliability, validity and applicability of cycle ergometry protocols as being suitable for assessment of RSA, the modality needs an analysis from the aspect of specificity. For the test results to be of practical significance, the exercise mode must be specific to the sport (MacDougall & Wenger, 1991). Although alternate modes may be available and highly reliable, their validity declines as the motor pattern becomes different (MacDougall & Wenger).

Cycling is a weight-supported activity and predominantly involves the lower body muscle mass as opposed to running which also involves the upper body muscle mass. Moreover, performance on all test protocols has an element of learning, and both motor co-ordination and individual skill levels in a given performance contribute to the test results (Baker & Davies, 2002). Apart from this, each test measuring a specific fitness attribute demands a skill component, and the required skill specificity causes individuals to perform differently on each of the tests (Baker & Davies, 2002). Although at times the relative RSA test performance may be reasonably indicated by a non-specific test, cycling tests should remain a second preference for running athletes and wherever possible, exercise-specific test formats should be utilised (Fitzsimmons et al., 1993).

1.14. *Repeated high-intensity running performance in soccer – future research*

The energy demands of soccer are complex and difficult to quantify. Repeated high-intensity exercise derives energy from all three energy systems in different proportions. Further, the lack of established 'gold-standard' criteria against which the responses elicited in the tests can be compared, make the assessment of this mode of exercise a greater challenge than the assessment of continuous modes of exercise. Studies on elite soccer players are largely limited to a cross-sectional design. As repeated high-intensity running performance extensively taxes both aerobic and anaerobic energy systems, soccer with its intermittent high-intensity activity pattern presents different performance demands according to the level of participation and the age group. A longitudinal assessment of repeated high-intensity running capability in different soccer playing populations is desirable to have greater insights into understanding of the functional bases of this performance capability. Moreover, a research study on elite younger age-group soccer players is encouraged to determine the effect of physical growth and development on this performance capability.

There is a relative scarcity of studies on different aspects of match performance in soccer. With respect to the performance of high-intensity exercise during soccer games, estimations are generally done by the monitoring the work-intensity or by the determination of the motion characteristics of the game in terms of number of high-intensity runs or sprints performed during the game. While the measures of intermittent high-intensity running are significantly correlated to high-intensity exercise performed during the soccer games, the measures of RSA showed a non-significant correlation (Mukherjee, 2008). This brings into question the criterion validity of the RSA tests. The RSA test structure in both the modes used in the present study can be said to have logical, content and construct validity. In this respect, it is surprising to find a non-significant correlation between RSA test performances and match performance.

All-out sprinting represents the extreme zone of high-intensity running efforts. It is observed that a strategic execution of all-out sprints, with or without the ball, often leads to decisive outcomes in soccer. Therefore, the importance of all-out sprinting efforts in soccer cannot be underestimated. Future studies therefore, should assess the translation of different measures of RSA into game performance.

Playing conditions in most Asian countries pose different environmental challenges (high temperature and high humidity) on the players compared to that in the European and Scandinavian countries. Therefore, the results of the studies in countries with colder climate may not be applicable in a straightforward manner on Asian soccer players. A relative paucity of studies on Asian elite soccer players make it imperative to conduct further research on this population under local weather conditions to evaluate the effect of playing conditions on the performance of repeated high-intensity exercise during soccer games.

References

1. Apor, P. (1988). Successful formula for fitness training. In T. Reilly, A. Lees, A. Davids, & W.J. Murphy (Eds.), *Science and Football* (pp. 95-107). New York: E & F.N. Spon.
2. Åstrand, P.O., Hultman, E., Juhlin-Dannfelt, A., & Reynolds, G. (1986). Disposal of lactate during and after strenuous exercise in humans. *Journal of Applied Physiology*. 61, 338-342.
3. Aziz, A.R., Chia, M., & Teh, K.C. (2000). The relationship between maximal oxygen uptake and repeated sprint performance indices in field hockey and soccer players. *Journal of Sports Medicine and Physical Fitness*. 40, 195-200.
4. Baker, J.S., & Davies, B. (2002). High intensity exercise assessment: Relationships between laboratory and field measures of performance. *Journal of Science and Medicine in Sport*. 5, 341-347.
5. Baker, J., Ramsbottom, R., & Hazeldine, R. (1993). Maximal shuttle running over 40 m as a measure of anaerobic performance. *British Journal of Sports Medicine*. 27, 228-232.
6. Balsom, P.D., Seger, S.Y., & Ekblom, B. (1992). Physiological evaluation of high-intensity intermittent exercise. *Journal of Sports Sciences*. 10, 160-161.
7. Bangsbo, J. (1993). *The Physiology of Soccer – with Special Reference to Intense Intermittent Exercise*. August Krogh Institute, University of Copenhagen. Denmark.
8. Bangsbo, J. (1994a). Energy demands in competitive soccer. *Journal of Sports Sciences,* 12, S5-S12.
9. Bangsbo, J. (1994b). *Fitness Training in Football: A Scientific Approach.* Denmark: HO+Storm.
10. Bangsbo, J. (1996). Regulation of muscle glycogenolysis and glycolysis during intense exercise: in vivo studies using repeated intense exercise. In R.J. Maughan & S.M. Shirreffs (Eds.), *Biochemistry of Exercise* (pp. 261-275). Champaign (IL): Human Kinetics.
11. Bangsbo, J., Krustrup, P., González-Alonso, J., & Saltin, B. (2001). ATP production andefficiency of human skeletal muscle during intense exercise: effect of previous exercise. *American Journal of Physiology, Endocrinology and Metabolism*. 280:E956-E964.

12. Barros, T., Valquer, W., & Sant'Anna, M. (1999). High intensity motion pattern analysis of Brazilian elite soccer players in different positional roles. *Medicine and Science in Sports and Exercise*. 31, S260.
13. Bangsbo, J., Nørregaard, L., and Thørso, F. (1991). Activity profile of competition soccer. *Canadian Journal of Sports Sciences,* 16, 110 – 116.
14. Bishop, D., Spencer, M., Duffield, R., & Lawrence, S. (2001). The validity of a repeated sprint ability test. *Journal of Science and Medicine in Sport*. 4, 19-29.
15. Bogdanis, G.C., Nevill, M.E., Boobis, L.H., Lakomy, H.K., & Nevill, A.M. (1995). Recovery of power output and muscle metabolites following 30 s of maximal sprint cycling in man. *Journal of Physiology (London)*. 482, 467-480.
16. Bogdanis, G.C., Nevill, M.E., Lakomy, H.K., & Boobis, L.H. (1995). Power output and muscle metabolism during and following recovery from 10 and 20 s of maximal sprint exercise in humans. *Acta Physiologica Scandinavica*. 163, 261-272.
17. Bishop, D., & Spencer, M. (2004). Determinants of repeated sprint ability in well-trained team-sport athletes and endurance-trained athletes. *Journal of Sports Medicine and Physical Fitness*. 44, 1-7.
18. Castagna, C., Impellizari, F.M., Chamari, K., Carlomagno, D., & Rampinini, E. (2006).
19. Aerobic fitness and Yo-Yo continuous and intermittent tests performances in soccer players: A correlational study. *Journal of Strength and Conditioning Research*. 20, 320-325.
20. Criswell, D., Powers, S., Dodd, S., Lawler. J., Edwards. W., Renshler. K. et al. (1993). High-intensity training-induced changes in skeletal muscle antioxidant activity. *Medicine and Science in Sports and Exercise*. 25, 1135-1140.
21. Dawson, B., Fitzsimons, M., & Ward, D. (1993). The relationship of repeated sprint ability to aerobic power and performance measures of anaerobic work capacity and power. *The Australian Journal of Science and Medicine in Sport*. 25, 88-93.
22. Di Salvo, V., Baron, R., Tschan, H., Calderon Montero, F.J., Bachl, N., & Pigozzi, F. (2007). Performance characteristics according to playing position in elite soccer. *International Journal of Sports Medicine*. 28, 222-227.
23. Doherty, M., Hughes, M.G., & Toms, H. (2007). The reliability of non-motorised treadmill sprint performance. *Journal of Sports Sciences*. 25, 259.
24. Drust, B., Reilly, T., & Cable, N.T. (2002). Metabolic and physiological responses to a laboratory-based soccer-specific intermittent protocol on a non-motorized treadmill. In W. Spinks, T. Reilly & A. Murphy (Eds.), *Science and Football IV* (pp. 217-225). London and New York: Routledge.

25. Drust, B., Reilly, T., & Rienzi, E. (1998). A motion-analysis of work rate profiles of elite international soccer players. *Journal of Sports Sciences*. 16, 460.
26. Dupont, G., Defontaine, M., Bosquet, L., Blondel, N., Moalla., & Berthoin, S. (2008). Yo-Yo intermittent recovery test versus the Université de Montréal Track test: Relation with a high-intensity intermittent exercise. *Journal of Science and Medicine in Sport*. doi: 10.1016/j.jsams.2008.10.007.
27. Edge, J., Bishop, D., Hill-Haas, S., Dawson, B., & Goodman, G. (2006). Comparison of muscle buffer capacity and repeated-sprint ability in untrained, endurance-trained and team-sport athletes. *European Journal of Applied Physiology*. 96, 225-234.
28. Ekblom, B. (1986). Applied Physiology of Soccer. *Sports Medicine*, 3, 50-60.
29. Fitzsimmons, M., Dawson, B., Ward, D., & Wilkinson, A. (1993). Cycling and running tests of repeated sprint ability. *The Australian Journal of Medicine and Science in Sport*, 25, 82-87.
30. Gaitanos, G.C., Williams, C., Boobis, L.H., & Brooks, S. (1993). Human muscle metabolism during intermittent maximal exercise. *Journal of Applied Physiology*. 75, 712-719.
31. Harris, R.C., Edwards, R.H.T., Hultman, E., Nordesjo, L.O., Nyland, B., & Sohlin, D. (1976). The time course of phosphoryl-creatine resynthesis during recovery of quadriceps muscle in man. *Pflugers Archives. European Journal of Applied Physiology*. 367, 137-142.
32. Helgerud, J., Engen, L.C., Wisløff, U., & Hoff, J. (2001). Aerobic endurance training improves soccer performance. *Medicine and Science in Sports and Exercise*. 33, 1925-1931.
33. Hirvonen, J., Rehunen, S., Rusko, H., & Harkoven, M. (1987). Breakdown of high energy phosphate-compounds and lactate accumulation during short supramaximal exercise. *European Journal of Applied physiology and Occupational Physiology*. 56, 253-259.
34. Holymard, D.J., Cheetham, M.E., Lakomy, H.K.A., & Williams, C. (1988). Effect of recovery duration on performance during multiple treadmill sprints. In T. Reilly, A. Lees, K. Davids & W.J. Murphy (Eds.), *Science and Football* (pp. 134-142). NewYork: E & FN Spon.
35. Hughes, M.G., Doherty, M., Tong, R.J., Reilly, T., & Cable, N.T. (2006). Reliability of repeated sprint exercise in non-motorised treadmill ergometry. *International Journal of Sports Medicine*. 27, 900-904.
36. Hultman, E., & Sjöholm, H. (1983). Energy metabolism and contraction force of human skeletal muscle in situ during electrical stimulation. *Journal of Physiology*. 3454, 525-532.

37. Jansson, E., Dudley, G.A., Norman, B., & Tesch, P.A. (1990). Relationship of recovery from intense exercise to the oxidative potential of skeletal muscle. *Acta Physiologica Scandinavica.* 139, 147-152.
38. Krustrup, P., Mohr, M., Amstrup, T., Rysgaard, T., Johansen, J., Steensberg, A. et al. (2003). The Yo-Yo Intermittent Recovery Test: Physiological response, reliability, and validity. *Medicine and Science in Sports and Exercise,* 35, 697 – 705.
39. Krustrup, P., Mohr, M., Nybo, L., Jensen, J.M., Nielson, J.J., & Bangsbo, J. (2006). The Yo-Yo IR2 test: physiological response, reliability, and application to elite soccer. *Medicine and Science in Sports and Exercise.* 38, 1666-1673.
40. MacDougall, J.D., Wenger, H.A. (1991). The purpose of physiological testing. In J.D. MacDougall, H.A. Wenger & H.J. Green (Eds.), *Physiological Testing of the High-Performance Athlete* (pp. 1-5). Illinois: Champaign.
41. Mayhew, S.R., & Wenger, H.A. (1985). Time-motion analysis of professional soccer. *Journal of Human Movement Studies.* 11, 49-52.
42. McMahon, S., & Wenger, H.A. (1998). The relationship between aerobic fitness and both power output and subsequent recovery during maximal intermittent exercise. *Journal of Science and Medicine in Sport.* 1, 219-227.
43. McCartney, N., Spriet, L.L., Heigenhauser, G.J.F., Kowalchuk, J.M., Sutton, J.R., & Jones, N.L. (1986). Muscle power and metabolism in maximal intermittent exercise. *Journal of Applied Physiology.* 60, 1164-1169.
44. Mohr, M., Krustrup, P., & Bangsbo, J. (2003). Match performance of high-standard soccer players with special reference to development of fatigue. *Journal of Sports Sciences.* 21, 519-528.
45. Mukherjee, S. (2008). *Assessment of the capability to perform repeated high-intensity running in youth profesional soccer players.* Unpublished doctoral dissertation, National Institute of Education, Nanyang Technological University, Singapore.
46. Newman, M.A., Tarpenning, K.M., & Marino, F.E. (2004). Relationships between isokinetic knee strength, single-sprint performance, and repeated sprint ability in football players. *Journal of Strength and Conditioning Research.* 18, 867-872.
47. Nieman, D.C., Miller, A.R., Henson, D.A., Warren, B.J., Gusewitch, G., Johnson, R.L., et al. (1993). Effects of high-vs moderate-intensity exercise on natural killer cell activity. *Medicine and Science in Sports and Exercise.* 25, 1126-1134.
48. O'Donoghue, P.G. (2003). Analysis of the duration of periods of high-intensity activity and low-intensity recovery performed during English FA Premier League soccer. *Journal of Sports Sciences.* 21, 285-286.

49. O'Donoghue, P., Rudkin, S., Bloomfield, J., Powell, S., Cairns, G., Dunkerley, A. et al. (2005). Repeated work activity in English Premier League soccer. *International Journal of Performance analysis in Sport.* 5, 46-57.
50. Pyne, D.B., Saunders, P.U., Montgomery, P.G., Hewitt, A.J., & Sheehan, K. (2008).Relationship between repeated sprint testing, speed, and endurance. *Journal of Strength and Conditioning Research.* 22, 1633-1637.
51. Racinais, S., Bishop, D., Denis, R., Lattier, G., Mendez-Villaneuva, A., & Perrey, S. (2007). Muscle deoxygenation and neural drive to the muscle during repeated sprint cycling. *Medicine and Science in Sports and Exercise.* 39, 268-274.
52. Rampinini, E., Bishop, D., Marcora, S.M., Ferrari Bravo, D., Sassi, R., & Impellizeri, F.M. (2007). Validity of simple field tests as indicators of match related physical performance in top-level professional soccer players. *International Journal of Sports Medicine.* 28, 228-235.
53. Rebelo, N., Krustrup, P., Soares, J., & Bangsbo, J. (1998). Reduction in intense intermittent exercise performance during a soccer match. *Journal of Sports Sciences.* 16, 482-483.
54. Reilly, T. (1994). Physiological profile of the player. In B. Ekblom (Ed.), *Football* (pp. 78-94). Oxford: Blackwell scientific.
55. Reilly, T. (1997). Energetics of high-intensity exercise (soccer) with particular reference to fatigue. *Journal of Sports Sciences.* 15, 257-263.
56. Reilly, T., Bangsbo, J., & Franks, A. (2000). Anthropometric and physiological predispositions for elite soccer. *Journal of Sports Sciences.* 18, 669-683.
57. Reilly, T., & Thomas, V. (1976). A motion analysis of work rate in different positional roles in professional football match-play. *Journal of Human Movement Studies.* 2, 87-97.
58. Serresse, O., Lortie, G., Bouchard, C., & Boulay, R. (1988). Estimation of the contribution of various energy systems during maximal work of short duration. *International Journal of Sports Medicine.* 9, 456-460.
59. Smith, M., Clarke, G., Hale, T. & McMorris, T. (1993). Blood lactate levels in college soccer players in match play. In T. Reilly, J. Clarys & A. Stibbe (Eds.). *Science and Football II* (pp 129-134). London: E & FN Spon.
60. Spriet, L.L., Lindinger, M.I., McKelvie, R.S., Heigenhauser, G.J.F., & Jones, N.L. (1989). Muscle glycogenolysis and H+ concentration during maximal intermittent cycling. *Journal of Applied Physiology.* 66, 8-13.
61. Strøyer, J., Hansen, L., & Klausen, K. (2004). Physiological profile and activity pattern of young soccer players during match play. *Medicine and Science in Sports and Exercise.* 36, 168-174.

62. Tesch, P.A., Thorsson, A., & Fujitsuka, N. (1989). Creatine Phosphate in fibre types of skeletal muscle before and after exhaustive exercise. *Journal of Applied Physiology*. 66, 1756-1759.
63. Tong, R.J., Bell, W., Ball, G., & Winter, E.M. (2001). Reliability of power output measurements during repeated treadmill sprinting in rugby players. *Journal of Sports Sciences*. 19, 289-297.
64. Tumilty, D. (1993). Physiological characteristics of elite soccer players. *Sports Medicine*. 16, 80-96.
65. Tumilty, D., Hahn, A.G., Telford, R.D., & Smith, R.A. (1988). Is lactic acid tolerance an important component of fitness for soccer? In T. Reilly, A. Lees, K. Davids, & W.J Murphy (Eds.), *Science and Football* (pp. 81-86). London: E & FN Spon.
66. Van Gool, D., Van Gerven, D., & Boutmans, J. (1988). The physiological load imposed on soccer players during real match play. In T. Reilly, A. Lees, K. Davids, & W.J Murphy (Eds.), *Science and Football* (pp. 51-59). New York: E & F.N. Spon.
67. Wisloff, U., Helgerud, J., & Hoff, J. (1998). Strength & endurance of elite soccer players. *Medicine and Science in Sports and Exercise*. 30, 462-467.
68. Wadley, G., & Le Rossignol, P. (1998). The relationship between repeated sprint ability and the aerobic and anaerobic energy systems. *Journal of Science and Medicine in Sport*. 1, 100-110.
69. Wells, C.M., Drust, B., Winter, E.M., & Fysh M. (2005). Performance of professional and amateur soccer players on Yo-Yo Recovery test level-2. *Journal of Sports Sciences*. 23, 132-133.
70. Withers, R.T., Maricic, Z., Wasilewski, S., & Kelly, L. (1982). Match analysis of Australian professional soccer players. *Journal of Human Movement Studies*. 8, 159-176.
71. Wragg, C.B., Maxwell, N.S. & Doust, J.H. (2000). Evaluation of the reliability and validity of a soccer-specific field test of repeated sprint ability. *European Journal of Applied Physiology*. 83, 77-83.

RELATIONSHIP BETWEEN COMPOSITE TORQUE AND SPRINT CYCLING POWER IN ADULTS

MICHAEL CHIA

Physical Education and Sports Science, National Institute of Education, Nanyang Technological University, Singapore

The purpose of the study was to examine the relationships between composite concentric isokinetic torque (CCIT), peak power (PP) and mean power (MP) of male and female adults using allometric scaling. Eighteen male (age: 21.3±1.9yrs, stature: 1.71±0.05m & body mass: 64.5±5.4kg) and 20 female adults (age: 20.2±2.0y, stature: 1.62±0.06m & body mass: 51.3±7.9kg) participated in the study. Lower limb muscle mass (LLMM) of the participants was determined using a dual energy X-ray absorptiometric (DXA) procedure. Peak leg extension and flexion torque at 1.05, 3.14 and 5.20 rad/s were determined using an isokinetic dynamometer (Cybex 6000), and were summed to derive CCIT. PP and MP were derived from a 30-s Wingate Anaerobic Test (WAnT) on a cycle ergometer (Monark 814*E*). Data allometrically scaled to LLMM, respectively, were for PP (77.6±7.4 vs. 72.9±8.4 W/kg $LLMM^{0.72}$, p>.05) and MP (57.2±5.7 vs. 55.1±4.8, W/kg $LLMM^{0.76}$ p>.05). Equivalent data for CCIT, respectively, were at 1.05 rad/s (19.7±3.0 vs. 18.4±2.1 Nm/kg $LLMM^{0.93}$, p>.05), at 3.12 rad/s (6.7±1.3 vs. 6.7±1.1 Nm/kg $LLMM^{1.18}$, p>.05) and at 5.20 rad/s (6.2±1.2 vs. 6.6±1.0 Nm/kg $LLMM^{1.12}$, p>.05). Significant correlations (male: r=0.50-0.66, p<.05; female: r=0.53-0.84, p<.05) were established between PP (W/kg $LLMM^{0.72}$) and MP (W/kg $LLMM^{0.76}$), and CCIT at 1.05 rad/s (Nm/kg $LLMM^{0.93}$), at 3.14 rad/s (Nm/kg $LLMM^{1.18}$) and at 5.20 rad/s (Nm/kg $LLMM^{1.12}$). Correlations between LLMM-independent variables- PP and CCIT, were higher at 5.20 rad/s than at 1.05 rad/s (r=0.61 vs. r=0.65) but not for MP and CCIT (r=0.64 vs. r=0.61). Data showed that LLMM-independent power and torque variables shared moderate common variances.

1. Introduction

Studies on isokinetic torque and power in adults are diverse in research foci. They include: the collection of normative values for different muscle groups from different subject populations, investigations on the relationships between torque or power measurements and body size descriptors and measurements obtained from other tests (Davies, Heiderschet & Brinks, 2000; Inbar, Bar-Or &

Skinner, 1996). Despite considerable attention from researchers, Jaric (2002) argues that the appropriate torque-power relationships are often ignored or are incorrectly taken into account when torque and power results are compared. For example, it is common for researchers to make comparisons between groups or sex, based merely on results that are in absolute values of strength or power, without accounting for the significant body size differences. Jaric (2002) contends that in studies where data are normalized (e.g. ratio scaling, linear adjustment techniques or allometric scaling), they may have been done so indiscriminately, without first verifying that the scaling method used is appropriate based on the characteristics of the data set (e.g. heteroscedascity). The erroneous use of scaling approaches may obscure the real relationships between performance measures that are purportedly free from the influence of body size (Chia & Aziz, 2008).

Performances in isokinetic concentric torque of the lower limbs have commonly focused on knee extension alone (Baltzopoulos, Eston & Maclaren, 1988) or knee extension and flexion (Davies & Dalsky, 1997), at either single (Baltzopoulos, Eston & Maclaren, 1988) or multiple angular velocities (Davies & Dalsky, 1997). There are fewer studies, which are based on the concept of total leg strength or composite concentric isokinetic torque (CCIT), where several tests of lower extremity muscles (e.g. knee extension and flexion) are performed and the data are summated to give a composite score (Boltz & Davies, 1984). The concept of a composite value for isokinetic torque allows researchers to evaluate the entire lower extremity as a total isokinetic chain (Feiring, Ellenbecker & Dersheid, 1990). A measure of composite torque is more useful when correlating constant velocity torque to power generated during sprint cycling since the cycling movement involves both flexion and extension of the muscles of the lower limbs (Too, 1990).

In adults, the capability to generate muscle torque or power can be explained to a great degree by the muscle mass that is actively involved in the movement (Chia, 2003).

In order to compare results between groups of different body sizes in weight bearing exercises such as treadmill sprinting and jumping, it is arguably defensible to express the performance in relation to body mass or stature, rather than total muscle mass since adults must function with total body mass and not just total muscle mass (Davies & Dalsky, 1997). However, Chia (2003) proposed that in seated assessments involving the lower limbs such as isokinetic torque determination or power determination during sprint cycling, where the body mass of the participant is supported, it may be more suitable to relate the performance (i.e. torque or power) to some indicator of muscle size (e.g. lower limb muscle mass or LLMM) that are involved during the assessments. In his study, which examined PP and MP of 48 boys and 38 girls aged 14-15 years, stepwise regression analysis revealed that among body size descriptors, body mass, stature and LLMM, LLMM was the best predictor in boys and girls for PP ($r=0.78$ & $r=0.82$, $p<0.05$) and for MP ($r=0.66$ and $r=0.82$, $p<0.05$). However, the situation in adults needs elucidation and confirmation.

Researchers commonly use the ratio method to address differences in body size but there is a growing conviction that the ratio method may not appropriately normalise exercise data or produce size-independent variables that appropriately take into account differences in body size (Welsman & Armstrong, 2000). The main aim of using the simple ratio method is that it is assumed that the simple division of the variable of interest (e.g. CCIT or PP) by a body size descriptor (e.g. LLMM) will provide a size-free variable in watts per kg $\text{LLMM}^{b=1.0}$.

However, in most situations involving exercise data, the simple ratio method often fails to achieve this. For instance in group of 25 boys and 25 girls aged 10 years, Chia (2003) reported common *b* exponents of 0.91 and 0.88 for PP and MP expressed in relation to body mass. In using the simple ratio standard where the *b* exponent is 1.0, this has the potential error of penalizing participants with greater body mass while at the same time inflating the values of participants with smaller body mass (Welsman & Armstrong, 2000). Moreover, the use of body mass in ratio scaling may also obscure the actual outcome since they could be differences in body composition (i.e. lean muscle mass). The use of active muscle mass (e.g. LLMM) as the body size descriptor of choice, for example in lower limb exercise performance, may provide additional insights to issues in performance. It is critical that the appropriate normalization of exercise data for differences in body size is used as it will allow researchers to correctly interpret the results of the research. An inappropriate use of the scaling method can lead to erroneous interpretations or spurious relationships and consequently cloud our understanding of performances of different groups of participants (e.g. male vs. female, children vs. adults, and athletes vs. non-athletes) who differ in body size.

Allometric (log-linear) methods are recommended as more appropriate in accounting for body size effects as they are able to accommodate data that are heteroscedastic (Welsman & Armstrong, 2000) in nature, that is, as body size increases (e.g. LLMM), so does the variability of the performance variable of interest (e.g. CCIT, PP or MP). Allometric modeling is also particularly useful for exercise data (e.g. CCIT, PP or MP) as the technique incorporates a multiplicative rather than an additive error term (Welsman & Armstrong, 2000). In essence, the technique requires the derivation of a common *b* exponent for two different groups, only when it is appropriate, by applying the least-squares regression to logarithmically transformed data (e.g. Ln CCIT and Ln LLMM) (Welsman & Armstrong, 2000) and solving for numerical values of *a* and *b* (where *a* is the Y-intercept, and *b* is the slope coefficient) from the linear form of the allometric model, loge Y= loge $a + b \cdot$loge X.

Allometric modeling of torque data has been successfully applied to adult (Vanderburg, Mahar & Chou, 1995) and paediatric (De Ste Croix, Armstrong & Welsman, 1999) populations, as has been the case for the allometric expression of PP and MP of young people in relation to body mass, thigh muscle volume (Chia, 2003) and LLMM (Chia, 2003), albeit the cited studies were focused on boys and girls and not adults. Jaric (2002) reported that allometric scaling of exercise data appears to be the exception rather than the rule, even though the statistical practice is widely accepted in the biological sciences (Welsman & Armstrong, 2000). Therefore the use of the method in exercise science should be encouraged as it may provide fresh insights to exercise data that have been inappropriately normalized for body size.

Isokinetic torque for knee extension and flexion in adults have been correlated with vertical jump (r=0.80-0.81, i.e. 12), swimming performance (r=0.45-0.52, i.e. Magnusson et al, 1995), various jumps (r=0.61-0.84, i.e. Wilklander & Lysholm, 1987), leg press (r=up to 0.83, i.e. Sleivert, Backhus & Wenger, 1995), short distance speed skating (r=-0.60, i.e. Liebermann, Maitland & Katz, 2002) and Wingate Anaerobic Test performance (r=0.50-0.68, i.e. Inbar, Bar-Or & Skinner, 1996; r=0.93, i.e. Tsaklis, 2002). The relationships between power and torque are insightful in that the two variables are inherently linked to aspects of maximal exercise performances that are amenable to specific training and can also provide useful information about the validity of novel ways of expressing performance such as the concept of composite torque used in the present study.

In the majority of cited studies, the correlations were derived between isokinetic torque in absolute values or ratio-scaled to body mass and the absolute values of the movement performance. However, in most situations the movement performance (e.g. PP and MP in the WAnT) is also body size-dependent (Chia, 2003) and this could also affect the results of power-torque correlations (Jaric, 2002). Correlations between power and torque are affected by the influence of body size and do not give a true picture of the real relationships between power and torque, with body size appropriately partitioned out. Apparently, there are no data on the relationships between power and isokinetic torque that have been allometrically scaled in relation to LLMM. Data that are unaffected by the effects of body size are needed so as to facilitate a greater understanding of the relationships between generated power and torque in adults. Since muscle mass is the common denominator for power and torque generation and as power and torque do not have identical relationships with muscle mass, examining the body-size free relationships between power and torque will help researchers and trainers to better plan intervention or training programs to enhance muscle power or torque in healthy adults.

It is hypothesized that in applying statistically sound allometric scaling to power and torque generated by untrained male and female adults, a clearer picture of the relationship between power and torque, and LLMM would emerge. Therefore the study was conducted with a two-fold objective: (i) to describe CCIT, PP and MP of male and female adults in relation to muscle mass using conventional ratio standards and allometric modelling (ii) to examine the relationships between body size-free variables- PP and MP, and CCIT which have been allometrically-scaled in relation to muscle mass in male and female adults.

2. Method

2.1. *Participants and test arrangement*

Institutional ethical approval for all testing procedures was obtained from the National Institute of Education Physical Education and Sports Science Group. Sixteen adult males and 18 adult females with written informed consent participated in the study. All participants were untrained and did not engage in any form of structured exercise or training over the last six months prior to testing. All participants had visited the laboratory before and were habituated to the test procedures, which were conducted over two sessions. Research has shown that one to two habituation and practice sessions before actual testing increases the reliability of WAnT performance (Barfield et al, 2002), and isokinetic testing (Brown, 2000).

The order of the assessments was: (i) determination of lower limb muscle mass (LLMM) using dual energy X-ray absorptiometry (DXA), (ii) determination of peak power (PP) and mean power (MP) using the 30-second Wingate Anaerobic Test (WAnT) and (iii) determination of composite concentric isokinetic torque (CCIT). All assessments were conducted between 0900 hours and 1200 hours in the laboratory and at least a day's rest separated the test occasions. A principal investigator was present for all the assessments.

2.2. *Determination of lower limb muscle mass (LLMM) using dual energy X-ray absorptiometry (DXA)*

The DXA equipment used was an X-Ray Bone Densitometer (QDR 4500 Elite Hologic). The machine was equipped with a patented Hologic continuous calibration system and was operated by a trained and licensed technician. The use of DXA, in particular machines that uses high speed fan-beam technology (Kelly et al, 1997) to derive accurate measurements of body mass and lean mass in human subjects is becoming more popular among researchers. The scanning procedure for DXA involved the participant, dressed in shorts and a T-shirt, lying still in a supine position on the scanning table with both feet rotated inward toward each other, and with arms placed by the side with the palms pronated. The participant was instructed to remain still throughout the scan, which took about seven minutes. The lights were switched off and soothing music was played to help the participant remain relaxed and still throughout the scan. The radiation dose for each DXA scan was less than 1 mrem. Participants were scanned with protons produced by an X-ray source at two energy levels. Bone ash tissue and soft tissue were differentiated according to the degree of photon attenuation. The differential absorption within soft tissues was measured and the ratio of absorbency of the two energy level photons (RST) was linearly related to the percentage of fat in these tissues (Jensen et al, 1993). Bone-free lower limb muscle mass (LLMM), which was assumed to be equivalent to appendicular skeletal mass (Heymsfiled et al, 1990) was then calculated as the total limb mass minus the sum of limb fat and bone mass. The precision error for fat and lean tissue using fan beam technology is reported as 300g and the reproducibility coefficient in replicate measurements is reported as r= 0.90 or higher (Kelly et al, 1997). After the scan, image adjustment (pixel size 2mm by 3mm) and region selection was carried out to generate the required reports. LLMM was subsequently derived from the computer software (Hologic Version 9.80).

2.3. *Determination of composite concentric isokinetic torque (CCIT)*

Concentric isokinetic knee extension and flexion were measured using a Cybex 6000 dynamometer. Proper positioning and body stabilization of the seated participant was carried out using straps at the waist and across the chest, which were individually adjusted for each participant. This was done to isolate the muscle groups of the lower limbs during testing and also to minimize the contribution from accessory muscle groups.

A standardized warm-up consisting of hamstring and quadriceps muscle stretches combined with three sub-maximal repetitions followed by three maximal repetitions. Such a warm-up protocol has been shown to provide good reliability of isokinetic measurement of knee extension and flexion torque (Brown, 2000). Testing of the dominant lower limb, as determined by kicking preference was performed at 1.05 rad/s, 3.14 rad/s and 5.20 rad/s, representing slow, intermediate and fast isokinetic test velocities (Brown, 2000). Research has established high reliability coefficients of greater than 0.95 for peak isokinetic torques for knee extension and flexion for angular velocities of between 1.05 and 5.20 rad/s (Feiring, Ellenbecker & Dersheid, 1990) and for intra-day replicates of isokinetic torques (Bohannon & Smith, 1985).

The test velocity for each participant was randomly assigned by a principal investigator. With the participant seated upright, the lever arm of the dynamometer was aligned with the lateral epicondyle of the knee, with the knee flexed at an angle of 90 degrees. The range of motion during testing was set so that the working range constituted 90 degrees. The force pad was consistently placed 3-5cm superior to the medial malleous with the foot in a plantigrade position (De Ste Croix, Armstrong & Welsman, 1999). Gravity correction procedures were carried out for each participant prior to each test in accordance to the procedures described by De Ste Croix, Armstrong & Welsman, (1999). In essence the procedures involved the determination of the angle-specific torque data generated during passive knee flexion of the participant and the weight of the input accessories, including the lever arm. The computer software for gravity correction recorded these data over the full range of motion for knee extension and knee flexion.

Gravity correction procedures are recommended during assessments of isokinetic torque in a seated position to avoid the underestimation knee extension torque and the overestimation of knee flexion torque (Brown, 2000). The participants were instructed to push and to pull the lever arm up and down as hard and as fast as they could for three maximal efforts at each test velocity, with knee extension always undertaken first. Three maximal trials at each test velocity were performed as multiple trials are necessary to obtain a true maximal value of torque (Brown, 2000). Strong verbal encouragement was provided by the same group of testers and a 90-second rest period was allowed between test velocities.

Research has documented that an interval of rest of between 30 and 60 seconds after four maximal efforts at any test velocity is sufficient for ensuring maximal efforts between trials (Brown, 2000). The three highest concentric isokinetic torques for knee extension and flexion achieved at each test velocity were averaged and reported as average peak knee extension torque and average peak flexion torque for each test velocity (Brown, 2000). Composite concentric isokinetic torque (CCIT) for each participant was obtained by summing the average peak extension and average peak flexion torque. The CCIT concept allows researchers to evaluate the lower limb as a total kinetic chain (Davies, Heiderscheit & Brinks, 2000), and its use has been supported by others (Boltz & Davies, 1984).

2.4. *Wingate Anaerobic Test (WAnT)*

Participants completed a 30-second WAnT (Inbar, Bar-Or & Skinner, 1996) on cycle ergometer (Monark model 814 *E*). The friction-loaded cycle ergometer was interfaced with a microcomputer and was calibrated for pedal velocity and for static applied force in accordance with the manufacturer's instructions. Saddle height was individually adjusted and toe-clips were used to secure the feet of participants to the pedals.

The test proceeded with a standardised warm-up, which consisted of four minutes of constant pedalling at 70 revolutions per min (rpm) against a minimum applied force (with the weight basket supported). This was interspersed with three maximal intensity sprints of two to three seconds against the test-applied force, which was set equivalent to 0.74 N/kg BM (Inbar, Bar-Or & Skinner, 1996).

Participants completed a series of stretches for the quadriceps and hamstring group of muscles, which took two minutes. The sprint cycle test commenced from a rolling start of 70 rpm and participants were verbally encouraged to cycle as fast as they could against the applied force.

Inertia-adjusted 1-second peak power (PP) and mean power over 30s (MP) were the variables of interest that were derived from the WAnT. The procedure for the direct determination of flywheel inertia and computation for inertia-adjusted power are described in detail elsewhere (Chia, 2003). In healthy adult populations, the reliability of the WAnT has been established in many instances as $r>0.94$ (Inbar, Bar-Or & Skinner, 1996).

2.5. *Statistical analysis*

All relevant data were stored and analysed using SPSS for Windows (Version 15.0). The normality of data distributions (examined by the Shapiro-Wilks statistic) and homogeneity of variances (examined by the Levene test statistic) in the power and torque data sets (i.e. PP and MP, and CCIT at 1.05, 3.14 and 5.20 rad/s) were investigated.

Descriptive statistics (mean±SD) of the participants and their performances on the cycle ergometer and isokinetic dynamometer were generated. Linear regression analyses were applied to the data with stature, BM and LLMM entered in turn, as the covariate and with CCIT, PP and MP entered in turn, as the dependent variable, to determine, which among the body size descriptors was the best predictor for CCIT, PP and MP.

A repeated measures analysis of variance (RM-ANOVA) was used to investigate differences in CCIT at 1.05, 3.14 and 5.20 rad/s in male and female participants. Multivariate analyses of variance (MANOVA) were run for anthropometric data (i.e. age, stature, body mass, body mass index and lower limb muscle mass) and for absolute values of test performance (i.e. PP, MP and CCIT at 1.05, 3.14 and 5.20 rad/s), and also for power and torque variables that have been adjusted for differences in LLMM (i.e. torque or power/LLMM or torque or power/LLMM$^{b\ \text{exponent}}$), to examine male and female characteristics in the data sets.

Peak power and MP, and CCIT, were expressed allometrically in relation to LLMM by deriving the exact common *b* exponent that described the relationship between PP or MP or CCIT and LLMM, for male and female participants.

Common *b* exponents that described the allometric relationships between CCIT and LLMM, PP and LLMM and MP and LLMM were obtained by running simple linear regression on natural logarithmic-transformed data, with Ln CCIT, Ln PP and Ln MP entered in turn as the dependent variable, and with Ln LLMM entered in all cases as the covariate.

In all cases, the common *b* exponents or slope coefficients (i.e. applicable to male and female participants) were derived only after ensuring that the sex-specific derived *b* exponents were not significantly different (i.e. all Sex*Ln LLMM interactions, $p>0.05$).

Power function ratios (Welsman & Armstrong, 2000) or body-size free variables (e.g. Power/LLMM$^{b\ \text{exponent}}$ or CCIT/LLMM$^{b\ \text{exponent}}$) were subsequently computed. Pearson Product Moment correlations were used to examine the relationships between body size-free variables of CCIT, PP and MP and also to check if allometric modelling of the data appropriately normalised the data for differences in LLMM. The level of statistical significance was set at $p<.05$.

3. Results

3.1. *Normality of distribution and homogeneity of variance of the data sets*

Statistical checks for normality of distribution and homogeneity of variances for PP and MP, and CCIT showed that there was normality of distribution (Shapiro-Wilks statistics, $p>0.05$) and homogeneity of variance (all Levene test statistic, $p>.05$).

3.2. *Anthropometric and descriptive data of male and female participants*

Table 1 is a summary of the anthropometric and descriptive data of the participants. In essence, the data show that there were sex differences for age, stature, body mass, body mass index and muscle mass of the lower limbs. Importantly, there were no sex differences for PP, MP and CCIT, when the performances were expressed allometrically in relation to LLMM.

Table 1: Anthropometric data, peak power, mean power and composite concentric isokinetic torque of men and women

Variable	Male adults (n=18)	Female adults (n=20)
Age (yrs)	21.3±2.4	20.2±2.0*
Stature (m)	1.71±0.05	1.62±0.07*
Body mass (kg)	64.5±5.4	51.3±7.9*
Lower limb muscle mass (kg)	20.1±3.3	12.4±1.7*
Peak power (W)	671±72	468±85*
Mean power (W)	557±59	372±52*
Peak power (W/kg LLMM)	33.7±4.2	37.7±3.3*
Mean power (W/kg LLMM)	27.9±3.5	30.2±2.8*
Peak power (W/kgLLMM$^{0.72}$)	77.6±7.4	72.9±8.4
Mean power (W/kg LLMM$^{0.76}$)	57.2±5.7	55.1±4.8
Composite torque (Nm) at 1.05 rad/s	320±54	191±32*
Composite torque (Nm) at 3.12 rad/s	230±45	131±30*
Composite torque (Nm) at 5.20 rad/s	177±33	110±23*
Composite torque (Nm/kg LLMM) at 1.05 rad/s	16.0±2.5	15.5±1.7
Composite torque (Nm/kg LLMM) at 3.12 rad/s	11.5±2.1	10.6±1.7
Composite torque (Nm/kg LLMM) at 5.20 rad/s	8.9±1.6	8.9±1.3
Composite torque (Nm/kg LLMM$^{0.93}$) at 1.05 rad/s	19.7±3.0	18.4±2.1
Composite torque (Nm/kg LLMM$^{1.18}$) at 3.12 rad/s	6.7±1.3	6.7±1.1
Composite torque (Nm/kg LLMM$^{1.12}$) at 5.20 rad/s	6.2±1.2	6.6±1.0

* Differences significant at $p<.05$. Values are mean±standard deviation. LLLM: lower limb muscle mass.

3.3. *Body size descriptor of choice*

In all cases for PP and MP, CCIT and LLMM, linear regression analyses carried out separately for male and female data confirmed that LLMM was the best significant predictor for the generated power and composite torque. The addition of stature or BM did not make an additional significant contribution (i.e. $p>0.05$) to the regression equation. Correlations between CCIT, PP and MP and LLMM in absolute terms for male adults were $r=0.31\text{-}0.60$ (all $p<0.05$) and $r=0.62\text{-}0.75$ (all $p<0.05$) for female adults.

3.4. *Common b exponents*

The *b* exponents in all cases for CCIT, PP and MP in male and female participants, were not significantly different from each other (i.e. Sex*Ln LLMM, $p>0.05$). Common *b* exponents were therefore used to describe the allometric relationships between CCIT and LLMM, and also PP and LLMM and MP and LLMM, respectively. The specific power function ratios computed for CCIT, PP and MP are shown in Table 1.

3.5. *Checks for appropriate normalization power and composite torque for body size*

There were no significant correlations between power function ratios derived for CCIT, PP and MP, respectively (i.e. PP or MP/LLMM$^{b\ \text{exponent}}$ or CCIT/LLMM$^{b\ \text{exponent}}$) and LLMM (i.e. $r=0.06$ to 0.18, all $p>0.05$). However, significant negative correlations were obtained between ratio-scaled PP and MP (i.e. Power/LLMM) ($r=-0.60$ to -0.62, $p<0.05$) and LLMM, but not for CCIT (i.e. CCIT/LLMM) and LLMM ($r=-0.16$ to 0.09, $p>0.05$). The above results demonstrated that the use of allometric techniques produced power function ratios for power and torque that were free from the effects of body size whereas simple ratio-scaling produced a variable that was still significantly related to LLMM.

3.6. *Torque generated at different angular velocities*

Results of RM-ANOVA revealed significant differences in CCIT generated at 1.05, 3.14 and 5.20 rad/s for female participants (Greenhouse-Geiser, $F=170.0$, $p<0.05$) and for male participants (Greenhouse-Geiser, $F=263.3$, $p<0.05$). In male participants, CCIT at 1.05 rad/s was 1.80 times that of CCIT at 5.20 rad/s and in female participants CCIT at 1.05 rad/s was 1.73 times that of CCIT at 5.20 rad/s (see Table 1).

3.7. *Relationships between power and composite torque*

Figures 1 to 6 depict the relationships between PP and MP and CCIT for pooled data of male and female participants. While the correlations between PP and MP, in watts and CCIT in Newton-metre, were 0.88 or greater, the correlations between PP and MP, and CCIT that were allometrically-scaled to LLMM (see Table 2) ranged between r=0.55 and r=0.65.

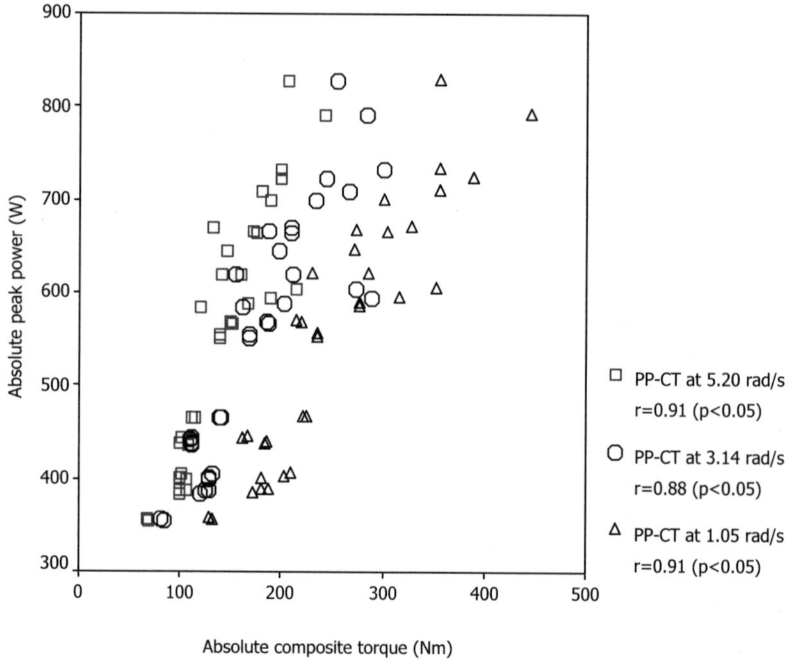

Figure 1: Relationships between peak power and composite torque in male and female adults. PP: peak power and CT: composite torque. (N=34).

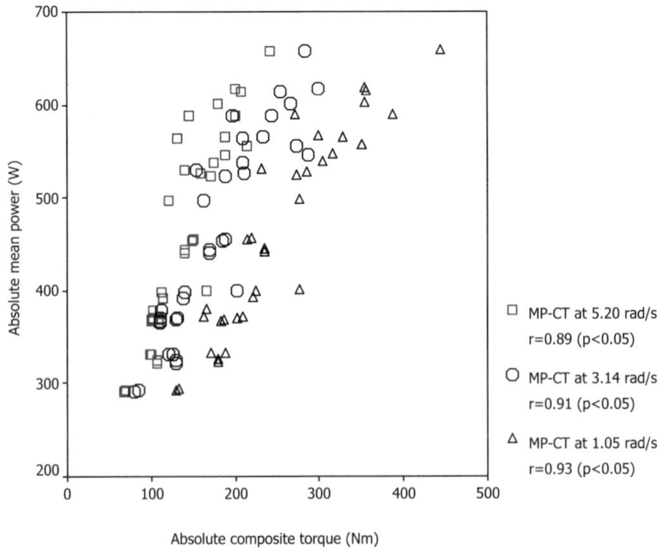

Figure 2: Relationships between mean power and composite torque in male and female adults. MP: mean power and CT: composite torque. (N=34).

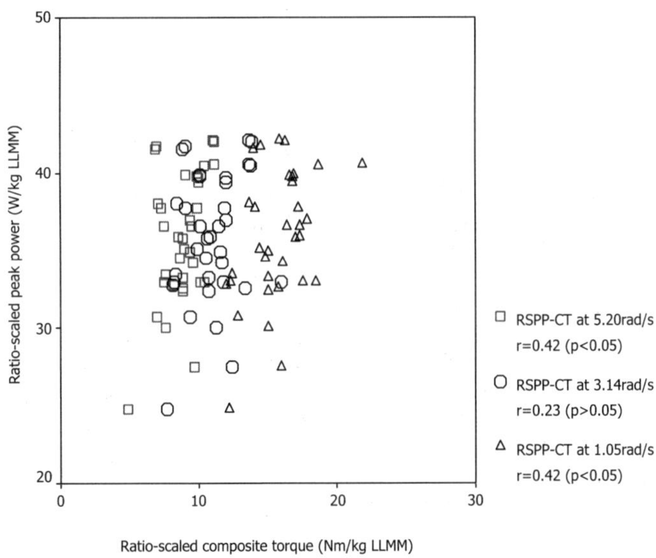

Figure 3: Relationships between ratio-scaled peak power and ratio-scaled composite torque, expressed to lower limb muscle mass in male and female adults. RS: ratio-scaled, PP: peak power, CT: composite torque and LLMM: lower limb muscle mass. (N=34).

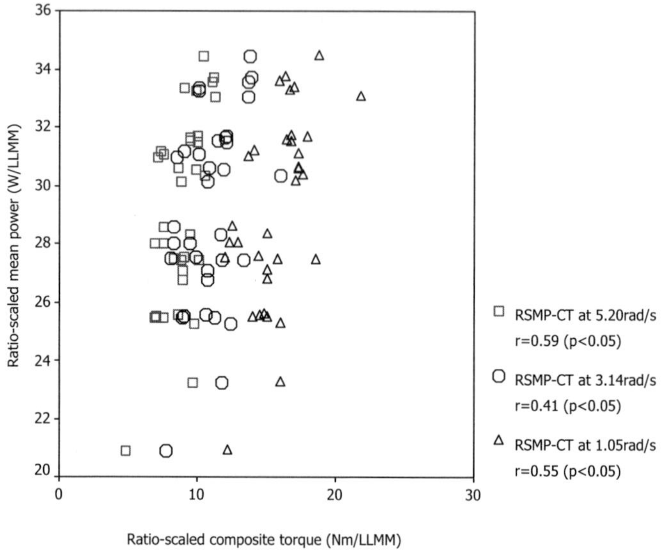

Figure 4: Relationships between mean power and composite torque, ratio-scaled to lower limb muscle mass in male and female adults. RS: ratio-scaled, MP: mean power, CT: composite torque and LLMM: lower limb muscle mass. (N=34).

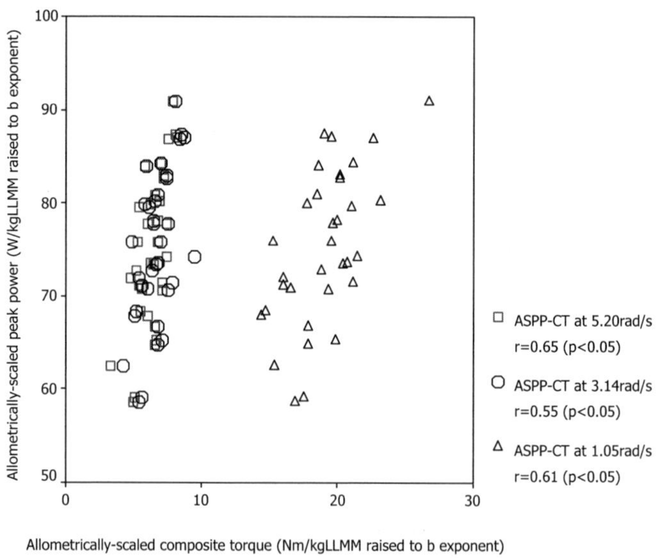

Figure 5: Relationships between peak power and composite torque, allometrically-scaled to lower limb muscle mass in male and female adults. AS: allometrically-scaled, PP: peak power, CT: composite torque and LLMM: lower limb muscle mass. (N=34).

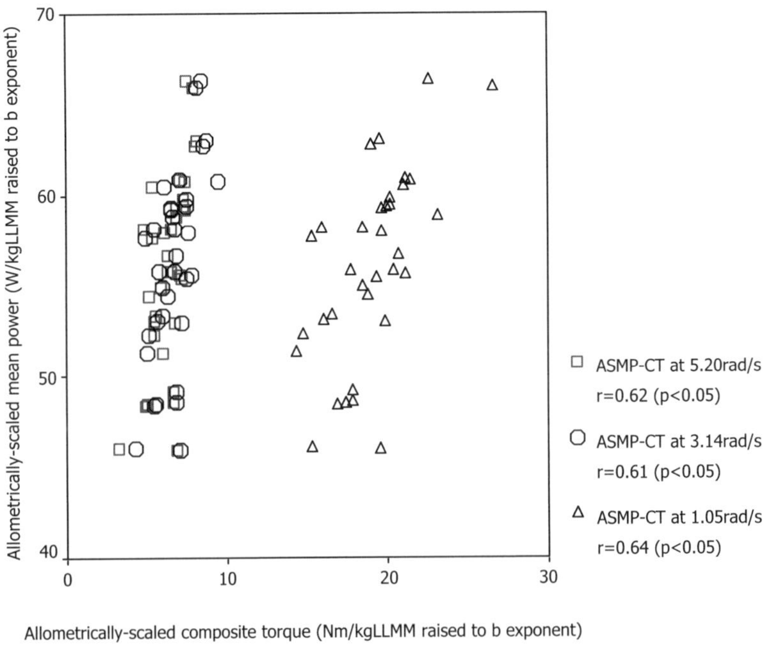

Figure 6: Relationships between mean power and composite torque, allometrically-scaled to lower limb muscle mass in male and female adults. AS: allometrically-scaled, MP: mean power, CT: composite torque and LLMM: lower limb muscle mass. (N=34).

Table 2 shows the correlation matrix for power function ratios for PP and MP and CCIT, segregated by sex. Correlations were higher for female adults than for male adults, between PP and MP, and CCIT at 3.14 rad/s and 5.20 rad/s. However, the correlations between PP and MP, and CCIT, allometrically-scaled to LLMM, were higher at 5.20 rad/s than at 1.04 rad/s for female participants but not for the male participants.

Table 2: Correlation matrix for body size-free torque and power for male and female adults. (N=34).

Power function ratio	Torque at 1.05 rad/s (Nm/kg LLMM$^{0.93}$)	Torque at 3.14 rad/s (Nm/kg LLMM$^{1.18}$)	Torque at 5.20 rad/s (Nm/kg LLMM$^{1.12}$)
Peak power (W/kg LLMM$^{0.72}$)	0.66* [0.53*]	0.54* [0.74*]	0.64* [0.84*]
Mean power (W/kg LLMM$^{0.76}$)	0.64* [0.62*]	0.50* [0.72*]	0.55* [0.81*]

Correlations within brackets [] refer to female data.
* Correlation (2-tailed) significant at p<0.05.

4. Discussion

4.1. *Anthropometric characteristics*

The participant characteristics in terms of stature, BM and BMI are in agreement with that of the National Health Survey conducted in Singapore (NHS, 1998). However, the percentage of LLMM to BM in male participants (i.e. 31 %) and in female participants (i.e. 24 %) appears to be less than those reported elsewhere (Murphy & Wilson, 1997). This difference could be attributed to differences in body built and composition between Asian and Western populations.

4.2. *Body size descriptor of choice*

A key finding of the present study was that for CCIT, PP and MP, LLMM was confirmed as the best predictor for power and composite torque performance in male and female adults, albeit the correlations between CCIT, PP and MP, and LLMM were higher in female than in male participants (i.e. r=0.64-0.75 vs. r=0.31-0.60, all p<.05). This is in agreement with data reported by Chia (2003) where LLMM was the best predictor for PP and MP, albeit in a paediatric population of 48 boys and 38 girls aged 14-15 years old. Buttressing the present results, Mameletzi et al, (2003) reported significant pooled correlations of r=0.77-0.89 for 31 male and 22 female competitive swimmers, aged 10-12 years old for peak isokinetic knee extension and flexion torque at 1.05, 2.01 and 3.14 rad/s and lean body mass (LBM). The present results supported the view that in BM-supported exercise, the use of LLMM, rather than BM or stature, as the body size descriptor of choice for normalization purposes has merit, but the ultimate decision should be based on informed decision that is confirmed by statistical analysis (Chia, 2003), as was the case in the present study.

This proposal is corroborated by Jaric (2002) who argued that although BM is most frequently used as the body size descriptor of choice, it may not be as effective as bone-free lean tissue mass (Davies & Dalsky, 1997) or bone-free lean leg mass (Neder et al, 1999) when adjusting strength for body size. Despite these compelling evidence, the use of total body mass in scaling for body mass-supported exercise such as sprint cycling and rowing continue to be frequently reported (Chia, 2003).

4.3. *Ratio standard versus allometric scaling*

Another significant finding was that ratio scaling for PP and MP in relation to LLMM did not adequately account for differences in LLMM. The use of ratio standards to normalize exercise data in relation to body size assumed that the *b* exponent that described, in a given study, the relationships between PP and LLMM and MP and LLMM, was equal to 1.0.

For the present data set, the use of ratio standards in expressing PP and MP in relation to LLMM still resulted in significant negative relationships between PP/LLMM and LLMM and MP/LLMM and LMMM. This demonstrated that the use of the ratio standard 'over-scaled' the power data (Welsman & Armstrong, 2000). The practical implication of this tendency to 'over-scale' is to penalize participants with greater LLMM whilst advantaging participants with lower LLMM, a situation to be avoided if valid comparisons in performances are to be made.

The fallacy of using ratio standards indiscriminately to scale exercise data is reported by Welsman and Armstrong (2000) where the use of ratio standards in normalizing peak V02 data in relation to BM for 106 boys and 106 girls, still remained size-dependent with negative slope coefficients of –0.35 and –0.39 in boys and girls respectively. Allometric modeling of CCIT, PP and MP in relation to LLMM on the other hand, produced variables for power and composite torque that were free from the effect of LLMM. Correlations between CCIT/LLMM$^{0.93,\ 1.18\ \&\ 1.12}$, PP/LLLMM$^{0.72}$ and MP/LLMM$^{0.76}$, and LLMM were non-significant. This, according to Welsman and Armstrong (2000) confirmed that allometric modeling of the data, most appropriately normalized CCIT, PP and MP for differences in LLMM.

4.4. *Common b exponents for PP, MP and CCIT*

In the present study, the common *b* exponents identified for CCIT, PP and MP in relation to LLMM, using allometric scaling, were *b*=0.93, 1.18 and 1.12, *b*=0.72 and *b*=0.76 respectively. In essence the results showed that for CCIT at 3.14 and 5.20 rad/s, CCIT increased faster than the increase in LLMM for both sexes. The present result compares with sex-specific *b* exponents (i.e. *b*=0.91 for 34 males and *b*=1.10 for 37 females) for concentric knee extension peak torque at 1.05 rad/s that was expressed in relation to bone-free lean leg mass (Neder et al, 1999). In the cited study, separate *b* exponents were derived, rather than a common *b* exponent, because the separate slope coefficients for male and female participants were significantly different from each other.

In another study, Batterham and Birch (1996) allometrically scaled PP derived from a 30-second WAnT in relation to fat-free mass (FFM) that was anthropometrically determined from skinfold calculations in a group of 12 males and 12 females, aged 18-24 years. The identified common *b* exponent between PP and FFM was reported as 1.5. However, it should be noted that in the latter study, total body FFM was used as the body size descriptor rather than LLMM, even though sprint cycling involves predominantly muscles of the lower limbs (Too, 1990).

Peak power and MP in males and females in the present study, did not increase in exact proportion to an increase in LLMM. It is of interest that Chia (2003) reported common *b* exponents of 0.65 for PP and 0.79 for MP, in relation to LLMM in a group of 48 boys and 38 girls, aged 14-15 years. Juxtaposing the results of the present study and that of Chia (2003), it appears that for both adolescents and adults, PP and MP increased in tandem with LLMM but not by the same magnitude.

As in the present and previous studies that have employed allometric modeling, the principle of its use is based on 'geometric similarity' of the participants tested- that is participants are similar in shape and body composition (Jaric, 2002). In the present study of male and female adults where the mean age was 22.5 years and where the body size descriptor of choice was LLMM and not body mass, where differences in body composition might be an influencing factor (Jaric, 2002), the participants in the present study were less likely to be 'geometrically dissimilar'.

According to geometric similarity theory and assuming complete compliance with the assumptions for the use of allometric scaling, power should scaled to body size descriptor$^{0.67}$ and torque should scale to body size descriptor$^{1.0}$ (Jaric, 2002). Results of the present study showed that common *b* exponents identified for CCIT, PP and MP expressed in relation to LLMM were in general agreement with those, which are predicted from geometric similarity theory. Nonetheless, the way forward is to derive the exact *b* exponents for each specific data set, rather than to use a fixed predicted *b* exponent to normalize exercise data (2002). Although it has been advocated (Chia, 2003; Welsman & Armstrong, 2000), researchers should be cautioned against using fixed predicted *b* exponents since there are limitations in using allometric scaling because human beings do not always meet the criteria of geometric similarity- that is there are systematic differences in the body shape and body composition of males and females, athletes and non-athletes or in the quality of muscle during growth, maturation and aging (Jaric, 2002). These factors can affect the identified *b* exponents.

4.5. *Correlations between computed power function ratios for PP and MP, and CCIT*

The present study was apparently the first to examine the relationships between computed power function ratios for PP and MP, and CCIT. Data for female participants showed that the significant correlations between PP and MP, and CCIT increased with an increase in angular velocity while the situation for male participants was less certain. Female participants also showed higher correlations between PP and MP, and CCIT than male participants. As higher values of isokinetic torque are usually obtained at the slower angular velocities (Brown, 2000) it is important for researchers to consider testing CCIT at higher angular velocities when correlating with sprint cycling performance (e.g. PP and MP).

In a review paper, Jaric (2002) suggested that no study had considered the role of body size in both muscle and movement performance tests. Correlations between muscle strength and movement performance reported in the literature are confounded by the effects of body size, thereby obscuring the true relationships. Barring that, in the majority of studies, authors have reported relatively high correlations (i.e. $r>0.60$, $p<.05$) between isokinetic torque and power, expressed in absolute terms and derived from cycle ergometry (1). Data from the present study showed that significant correlations between PP and MP, and CCIT, allometrically-scaled to LLMM, ranged between 0.55 and 0.65. With a shared variance of 30-42 % between PP, MP and CCIT, where the variables were independent of the effect of LLMM, trainers and coaches should be mindful of the expected potential gains when using an isokinetic training model to improve power performances in sprint cycling, and vice versa. Future studies should consider appropriately creating body size-free measures of strength and power before correlating them so that the true relationship between CCIT, PP and MP can be elucidated in various populations.

5. Conclusion

The present study focused on exercise performances, namely CCIT, PP and MP generated by untrained male and female adults. Performance data were normalized for differences in body size using ratio standards and allometric modeling. Among the body size descriptors, LLMM emerged as the best predictor for composite torque and power. Results showed that the use of ratio standards did not appropriately account for differences in LLMM for PP and MP, and that allometric modeling of CCIT, PP and MP data, more appropriately accounted for the characteristics of the data sets. Common *b* exponents derived for CCIT, PP and MP expressed in relation to LLMM, were close to those predicted from geometric similarity theory but sample-specific allometric modeling of data is recommended to derive the exact *b* exponents. Significant correlations were obtained between CCIT and PP and MP that were independent of LLMM, in male and female adults.

References

1. Baltzopoulos, V., Eston, R.G. & Maclaren, D. (1988). A comparison of power outputs on the Wingate test and a test using isokinetic device. *Ergonomics, 3,* 1693-1699.
2. Barfield, J.P., Sells, P.D., Rowe, D.A. et al. (2002). Practice effect of the Wingate Anaerobic Test. *Journal of Strength and Conditioning Research, 16,* 472-473.
3. Batterham, A.M. & Birch, K.M. (1996). Allometry of anaerobic performance: a gender comparison. *Canadian Journal of Applied Physiology, 21,* 45-62.
4. Bohannon, R.W. & Smith, M.B. (1985). Intra-session reliability of angle-specific knee extension torque measurements with gravity corrections. *Journal of Orthopedics and Sports Physiotherapy, 11*, 155-157.
5. Boltz, S. & Davies, G.J. (1984). Leg length differences and correlation with total leg strength. *Journal of Orthopedics and Sports Physiotherapy, 8,* 484-488.
6. Brown, L. (2000). *Isokinetics in Human Performance* (pp. 20). Human Kinetics, Champaign, IL.
7. Chia, M, & Aziz, R. (2008). Modelling maximal oxygen uptake to body size in trained adult athletes: ratio versus allometric scaling. *Annals Academy of Medicine Singapore*, *37,* 300-306.

8. Chia, Y.H.M. (2003). Wingate Anaerobic Test power of boys and girls expressed in relation to lower limb muscle mass as determined using dual energy x-ray absorptiometry. *Advances in Exercise and Sports Physiology, 9,* 55-59.
9. Davies, G.J., Heiderscheit, B. & Brinks, K. (2000). Test Interpretation In: *Isokinetics in Human Performance.* (pp 3-24). L.E. Brown (Ed). Champaign: Human Kinetics.
10. Davies, M.J. & Dalsky, G.P. (1997). Normalising strength for body size differences in older adults. *Medicine and. Science in Sports and Exercise, 29,* 713-717.
11. De Ste Croix, M.B.A., Armstrong, N. & Welsman, J.R. (1999). Concentric isokinetic leg strength in pre-teen, teenage and adult males and females. *Biology of Sport, 16,* 75-86.
12. Feiring, D.C., Ellenbecker, T.S. & Dersheid, G.L. (1990). Test-retest reliability of the Biodex isokinetic dynamometer. *Journal of Orthopedics and Sports Physiotherapy, 8,* 480-483.
13. Hakkinen, K. (1991). Force production characteristics of leg extensor, trunk flexor and extensor muscles in male and female basketball players. *Journal of Sports Medicine and Physical Fitness, 31,* 325-331.
14. Heymsfiled, S.B., Smith, R., Aulet, M. et al. (1990). Appendicular skeletal mass: measurement by dual-photon absorptiometry. *American Journal of Clinical Nutrition, 52,* 214-218.
15. Inbar, O., Bar-Or, O. & Skinner, J.S. (1996). *The Wingate Anaerobic Test.* Champaign: Human Kinetics.
16. Jaric, S. (2002). Muscle strength testing: use of normalization for body size. *Sports Medicine, 32,* 615-631.
17. Jensen, M.D., Kanaley, J.A., Roust, L.R. et al. (1993). Assessment of body composition with use of dual-energy x-ray absorptiometry: evaluation and comparison with other methods. *Mayo Clinical Proceedings, 68,* 867-873.
18. Kelly, T., Shepherd, J., Steger, P. et al. (1997). Accurate body composition assessment using fan-beam DXA: technical and practical considerations. *Journal of Bone Mineral Research, 12,* s269.
19. Liebermann, D.G., Maitland, M.E. & Katz, L. (2002). Lower-limb extension power: how well does it predict short distance speed skating performance? *Isokinetic. Exercise Science, 10,* 87-95.
20. Magnusson, S.P., Constantantini, N.W., McHugh, M.P. et al. (1995). Strength profiles and performance in masters' level swimmers *American Journal of Sports Medicine, 23,* 626-631.
21. Mameletzi, D., Siatras, T., Tsalis, T. et al. (2003). The relationship between lean body mass and isokinetic peak torque of knee extensors and flexors in young male and female swimmers. *Isokinetics Exercise Science, 11,* 159-163.

22. Murphy, M.M., Patton, J.F. & Frederick, F.A. (1984). A comparison of anaerobic power capacity in males and females accounting for differences in thigh volume, body weight and lean body mass. *Medicine and Science in Sports and Exercise, 16,* 108.
23. Murphy, A.J. & Wilson, G.J. (1997). The ability of tests of muscular function to reflect training induced changes in performance. *Journal of Sports Science, 15,* 191-200.
24. *National Health Survey.* Ministry of Health. Singapore. 1998.
25. Neder, J.A., Nery, L.E., Silva, A.C. et al. (1999). Maximal aerobic power and leg muscle mass and strength related to age in non-athletic males and females. *European Journal of Applied Physiology, 79,* 522-530.
26. Sleivert, C.G., Backhus, R.D. & Wenger, H.A. (1995). Neuromuscular differences between volleyball players, middle distance runners and untrained controls. *International Journal of Sports Medicine, 16,* 390-398.
27. Tsaklis, P. (2002). Isokinetic evaluation of the knee extensors and flexors anaerobic capacity. *Isokinetic Exercise Science, 10,* 69-72.
28. Too, D. (1990). Biomechanics of cycling and factors affecting performance. *Sports Medicine, 5,* 268-302.
29. Vanderburg, P.M., Mahar, M.T. & Chou, C.H. (1995). Allometric scaling of grip strength by body mass in college-age men and women. *Research Quarterly in Exercise and Sport, 66,* 80-84.
30. Welsman, J.R. & Armstrong, N. (2000). Scaling performance for differences in body size. In: *Paediatric Exercise and Sport Medicine* (pp. 7-23). N. Armstrong & W.V. Mechlen (Eds) London: Oxford University Press.
31. Wilklander, J. & Lysholm, J. (1987). Simple tests for surveying muscle strength and muscle stiffness in sportsmen. *International Journal of Sports Medicine, 8,* 50-54.

THE DEVELOPMENT OF SPORT BIOMECHANICS IN TAIWAN

TZYY-YUANG SHIANG

Graduate Institute of Exercise and Sports Science, National Taiwan Normal University, Taiwan

As more people become involved in sport, it is essential that both athletes and coaches make use of biomechanics to further sport performance and also to keep sport injury at bay. In Taiwan, sports biomechanics plays an important role in athlete preparation for major international competitions. The chapter provides an overview of how biomechanics is used in variety of sports.

1. Introduction

To achieve the Olympic goal of "faster, higher, stronger", athletes must move their bodies in the most accurate, efficient and safest ways. By utilizing scientific methods, sport biomechanics can make people understand each movement of the human body, and then modify the ways of movement, improve performance and prevent sports injuries. Sport biomechanics is a science that combines biology and mechanics. The main objective of sport biomechanics is, in the active aspect, to enhance sport performance and, in the passive aspect, to prevent injury. Why do we need sport biomechanics and technical analysis? Many people consider that body movement is produced naturally. In fact, each part of the human body that is involved in movement follows the principles of mechanics and physiology to produce movement. Physical education teachers, coaches, and athletes may know how to perform a specific movement but may not know how to explain the movement in scientific terms. This gap may impede further improvement in sport competition and cause otherwise excellent athletes to stagnate. More seriously, the gap in knowledge may cause sport injury. Thus, it is essential for the coaches, athletes, PE teachers and sport science researchers to better understand sport biomechanics and what it can offer.

Human movement is getting scientists' attention in recent years. At the beginning, kinesiology represented the science of human movement. In kinesiology, the human body is regarded as a machine where the performance of a movement could be discussed. The theoretical basis of kinesiology includes issues of movement science, anatomy and engineering. As research of human movement continues to expand, the principles of mechanics are also expanded. Other compound nouns other than kinesiology such as, biodynamics and anthropomechanics, among others were used to describe the study of human movement but none of these terms were used extensively until the emergence of biomechanics. Scientists consider biomechanics as most appropriate in describing the study of human movement, the term biomechanics is then used to represent the biology-related mechanics.

There are two major international societies involving the study of biomechanics with different focii. The International Society of Biomechanics (ISB) is the first international society that focused research in biomechanics in more general terms. The International Society of Biomechanics in Sports (ISBS) is the other international society that focuses on one specific area- sports biomechanics. Nowadays, biomechanics is a well established scientific discipline which is intertwined with research in other fields such as medicine, physiology, neuroscience, physics, mathematics and engineering. Biomechanics research encompasses a very wide scope of issues: animation, anthropometry, biofluid dynamics, bioheat transfer, biomaterials & medical devices, bone structure/remodeling, cardiovascular biomechanics, cell mechanics/engineering, clinical biomechanics, dental biomechanics, ergonomics, gait and locomotion, hearing mechanics, human movement, injury biomechanics, joint mechanics, medical vision and optometry, microcirculation, microelectromechanical systems, modeling techniques, molecular biomechanics, muscle mechanics, neuromuscular mechanics, orthopaedics, rehabilitation, respiratory biomechanics, spine biomechanics, tissue mechanics/engineering, sports biomechanics and sports equipment design.

Sports biomechanics on the other hand, is an indispensable division of biomechanics. In the early days, sports biomechanics was mainly focused on sports competition and physical education, where the research scope was primarily movement analysis. Movement analysis started with animal and human gait analysis, then simple locomotion analysis such as walking, running and jumping. Finally, complex sport technique was also analyzed with the primary purpose of enhancing sport performance and reducing sport injury during training and competition. Another objective in the use of sport biomechanics research is also to make physical education more effective. Due to the wide scope of applications, sports biomechanics evolved more research fields that primarily covers the internal part of human body (musculoskeletal biomechanics), performance of human body (movement analysis) as well as the external part of human body (sport equipment design). In order to know the internal reasons of a good or bad movement, sports biomechanics research started to further probe into the function of musculoskeletal system. Scientists combined sports biomechanics with the sports medicine such as rehabilitation and orthopedics with the intent of better understanding how the biomechanics principles of the internal body affect movement. As technology keeps progressing and is applied to sport training and competitions as well as affecting human movement, sports biomechanics has also evolved into research of sports equipment design and analysis. Figure 1 provides a schematic representation of the major research branches of sports biomechanics.

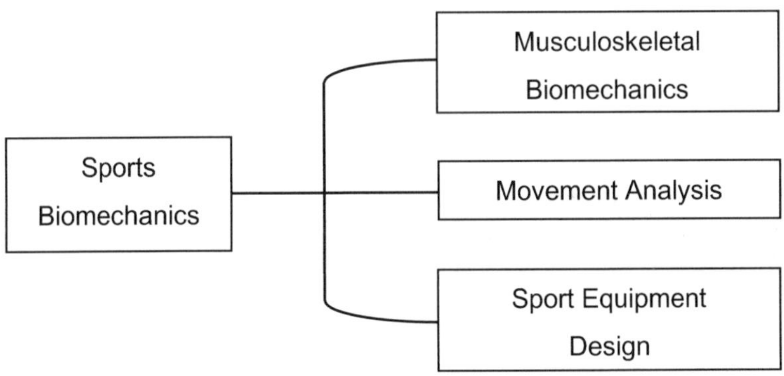

Figure 1: The major research areas in sports biomechanics

Research methodology in sports biomechanics also progressed when new advanced instrumentation was developed. Two-dimensional quantitative analysis was used in biomechanics when the 16mm video camera was developed. Then various two-dimensional and three-dimensional quantitative analyses were developed and applied to movement analysis. In 1960s, James Hay brought up the idea of using the tree diagram to demonstrate factor analysis of movement production, and founded the relation of mechanics equations between movement factors and so emerged the qualitative analysis model in sports biomechanics. Soon afterwards, many active and passive automated capture analysis systems joined the line of analysis and greatly increased the accuracy and speed. These advances allowed for the analysis of more sports techniques and more complex movement. In addition to the progress of movement analysis methods, the development of sensor made detecting body signals possible and led to the study of statics and kinetics. By using sensors from load cell-to-force plate, the force signals from different parts of the human body can be detected. Electromyography or EMG can sense muscle activity while goniometer, accelerometer, pressure sensors and other detectors can detect different analog signals from the human body. All these signals can be used with movement analysis simultaneously to provide greater research scope in sport biomechanics. The rapid progress of computer technology allowed for computer simulations to be used in biomechanics. These required faster computation speeds when analyzing complex structures and nonlinear properties of human movement.

2. Future research directions in sports biomechanics

The advancement of computer technology enhanced the width and depth of the study of sports biomechanics with more complex movement, more microcosmic changes, more precise analysis and more prompt feedback made possible. It is likely that in the future, the study of sports biomechanics will involve the following:

1. Far more accurate and complex computer simulation
2. More prompt information feedback analysis
3. More sensors with expanded applications being used
4. More multidisciplinary approaches
5. Greater collaborations with the sports industry.

3. Sports biomechanics in practice in Taiwan

The rest of the chapter provides a brief description on how sports biomechanics was used to enhance athlete performance in Taiwan. Recently, the National Training Center in Taiwan extensively used the real time video feedback system and the motion analysis system in the provision of sports science support. For example, during the training period for the 2008 Olympics Qualification Tournament, the pitching coach of the Taiwan Women's Softball Team actually used the real time video feedback system in the training field to garner data on the pitchers' squat angle and pitching timing. Pitching images are filmed using a digital video and transmitted through a 1394 interface to a laptop with the image replay software and connected to a big TV screen right by the field (as shown in

Figure 1). The coach and the team members can watch the pitching action immediately after each pitch on the big screen. Such a system has helped the coach to explain the pitching shortcomings as well as helped the pitchers to correct their pitching actions.

Sports biomechanists used the real time video feedback system to analyse movement and collect useful data in martial arts like karate for the 2006 Asian Games in Doha, in shooting, in weightlifting and during baton-changing in track relay training prior to the 2004 Athens Olympic Games and also in the Asian Games.

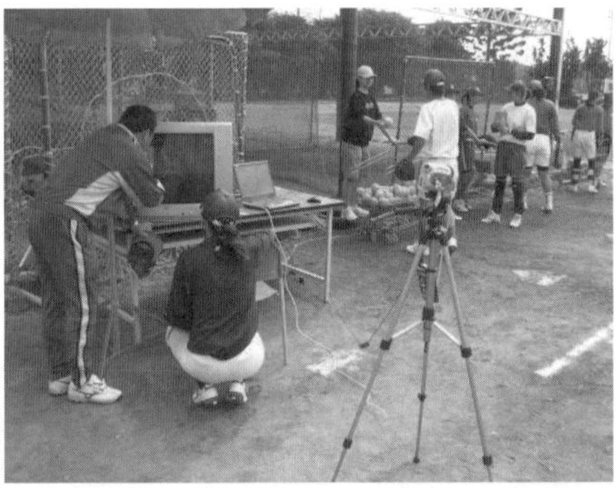

Figure 1: Use of the real time motion feedback system during training

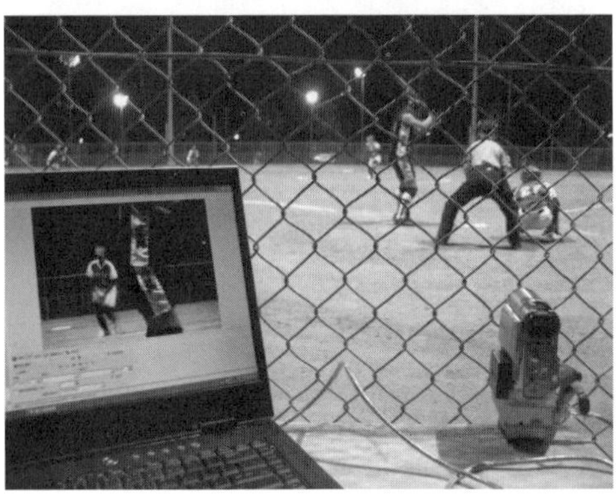

Figure 2: Qualitative analysis used in pitching

Besides video analysis, force signals are often used to analyze sport performances.

For example, a tensionmeter can be used to measure the pulling force for tug-of-war athletes or the paddling force of rowers in a canoe ergometer (as shown in Figure 3) (Shiang and Tsai, 1998). Such a device can also be applied in strength training to collect the ground reaction force (as shown in Figure 4).

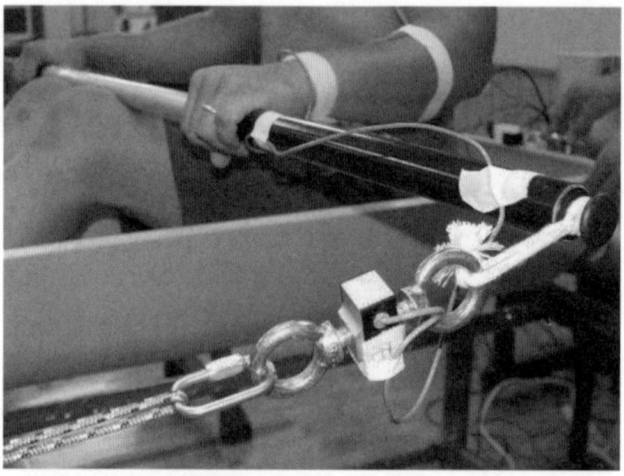

Figure 3: Use of a tensionmeter in a canoe ergometer

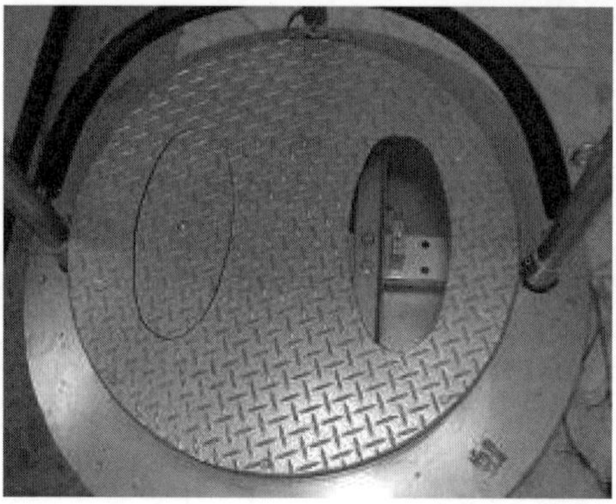

Figure 4: Use of a load cell in a strength training machine

Another major mission of the sports biomechanists in Taiwan is to develop new and effective strength training methods for the Taiwan National Sports Teams (as shown in Figure 5). Passive training involves stimulating the muscle groups of athletes passively in order to achieve a better training result. The theory base for this training is the stretch shortening cycle or SSC. Being driven by motors, the training platform allows muscles to stretch and contract rapidly in a passive way. It is reported that when muscles are stimulated to contract continuously at a constant velocity, a better training outcome is possible (Chen, et al., 2002). Such a technique has been applied during training to national athletes of track & field, taekwondo, baseball, basketball, canoe, soccer, women's softball and rowing.

Another training method is to give muscle belly or tendons some vibration stimulation so as to make the muscles contract involuntarily and to induce a vibration training effect of the tonic vibration reflex, TVR. Such whole body vibration training is proven to be effective for sports performance (Delecluse et al, 2003, Chen, et al., 2004). Therefore, the whole body vibration training would possibly be widely used in sports training in the future.

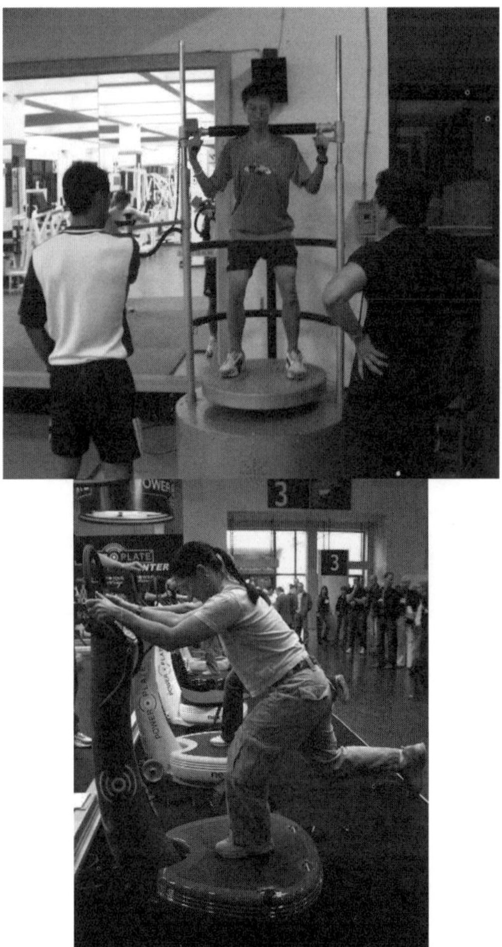

Figure 5: Strength training- using passive and whole body vibration training approaches

Sport scientists also analyzed the EMG data of the Taiwan Archery Team for the 2004 Athens Olympics investigate the muscle groups used during archery for force exertion; to describe the force-exertion pattern; to compare the differences in muscle exertion patterns between fast and slow release, and to monitor the level of muscle fatigue. Results of the analysis showed that the archers' major working muscle is the trapezius muscle, the synergistic muscle is the deltoid, and the major working muscle upon releasing is extensor digitorum. These findings were used to strengthen the athletes' weaker muscle groups (Hung, et al., 2009). The experimental set up is shown in Figure 6.

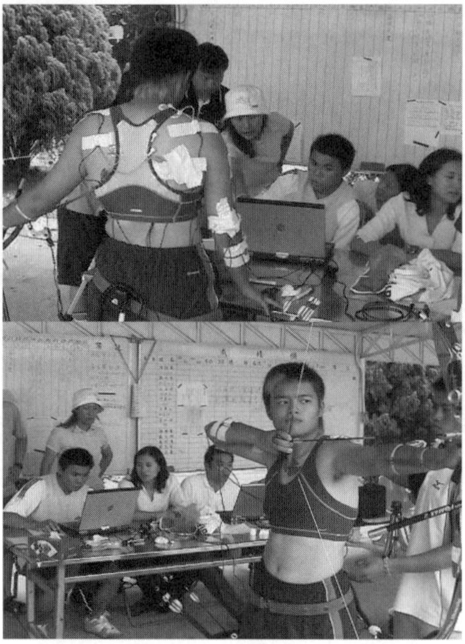

Figure 6: EMG analysis of the 2004 Athens Olympics archery team during training

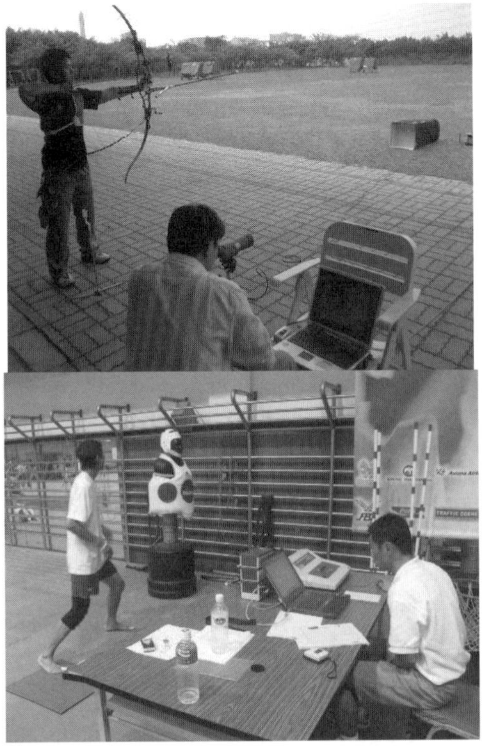

Figure 7: Taiwanese athletes had great successes with the assistance of biomechanics

Sports such as archery, taekwondo and table tennis are the potential medal-winning events for Taiwan in future Olympic Games. Biomechanics is playing a decisive role in helping these sports advance even further. Sports biomechanics continues to be of great service to the archers in analyzing the execution of the center of mass during archery shooting and the EMG efficiency of the muscle group when drawing the bow. Sports biomechanics is also helping the taekwondo athletes to gather useful data about the reaction time and help with lower-body training (as shown in Figure 7) (Shiang and Chou, 1998). It is also used in table tennis to collect information about competitors' action of serving, and the strategy of their first three strokes of the match. Sports biomechanics is science in practice and in Taiwan it plays an important role in heightening sports performance

References

1. Chen, C.S., Shiang, T. Y. and Liu, C. (2002). Research and development of a new muscular strength and power training machine: Passive Repeatedly Plyometric training machine. *The Book of the 4th International Conference on the Engineering of Sport* 2002/09/02-06, Kyoto, Japan, pp 140-143.
2. Chen, W. C. and Shiang, T. Y. (2004). Design of an upper arm isometric contraction platform with different vibration stimuli. *The Engineering of Sport, 5* Vol 1, pp 155-160.
3. Delecluse, C., Roelants, M. & Verschueren, S. (2003). Strength increase after whole-body vibration compared with resistance training. *Medicine and Science in Sports and Exercise, 35*(6), 1033-41.
4. Hay, J. G. (1978). *The Biomechanics of Sports Techniques,* Prentice Hall.
5. Hung, T. M., Tang, W. T. and Shiang, T. Y. (2009). A case study of integrated sport sciences for an Olympic archer. *Journal of Medical and Biological Engineering*, 29(4): 164-171.
6. Shiang, T. Y. and Tsai, C. B. (1998). The kinetic characteristics of rowing movement. *The Engineering of Sport,5,* 219-224.
7. Shiang, T. Y. and Chou, K.M. (1998). The quantitative measurement of Taekwondo movement". *The Engineering of Sport, 3,*481-486.

A MISUNDERSTOOD MUSCLE PROBLEM IN ATHLETES

JOSEPH LIN

Physical Medicine and Treatment Center, Gaithersburg, Maryland U.S.A

CHANG-ZERN HONG

Department of Physical Medicine and Rehabilitation University of California-Irvine, Irvine, California, U.S.A

JAMES RUSSELL

National Institute of Child Health and Human Development, National Institutes of Health, Bethesda, Maryland, U.S.A.

Myofascial pain is extremely common in athletes. It is a clinical syndrome caused by myofascial trigger points (MTrPs). MTrP is a highly localized and hyper-irritable spot in a palpable taut band of skeletal muscle fibre and/or its associated fascia. MTrP is usually caused by or associated with neuromuscular injuries, and can be perpetuated or aggravated by some medical conditions (perpetuating factors). There are certain characteristics of a MTrP; localized spot, tenderness, taut band, referred pain, local twitch response, reduced joint range of motion, symptoms waxed and waned, muscle weakness but without atrophy, and autonomic phenomena. Anybody can have MTrP and any one of the 696 skeletal muscles in the body can have MTrp. MTrPs might not exist in early life, but develop in later life due to soft tissue injuries. MTrP is more likely located at the site of dysfunctional endplates. The pathogenesis of MTrPs is probably related to an integrative mechanism in the spinal cord in response to sensitized sensory nerve fibers (nociceptors) associated with dysfunctional endplates.

1. Introduction

In 1922, the Nobel committee awarded Archibald Vivian Hill "for his discovery relating to the production of heat in the muscle," and Otto Meyerhof "for his discovery of the fixed relationship between the consumption of oxygen and the metabolism of lactic acid in the muscle." Exactly 85 years ago today, on December 12, 1923, Archibald Hill delivered his Nobel prize lecture, "The mechanism of muscular contraction," and Otto Meyerhof delivered his speech "Energy conversions in muscle." Much progress has been made over the past 85 years in the field of muscular science. But in this chapter, I have nothing esoteric about muscles to propound to you. Instead, I am going to share with you an extremely common but frequently overlooked, misunderstood, and often neglected muscle problem.

2. A case of chronic myofascial pain

One day, several years ago, I went to a tennis tournament. Sitting next to me was a young man who did not seem to be able to sit still; he was either stretching his right elbow or rubbing his right forearm or shaking his right hand. So I asked him if he was ok. He said his right arm hurt. I asked him what had happened.

He told me that he was a semi-professional tennis player. One day several years ago, he first felt some pain on the outside of his right elbow when he was playing tennis. It got worse as the game progressed. Eventually, the elbow turned red and became swollen. It also felt hot. He stopped playing for a few days but it got worse. So, he went to his family doctor. The doctor told him that he had tennis elbow, most likely from over-using the elbow extensors, and had developed tendinitis. The doctor told him to rest, put ice on the elbow, use a brace, keep his right arm elevated, and the doctor prescribed non-steroidal anti-inflammatory medications and a muscle relaxant. He felt better, but when he returned to playing tennis, the problems recurred. The doctor then sent him to see an orthopedic surgeon. The surgeon told him that he had lateral epichondylitis and gave him a shot of cortisone. He felt better, but he still had pain in his forearm, wrist and hand. His forearm muscles also felt tight. So, he went back to his doctor.

The doctor sent him to have X-rays and an ultrasound. The X-rays showed bone spurs in the lateral epicondyle, and the ultrasound showed hypertrophy in the wrist extensor tendon. The doctor suggested surgery to repair the damage. So, he had elbow surgery. He felt pretty good after the surgery, but when he returned to the tennis court, he felt pain in the elbow, forearm, wrist and hand and his forearm muscles felt tight after only a few strokes. In addition, he felt numbness and weakness in the forearm and hand. So, he was sent to a neurosurgeon.

The neurosurgeon sent him for a neck MRI and ran some nerve tests. He told the man that he had two problems. First of all, he had a herniated disc between the 5th and the 6th cervical spines that compressed on the 6th cervical nerve root. Second, his radial nerve was entrapped by the supinator muscle at the elbow. Both problems could give rise to the symptoms in his arm, forearm and hand. The neurosurgeon suggested an operation to free the 6th cervical nerve root, and another surgery to relieve the radial nerve at the forearm under the supinator muscle. He was afraid to be cut in the neck, so he went to physical therapy to have cervical traction, but he had another elbow surgery to free his radial nerve at the elbow. He felt pretty good for about 2 months after the surgery, and then all the problems returned after just one game of tennis. He had pain in the elbow, forearm, wrist and hand; muscle tightness in the forearm; muscle twitch in the forearm; muscle weakness; reduced elbow mobility; and sensitive skin. The symptoms waxed and waned. He was very disappointed and very depressed. A doctor suggested that he should go see a psychiatrist. Instead, he went to Hawaii for a few weeks. Unfortunately, his symptoms remained.

One of his friends suggested that he should have acupuncture treatments, so he went to an acupuncturist. The acupuncturist told him that he had a "Qi" problem and treated him with acupuncture and Chinese herbs. His symptoms persisted, and now he had some new holes in his body. So there he was, sitting on the sideline watching other people playing and feeling sorry for himself.

"That's really terrible and I am very sorry to hear that," I said to him.

"Well, that's life I guess," he said.

"Do you mind if I take a look at your elbow?" I asked him.

"Do you have the same problem?" he asked me.

"No, I don't," I said.

"Are you a doctor?" he asked me.

"Yes, I am," I said to him, "and I take care of those players down there playing right now."

So we went to the dressing room to check his elbow. Other than the healed scars, everything looked and felt fine to me; there was no redness, swelling, joint instability, neurological deficit, or muscle atrophy. He had full range of motion in his shoulder, elbow, and wrist except that he had apparent weakness in his wrist extensors and supinator. When I pressed on his lateral epicondyle, he felt no pain at all. But, when I pressed on certain spots on his extensor carpi radialis longus, extensor carpi radialis brevis, brachioradialis, supinator, and even the distal triceps, he screamed and nearly peed in his pants. He had excruciating pain not only where I pushed, but also at the lateral epichondyle, his wrist and his hand, with some feelings of numbness. In addition, I also found several tender spots in his neck and upper back that also sent pain down his shoulders.

"That's exactly the kind of pain I have for the past few years. How did you reproduce that?" he said, looking amazed.

"Tell me," I asked him, "what would make your pain worse?"

"Playing tennis and turning a door knob," he said.

"What other conditions would make it worse?" I asked him.

He paused for a moment and said, "I feel terrible when the weather is cold or when the air conditioning is on; when I am sick or when I didn't sleep well or got upset."

"I thought so," I said to him.

"What's wrong with me? One doctor told me that I needed to see I psychiatrist, but I know I am not crazy."

"You are not crazy, but you have something called Myofascial Pain Syndrome (MPS)," I told the man.

"What's that?"

"Myofascial Pain Syndrome is a painful condition caused by Myofascial Trigger Points (MTrPs)."

3. Understanding Myofascial Trigger Points (MTrPs)

"What is a myofascial trigger point?"

"A myofascial trigger point is a highly localized and hyper-irritable spot in a palpable taut band of skeletal muscle fibers. Sort of like a tight knot in your muscles. The MTrPs in your muscles are responsible for your problems. Your muscles are laughing at you now!"

"Are you joking?"

"No," I said to him, "I am dead serious."

"But, they told me that I have problems in my elbow," he said.

"You did, but you don't have those problems now."

"Why does my elbow still hurt then?"

"It was referred pain from your wrist extensor muscles and supinator in the forearm," I said.

One recent study by Jay Shah and his co-workers (2008) at NIH, using microdialysis technique (immunocapillary electrophoresis and capillary electrochromatography), found that muscles with myofascial trigger points have higher level of bradykinin, serotonin, norepinephrine, substance P, calcitonin gene-related peptide(CGRP), tumor necrosis factor alpha(TNF-α),IL-1β, IL-6, and IL-8 levels. All these substances are pain sensitizing agents.

"Is this a new discovery?" he asked.

"No," I said to him. "The concept of myofascial pain is not new. If we look at the literature, way back in 1930s, we find terms such as muscular rheumatism, non-articular rheumatism, rheumatic myalgia, myalgia, myalgic spots, idiopathic myalgia, myofasciitis, muscular sciatica, fibrositis, interstitial myofibrositis, etc. All these terms mean the same thing. In 1940, Steindler used "myofascial" to describe the painful areas in muscles of the low back. In 1948, Rinzler and Travell used "myofascial" to describe the source of pain in pectoral muscles. In 1952, Travell and Rinzler described the most common patterns of pain referred from individual muscles.

Dr. Travell was considered "The Mother of MYOFASCIAL - TRIGGER POINT Knowledge." In 1955 she was called upon by the orthopedic surgeon for then-Senator John F. Kennedy, who had failed to recover from major back surgeries related to injuries he suffered in World War II. Dr. Travell was able to locate muscular sources for his chronic pain, and injected low-level procaine directly into the Senator's low back muscles to ease the pain. President Kennedy said that without Dr. Travell, his political career would end prematurely.

4. What causes Myofascial Trigger Points?

MTrPs are usually caused by or associated with neuromuscular injuries, and can be perpetuated or aggravated by some medical conditions (perpetuating factors). Following an injury, there is an increase in intracellular calcium. If uncontrolled muscle contraction occurs, such as with a defective neuromuscular junction, it may lead to an increase in metabolism; impaired circulation, oxygen, and nutrient; causing an energy crisis and perhaps lead to taut band formation. Taut band is a necessary precursor to the development of MTrPs (Simons, 1996) — based on the fact that taut bands commonly exist in pain-free individuals (Wolfe, 1992). People who are more prone to develop taut bands are also more likely to develop MTrPs (Pellegrino, Wayloins & Sommer, 1989).

5. Characteristics of Myofascial Trigger Points

Two important characteristics of MTrPs include Local Twitch Response (LTR) and referred pain. When a high pressure stimulation, such as needling, to the sensitive tiny locus (nociceptor) in an MTrP region, a sudden contraction of a small group of muscle fibers, LTR, can be elicited via spinal reflexes (Hong & Torigore, 1994; Hong, 1994; Hong & Simons, 1998). LTRs should be elicited during MTrP injection in order to obtain an immediate and complete pain relief. This is similar to the "De-Qi" effect during acupuncture therapy.

MTrPs are usually found in the endplate region based on the fact that endplate noise (EPN) can be recorded by needle electromyographic (EMG) examination on the MTrP region. The typical endplate potentials have a high frequency (10-12 Hz) repetitive spikes (endplate spikes – propagated action potentials), a continuous high frequency noise with low voltage (<100μV), and the EPN (non-propagated potentials) (Hong & Torigore, 1994). The pattern of endplate potentials in MTrP was thought to be due to excessive release of acetytcholine packets. The more active the MTrP, the easier it is to produce the twitch response. Superficial MTrP is more likely to produce twitch responses than deeper ones (Hong, 1994).

6. What is referred pain?

The referred pain phenomenon was probably first described in 1936, when Edeiken and Wolferth noticed many of their patients who had experienced a heart attack complained of persistent pain in the shoulder region following their heart attacks. In 1938, Kellgren reported many of his patients experienced remote pain from the injured area. In 1949, Kellgren injected 6 % hypertonic saline to many major muscles (including his own). He noticed pain often appeared in a remote portion of the same limb, even several spinal segments away from the site of injection. So, the pain was not transmitted by the peripheral nerves directly. The more active the MTrP, the less pressure is needed to produce referred pain. A very active MTrP may not need any pressure at all to produce referred pain.

7. Who gets MTrP?

Anybody can get it, and any one of the 696 skeletal muscles in the body can have MTrP. Sola AE and co-workers did a study in 1955 regarding MTrP in posterior shoulder muscles in asymptomatic college students. They found that 54 % of females and 45 % of males had MTrP (Sola, Rodenberger & Gettys, 1955).

Poor posture, direct physical trauma, over exertion, etc., can cause MTrPs. We all know that muscles are doing all the work and are extremely subject to wear and tear during physical activities. But physicians, for some reason, pay much more attention to tendons, ligaments, bones, joints, bursae and nerves. Perhaps it is because there is not a single diagnostic test that can detect MTrP; it is diagnosed solely by hands alone. The pathogenesis of MTrPs is probably related to an integrative mechanism in the spinal cord in response to sensitized sensory nerve fibers (nociceptors) associated with dysfunctional endplates (Simons, 1996; Hong, 1996). MTrPs can be active or latent. An active MTrP will cause pain spontaneously, while a latent MTrP produces pain only under physical pressure such as pressing on it.

"How do you get rid of the knots in my muscles?" the man asked me.

"Cut them loose! I think," I said to him.

"More surgery?" the man looked worried.

"No," I said to him, "fortunately, something simpler than that. MTrPs may be managed by medication(s), physical therapy, and injection therapy among other means. The most important thing is to treat the cause(s) and not just symptoms."

"Can you help me?" the man asked.

I told him what I was thinking and he agreed to give it a try.

He came to my office the following week. I brought out a 5cc syringe filled with 1 % Xylocaine and proceed to inject all the trigger points that I had found. I then sprayed some ethyl chloride vapor coolant to his radial forearm and elbow, followed with a moist heating pack and physical therapy, and sent him home with some instructions. He returned a week later, pain free.

"It's a miracle! I feel normal and I can play *my* backhand without any pain. How did you do that?" he asked me.

"Oh, it's an ancient Chinese secret!" I said to him.

Some frequently asked questions are: When can I go back to train? How hard, how long, and how often can I train? What kind of therapeutic exercises can I do?

The answer is "Case by case."

The general principles are to avoid heavy, rapid and prolonged exercises.

8. How do we know if someone has MTrPs?

There are certain characteristics in a MTrP (Hong & Simons, 1998).

1. First of all, it is localized and can be pointed out with one finger.
2. Another characteristic of a MTrP is tenderness. When you grab on a MTrP, the person will let you know that you have found one. For the very active TP, even pushing on the edge of the MTrP could produce intense pain.
3. MTrPs are only found in the taut band. The taut band felt like a rope!
4. Referred pain - It is a kind of pain that started in one place but can be felt somewhere else. Unlike radiating pain from a pinched nerve root, which produces neurological symptoms along the pathway of the nerve root, the referred pain produced by a trigger point does not follow any specific nerve root, but rather the specific PATTERN of that particular MTrP!

5. Local twitch response (LTR) - A local muscle contraction! Snapping or needling of a MTrP can elicit a local muscle contraction. The more active the MTrP, the easier it is to elicit a twitch response. Superficial MTrPs are more likely to produce twitch responses than deeper ones. In a local twitch response, it feels like you caught a fish. LTRs can be recorded from an EMG examination (Hong & Torigore, 1994).
6. Another characteristics of MTrP is reduced ROM because of the taut band (s).
7. The symptoms caused by MTrPs wax and wane. The intensity of the pain produced by any MTrP may be changeable and not constant. This may be because the factors that activate the pain mechanism in the central nervous system change in different environments and conditions.
8. Muscle weakness without atrophy. Because the pain caused by MTrP is not constant, therefore, the general physical activity is maintained.
9. Autonomic phenomena - When a MTrP is active, it may activate the autonomic nervous system and cause changes in endocrine functions, such as vasodilatation or vasoconstriction, diaphoresis or sweating, edema or dermagraphia. Some active MTrPs may lead to Reflex Sympathetic Dystrophy (RSD) with shiny and pale skin, sweating, intense pain, and osteoporosis. Of course, not all MTrPs would lead to RSD, as some RSD is a purely neuropathic phenomenon.

9. How to prevent MPS and MTrPs?

Prevention of MPS and MTrPs require a holistic approach. It involves biomechanics, coaching, exercise physiology, nutrition, psychology and practically all fields of medicine and science. In our lab at NIH, we are looking into the relationship between MTrP and Neuromuscular Junction (NMJ). NMJ is the junction of the axon terminal of a motoneuron with the motor end plate, the highly-excitable region of muscle fiber plasma membrane responsible for initiation of action potentials across the muscle's surface, ultimately causing the muscle to contract.

One of the objectives of our research is to understand the precise nature of neural activity-dependent glial cell signals and the consequence of such signals to nervous system function (Weerth, Holtzclaw & Russell, 2007). The glial cell is the "glue" of the nervous system. Glial cells modulate neurotransmission, surround neurons and hold them in place. They insulate one neuron from another, supply nutrients and oxygen to neurons, destroy pathogens, and remove dead neurons. The work involves the use of neural tissue and intact mice to record activity-dependent glial cell Ca2+ signals in Schwann cells – a type of glial cell, during normal function and pathological states. Schwann cells signaling occurs in the form of propagated Ca2+ waves that spread over long distances or in highly localized discrete microdomains.

Improvement in technology allows us to develop transgenic mice that express a genetically encoded fluorescent Ca2+ indicator protein in many tissues, which is very useful in studying NMJ (Livet et al., 2007). We have developed mice that express the genetically encoded fluorescent Ca2+ indicator protein discretely in glial cells. Our long-term goal is to understand the nature of the communication between neurons and glial cells in peripheral nervous systems and its role in MTrP formation.

References

1. Edeiken, J. & Wolferth, C.C. (1936). Persistent pain in the shoulder region following myocardial infarction. *American Journal of Medicine, 191*, 201
2. Hong, C-Z. & Simons, D.G. (1998). Pathophysiologic and electrophysiologic mechanisms of myofascial trigger points. *Archives of Physical Medicine and Rehabilitation, 79*, 863-872
3. Hong, C-Z. & Torigore, Y. (1994). Electrophysiologic characteristics of localized twitch responses in responsive bands of rabbit skeletal muscle fibers. *Journal of Musculoskeletal Pain, 2*(2), 17-43.
4. Hong, C-Z. (1996). Pathophysiology of myofascial trigger point. *Journal Formosa Medical Association, 95*, 93-104.
5. Hong, C-Z. (1994). Persistence of local twitch response with loss of conduction to and from the spinal cord. *Archives of Physical Medicine and Rehabilitation, 75,* 12-16.
6. Kellgren, J.H. (1938). A preliminary account of referred pains arising from muscles. *British Medical Journal, 1,*325-327.
7. Kellgren, J.H. (1949). Deep pain sensibility. *Lancet, 1*, 943-949.
8. Livet, J., Weissman, T.A., Kang, H., et al. (2007). Transgenic strategies for combinatorial expression of fluorescent proteins in the nervous system. *Nature, 450*, 56-62.
9. Pellegrino, M.J., Wayloins, G.W. & Sommer, A. (1989). Familiar occurrence of primary fibromyalgia. *Archives of Physical Medicine and Rehabilitation 70,* 61-63.
10. Shah, J.P., Danoff, J.V., Desai, M.J. et al (2008). Biochemicals associated with pain and inflammation are elevated in sites near to and remote from active myofascial trigger points. *Archives of Physical Medicine and Rehabilitation, 89*(1), 16-23.
11. Simons, D.G. (1996). Clinical and etiological update of myofascial pain from trigger points. *Journal of Musculoskeletal Pain, 4*, 93-121

12. Sola, A.E., Rodenberger, M.L. & Gettys, B.B. (1955). Incidence of hypersensitive areas in posterior shoulder muscles. *American Journal of Physical Medicine, 34*, 585-590.
13. Travell, J. & Rinzler, S.H. (1952). The myofascial genesis of pain. *Postgraduate Medicine, 11*(5), 425-34.
14. Weerth, S.H., Holtzclaw, L.A. & Russell, J.T. (2007). Signaling proteins in raft-like microdomains are essential for Ca2+ wave propagation in glial cells. *Cell Calcium 41*,155–167
15. Wolfe, F., Simons, D., Fricton, J., et al. (1992). The fibromyalgia and myofascial pain syndrome. *Journal of Rheumatology, 19,* 944-951.

SPORT
STUDIES

PHILOSOPHY AND LIFE: THE WISDOM OF A SUCCESSFUL LIFE

PETER CHEN

School of Health, Physical Education and Leisure Services,
University of Northern Iowa, U.S.A.

Philosophy can show us the power of creative thinking and effective wisdom. It can provoke us to constant questioning. Effective wisdom can overcome personal and professional problems. Philosophy searches the truth and wisdom is applied moral judgment. The two feed into each other and build on knowledge. Socrates said "True wisdom comes to each of us when we realize how little we understand about life, ourselves, and the world around us." Kant observed, "Science is organized knowledge. Wisdom is organized life." Of course we must acquire knowledge as these great men obviously did. But knowledge is little use without wisdom. Wisdom is to know what is appropriate to do in any situation: in the right time, to the right person, for the right reason, to the right extent. We need to cultivate wisdom. This requires many components including: vision, mission, inspiration, action and contribution. Combined with strong discipline we can generate an intuitive intelligence, a super sense to navigate our way through troubled waters and live a life, which is worthwhile and successful. With knowledge, philosophy and wisdom we can aim for the right goals, do the right things, live contented lives, inspire others and change the world for the better.

1. Introduction

Philosophy is derived from a Greek word, which means the love of wisdom. We are all philosophers to some extent since wisdom is necessary for our well-being and for living a worthwhile and successful life. Paul McLean explains, in his book *Great Western Thinkers* (1987), that philosophy:

"Teaches us how to think (logic), how to recognize beauty (aesthetics), how to conduct ourselves (ethics), how to organize ourselves (politics), and how to confront unknown (metaphysics and epistemology)...After all, philosophy is about life, it is about us."

The Oxford Dictionary (1999) defines philosophy as "the study of the fundamental nature of knowledge, reality, and existence", and wisdom as "the quality of being wise and the body of knowledge and experience that develops within a specified society or period." Philosophy is the way we search for truth, cultivate wisdom and give witness to value throughout our lives. It must be practiced in the context of our own cultures, customs, backgrounds, and personalities. Reinhold Niebuhr famously said in his 'Serenity Prayer': "God grant me the serenity to accept the things I cannot change, courage to change the things I can, and wisdom to know the difference." Life is much like the tides of the sea, coming in and going out. We cannot control the future but we can have the wisdom to know how to respond and to anticipate the consequences of our actions.

In the main, philosophy can accomplish the following:

1. It assists us to open our eyes, minds and hearts.
2. It develops our new vision, new mission and new life.
3. It helps to make a closer link in harmony with the universe.
4. It inspires us to value and appreciate other cultures and people.
5. It helps us to become a better citizen of the world now and future.

2. Wisdom in the successful life

2.1. *Contrasted with knowledge*

Wisdom is 1% instruction and 99% inspiration; 1% information and 99% imagination. Kant observed that: "Science is organized knowledge. Wisdom is organized life." Martin Fischer said: "Knowledge is a process of piling up facts; wisdom lies in their simplification." Einstein stated: "Imagination is more important than knowledge" and "wisdom is not a product of schooling but of the lifelong attempt to acquire it". A serious search for, and practice of, wisdom makes the world a more interesting place as we come to understand its ebbs and flows; to see, hear, feel, think, do and experience new things. It is inspiring and refreshing and it opens up exciting new possibilities that can continue to regenerate our lives.

2.2. *Holistic approach*

There are many roads to wisdom and wisdom has many fathers and mothers. We can continue to learn from the wisdom of great thinkers of the past and the present, from the East to West, from the sciences and the humanities, from music and the arts, from politics to philosophy, and from health to physical education. All are interrelated and connected in the web of life. An interdisciplinary approach and an active curiosity maximize our ability to acquire wisdom and live a successful and worthwhile life.

2.3. *External expression of wisdom*

Wisdom combines knowledge, experience, intuition and one's super senses. It is an attitude and a discipline to do the appropriate thing in every circumstance. It is an intuitive but developed intelligence to respond in the most fitting way to the expected and often unexpected twists and turns of life. It requires humility, action, creativity, contribution, and concern for others and for one's community. At its best it generates vision, mission, inspiration, leadership, and guidance for a consistent and principled lifestyle.

2.4. *Learning from great philosophers*

It is important we learn from great minds from the past and the present. For example, here are six very powerful, practical and useful examples from East and West:

Lau Tzu (570-490 B.C.) the Chinese philosopher stated:

1. "Know the universe as yourself and you can live anywhere in comfort."
2. "The softest thing in the universe freely controls the hardest thing."
3. "Teaching without words."

These statements may help us to think more about the way we approach our teaching and life as a whole.

Buddha (563-483 BC) founder of Buddhism highlighted that:

1. "The Noble Eightfold Path: right view, right aim, right speech, right action, right living, right effort, right mindfulness, and right contemplation."

This is a very good recipe for a good life. It encourages us to be well balanced and to be in harmony with the universe and people.

Confucius (551-479 BC) a Chinese philosopher and educator stressed:

1. "Everything has its beauty but not everyone sees it."
2. "Choose a job you love, and you will not have to work a day in your life."

This reminds us that we should never underestimate anyone's potential (something which is especially important for us as teachers) and to do what we love and love what we do.

Socrates (469-399 B.C.) a most well known Greek philosopher said:

1. "Know yourself."
2. "The unexamined life is not worth living."
3. "I am not an Athenian or a Greek, but a citizen of the world."

These statements remind us of the importance of continued review, reflection and renewal in our lives to improve ourselves.

Plato (427-347 BC) another great Greek philosopher advised educators of the importance of creative and indirect teaching:

> "That their main business was not put into the mind knowledge which was not there before, but to turn the mind's eye towards light so that it might see for itself."

Aristotle (384-322 BC) also a great Greek philosopher gives us a central example of wisdom in action. He said:

> "Anyone could become angry—that is easy. But to be angry with the right person, to the right degree, at the right time, for the right purpose, and in the right way- this is not easy."

These profound messages come down to us through the centuries to guide our lives. If we pay attention to them, we can avoid many mistakes and wrong turns in our quest for a more successful life.

3. Wisdom formulas in action

During 51 years of teaching in between the East and the West, I developed and practiced the following wisdom formulas in action as follows:

1. Last chance is the best chance
2. Never too late and never too early.
3. But, better be early than just on time.
4. Reflect, review and renew constantly.
5. Always give others a second chance.
6. Learn from the best is the best policy.
7. Make priority, take action and start now
8. Take an interdisciplinary approach in life.
9. Value every culture and learn from others.
10. Talk less, sense, feel, think and listen more.
11. Life is an art of beauty, heart and humanity,
12. Always ask questions and follow-up questions.
13. First time is the last time so makes the best of it.
14. Never underestimate others and overestimate self.
15. Learn to like those things are difficult but important.
16. Finding a good support system and network always.
17. Learn from anyone, anytime, anything and anywhere.
18. Learn to be an assistant coach rather than a head coach.

19. Turn negative to positive, change obstacle to opportunity.
20. Everyone is a good friend, even those who have never met.
21. Time doesn't mean anything unless one knows how to use it.
22. Fairness, justice, respect and dignity apply to all life situations.
23. Treat everyone equally regardless of his/her ability or disability.
24. Be aware of one's own strength may become one' own weakness.
25. Easier, quicker, safer and better are the simple policies in teaching.
26. To support, share and inspire others, which will inspire self in return.
27. Living locally but thinking globally or living globally and thinking locally.
28. Live with vision, mission, aspiration, inspiration, action and transformation.
29. Live life with adaptability, creativity, flexibility, responsibility and simplicity.
30. Live with 4 "C" of: communication, consultation, cooperation and contribution.

What are your own wisdom formulas?

4. Conclusion

In many ways, we are all philosophers. With modern technology, we have relatively simple access to learning from others around the world and over time. We live in a global village and we are brothers and sisters. History gives us many examples of people and situations we recognize, offering a close connection with people across cultures and times; showing us our common human spirit. There will be always differences among us but our many similarities are even more important. It is vital that we take an interdisciplinary approach to accelerate and stimulate our learning of new knowledge, technology, experience and wisdom to advance ourselves and to have a worthwhile and successful life.

References

Mclean, P. (1987). *Great Western Thinkers* (pp.1-2). London: Macmillan Publishers.

Pearsall, J. (1999). *Oxford Dictionary* Tenth Edition (pp.1073, 1641). London: Oxford University Press.

THE BODY FROM THE PERSPECTIVE OF THE HISTORICAL PHASE IN SOCIETY

KEIKO MIYAUCHI IKEDA

Faculty of Education, Yamaguchi University, Japan

The body of an individual in the military demonstrated the ultimate vigour exemplified by niku-dan— 'the human bullet' (also known as kamikaze and human being torpedo) that was used in Japan during World War II and exposed the contradiction between a body characteristic of the modern nation-state and that of a democracy in the past century. In view of this contradiction in the politics of various nation states, it was also difficult for the Modern Olympics to bridge this gap in politics to bring about peace. Then, Utopia was directed to the Pre-Modern Ages, and the idea that an inclusive body should be regained naturally was exaggerated among those who studied sport and body theory through this kind of contradiction. After all, the structure of military physical education in the modern nation states separated the body and the mind and provided a subjective element to the mind. It is likely that many countries have a similar military history. When it becomes necessary for us to regain the individual rhythm of our respective bodies, it is important that we consider what is required for the philosophy of the body in the context of implementing the motto of 'live'.

1. Introduction

Our body culture has changed dialectically over the years. In modern times, a rationally- trained body is needed to adjust to the modern army. For this purpose, even our way of walking has been modified. Before the modern era, there was more diversity in people's walking styles, as their walking styles varied with their style of living. For instance, a farmer had his own walking style, as did a fisherman and an aristocrat. However, in recent times, these different styles of walking came to be considered as indicative of an 'uncultivated body'.

Consequently, modern sports flourished in line with this rationalism, and this paralleled the training of individuals to develop a strong body that was required by the modern nation state. The mechanics of modernization consistently motivated us to train our bodies to resemble the bodies of top athletes so that we fit into the world of sports and sporting events such as the Olympics, thereby supporting the notion of the ideal super-modern body. However, on the other hand, the body of an individual in the military demonstrated the ultimate vigour exemplified by *niku-dan*— 'the human bullet' (also known as kamikaze and human being torpedo) that was used in Japan during World War II and exposed the contradiction between a body characteristic of the modern nation-state and that of a democracy in the past century, wherein one's body depended on one's lifestyle. In view of this contradiction in the politics of various nation states, it was also difficult for the Modern Olympics to bridge this gap in politics to bring about peace. Then, Utopia was directed to the Pre-Modern Ages, and the idea that an inclusive body should be regained naturally was exaggerated among those who studied sport and body theory through this kind of contradiction. Anthropological assertion grounded in 'cultural relativism', according to which every ethnic culture is entitled to being respected as a human culture, and criticism such as 'cultural genocide', etc., were included in the arguments on the theory of Modern Sports. Consequently, the idea of differentiation arose; for example, perspectives of 'an Oriental Body', 'multi-culturalism', or 'cultural pluralism' and alternatives like new sports for post-modernism were highlighted against modern competitive sports.

2. Theoretical Concepts

Before explaining the historical context, let me explain the following theoretical concepts below.

1. 'Bodily Democracy', a term used by Henning Eichberg, who states the following:
2. "The body constitutes fundamental conditions of human existence: therefore, the body is the base of our existence as human beings, a central unit in the struggle to identify 'what we are'".
3. A Japanese concept of '*Shin-Shin-Ichijo*' which literally means 'the Unity of the Mind and Body as a monism'
4. Our body is not a physical tool, nor an object as a flesh and
5. We have to avoid viewing our bodies from this perspective.

According to Henning Eichberg's study of the 'body culture-observing practice', the body is related to what is called 'people'. Playing and games, dancing and festivity, competition and fights are fundamental aspects of popular culture. In the movement culture, people develop identities. Thus, he states that people do not exist in themselves nor do they consider themselves, as it is made out by the authorities, an 'imagined community', an 'invented tradition' or even a 'false consciousness'. These points imply that 'the folk' were opposed to the structure of the nation state, because the imagined nation as a concept is nothing but a construct created by the propagandistic actions of some leaders of a political body. Therefore, the body was a central unit in the struggle to identify 'what we are'. We will attempt to understand a special term—namely, 'bodily democracy'—used by Eichberg in the context of this political and historical struggle in European history.[1]

The term 'bodily democracy' is reminiscent of the Japanese philosophical concept of 'the unity of the mind and body'. The unification of the body and mind is traditionally considered to be a monism because, according to Zen's preaching, in the context of the Japanese verb 'ichinyo-suru' (which means 'unify'), to ichinyo-suru the mind and body means to be 'nothing' in one's state of mind, which naturally brings one to the state of being in heaven.[2] However, Japanese history was far removed from the concept of 'bodily democracy'. The kind of physical education prevalent during wartime demonstrated that dualistic dimensions were the accepted ideas with respect to the body and mind, although the fascist leaders tactically emphasized the unity of mind and body despite it being contrary to the teachings of Zen. These leaders merely utilized Zen concepts in their endeavors to control people. The theory of the body at that time was embodied in the notion of totalitarianism in the context of Japanese fascism. The problem lay in the fact that in this case, the mind was considered as a subjective concept, in contrast to Zen's preaching that one should be 'nothing' in one's state of mind. Another widely accepted idea was that God's will was equal to the Emperor's will. This attitude would eventually lead to several tragic turns. The history of bodily democracy as well as that of the possibility of realizing the actual concept of Zen—the unity of the mind and body as a monism—shows how difficult it was to establish the body as a central unit in the struggle to identify 'what we are', free from the social and political context.

Friedrich Wilhelm Nietzsche appears to have taken note of this as well; in fact, this theoretical proposition may have been commonly considered by many philosophers in Europe and Asia. Nietzsche rejected the dualistic dimensions of the body and mind, stating in the chapter titled 'The Despisers of the body' in his *Thus Spoke Zarathustr* that "the body is a great wisdom, a plurality with one sense, a war and a peace, a flock and a shepherd. An instrument of your body is also your small wisdom, my brother, which you call the 'mind'—a little instrument and toy of your great wisdom".[3]

3. Resistance

There are historical instances exemplifying that people were opposed to this process of differentiating the mind and body as dualistic dimensions; consider the following examples.

1. The process of modernization through which the body is converted into a physical object to be perceived
2. The need to focus on the pre-industrial society, namely, the pre-Victorian era of British society
3. The contradiction of military physical education during the struggle to build the nation state

I have dealt with the subject of Britain's pre-Victorian sporting history for almost twenty years. My Ph.D. thesis was on the pre-Victorian British sports journalist Pierce Egan, the son of an Irish immigrant and born in London in 1774 [4]. Just before the Victorian period when modern sports began to flourish, there existed a pre-modern 'sporting' culture which was different from that in the modern era of sports. Egan persisted in preserving the traditional aspects of the sporting world. In this endeavour, he defended and supported popular sports among ordinary people. As a result of this, Egan became the first sports journalist, rendering sport journalism an independent existence. This traditional sporting culture that Egan tried to defend had peculiar characteristics. For example, sporting activities were referred to as 'Corinthian' or even came to have eponymic references based on the names of sporting persons such as 'Paul Pry' and 'Tom and Jerryism', and sportspersons came to be described by adjectives such as 'varmint' and 'swellish'. This shows that there existed an age where sports was esteemed in the state of unification of the body and mind.

Egan also used the rhetoric peculiar to the early nineteenth century radicals in his attempt to defend the old sporting world. The period was marked by a serious clash between the defenders of traditional popular sports and the opposition. The radicals of the late eighteenth century and early nineteenth century actually defended the culture of the 'people' and their rights from the perspective of 'British liberty'. In this case, the word 'people' was used as to distinguish the commoners from the elite or ruling class. The early radicals believed that it was important to understand the culture, customs and manners of the people in order to gain an understanding of human society. Therefore, they defended the culture of the people which encompassed, among other things, the sporting tradition, from the perspective of 'British Liberty'. This defense of popular sports influenced the writings of Pierce Egan, who went on to develop the grounds for this defense in his books. Through this argument, we understand that the sporting world before the Victorian era was linked with the notions of 'what constituted the people' and 'British Liberty'. In this sense, the efforts of the radicals and a pre-Victorian sport journalist to defend people's sports can be deemed, in a way, as part of the origins of bodily democracy.

People who began to be connected with sport journalism in the early nineteenth century were: those who questioned "what are the ordinary people?" or "what is the right of people?" Many of them were radical essayists, journalists and publishers. After investigating the rural culture of the lower class, they noticed the role of popular culture and described the need to defend popular sports, grounded in the theory of their early radical principle of 'British Liberty'. 'British Liberty' was the key concept in defending sports. There is the possibility that Radical essayists, William Cobbett, William Hazlitt, William Hone influenced the sport-journalist, Pierce Egan.

This attempt to defend traditional popular sports was also related to the verbalization of sporting matters as journalism. Starting in the late eighteenth century, with social changes such as urbanization, the need of writing down the characters of traditional popular pastimes increased, as utter extinction loomed, though there were some regional differences in the time and extent of the change. While there was an attempt to preserve them, many popular sports of the lower class were vehemently criticized and attacked for the reason of their savageness, or immorality and the concern for public disorder by the upper middle-class moralists and pious people. In refuting the above criticism, the verbalization of sporting matter was started in radical journalism. Through the refutations, the existence of sports in society was emphasized and their need and virtue were described in order to counter the criticism. The assertion of people's right to their sports, and social significance made up the rhetoric of defending sports. Therefore it may be said that sport journalism itself was the involved with the process of earlier case of 'bodily democracy'.

Thirdly, the notions such as 'fair play', 'courage', 'chivalrous honour', 'devotion' and 'prowess' thought to be peculiar to the sporting world were described as a social code. Although still showing pre-modern taste and far from the modern essence of athletic sports, it was philosophically grounded in the significance of sports. With it, newspaper columns dealing with social and cultural matters increased, including many criminal reports, and mixing pastimes and popular political journalism. In this sense the early sporting press was as if roots of the tabloids. This character was formed in the mixing of traditional popular broadsides, chapbooks and earlier radical popular journalism.[5]

Returning to the Japanese case, there was also some resistance against modern sports. Although this was after the pre-Victorian era when the Emperor's will dictated the militaristic physical education prevalent during World War II, the idea was borrowed from the traditional Zen philosophy; Zen preached sporting ideas similar to pre-Victorian sports in Britain, emphasizing that sports constituted a wholesome activity performed with the combined power of the mind and body. Kurakichi Hirata's theory exemplifies this notion; he stressed 'the posture of the lumbar-region abdominal-training method for the Righteous Centre'. Hirata (1901–1945) was an elite medical doctor, a Second Lieutenant and poet, who stated that military physical education, enables one to paradoxically consider the above statement in the context of bodily democracy. His writings not only describe the Japanese Fascist System but also present a notable aspect based on his scientific knowledge on the Asian anatomy—namely, 'the *topos*' of the Emperor in a personal body mechanism.

Hirata was the author of many books on philosophy, national physical education, military physical education and oriental medicine. Furthermore, he showed a talent for literature, started to write poems energetically, published his own collected works. One of his poems, "'Body': On the blade, there is a butterfly, and the light, the sun blessed." was etched on his tombstone according to Kurakichi's wish by his son after 1993, long after his death at the battle of Okinawa in 1945. Hirata created "the posture of lumbar-region abdominal-training-method for the Righteous Centre", which clearly shows the influence of oriental medical anatomical science. His way of the mixture of western, oriental, traditional folk medicine and the spirit of the age were particularly concerned with the answer to the question how the inheritance of democratic liberal physical education in the Taisho period, during 1912-26 and rising fascism could locate the Emperor of Japan at the core of the world and make him a human God. Japanese traditional martial art had been putting a stress on the lumbar region (loins) and the abdomen, especially the hypogastric region, which has given a special term, *tanden*. Japanese folk medicine also had thought this part as a very significant part of the autonomic nervous system, especially, in respiration. The significance of *tanden* in Hirata's idea was not the exception in this context. He assumed a horizontal line to the *tanden* and, in explaining the proper posture and the proper way of sitting, stressed its position. Another important line ran perpendicular direction from the *tanden* to the brain-stem cross formed by the brain stem and this horizontal line and this cross was called the brain-stem sacred point. It was believed that if the *tanden* as the physically imagined part functioned properly, its work would be transferred to the brain-stem sacred point and proper idea and action were accompanied autonomically. And that it was thought that this process was accomplished as the result of the voluntary expression, and such a phrase corresponded closely to an educational term emphasized as the result of the Taisho liberal education, which had insisted that the learning should be based on internal motivation, because freedom of the expression existed at that time. Such a freedom, however, was no more than "making a complete expressed will through physical body" or "making the unification of physical body and its will" in the statement of the fashion of the Taisho periods, which was accented by the educationalists of the day. This fact formed an ironic connection with the ideology of fascism because what should be transferred and what should be proper had been already prepared in the spirit of the age. Nobody questioned that it was an agency of the hegemony. Therefore what should be transferred to the brain-stem sacred point meant was the directed issue in Japanese fascism. Through this mechanism, the *topos* of the Emperor was confirmed by providing the physical and philosophical place understood for that purpose. That a link should have been drawn between the concept of the *tanden* and loyalty was inevitable. The logic of such a connection can be explained as follows. Physical training, to be conscious of the *tanden,* was conceived of as resulting in voluntary loyalty to the Emperor, freely given. Nowhere was it written that this loyalty arose as a result of physical or ideological coercion. Many people genuinely believed in this and even discovered an aesthetic side to it or that it inspired missionary zeal to give voluntary service to the Emperor in this process. Hirata himself was no exception in this. He advocated the role of the body, especially, the *tanden* in the normal moral and national consciousness, and expressed this theory in his *National Physical Education* [*Kokumin-Taiiku*] published in 1937 and his *Study of Military Physical Education* [*Guntai-Taiiku-no-Kenkyu*] published in 1943 etc., and devoted himself to the God, Emperor and died in the war. It is clear that a critical mistake was committed to giving the Emperor the authority over voluntary service.

For a long time after the war, because of the detestation of that period, and of fascism, imperialism, Hirata's works were neglected because they were thought as deliberate products of militarism and super-nationalism. Recently, however, these works have come to be re-examined and from the point of view of oriental medicine. The elaborate analysis of his writings brought another insight into his physical philosophy. Odd though it may seem, he prized physical education beyond other subjects and advocated the view that if it were treated lightly in education and society, people would be readily kill each other while at the same time becoming decadent:

Thus, the ideal of physical education is to directly and more straightly link the centre of the power of all minds, the brain stem, sincerity and whole heartedness, with the 'Righteous Centre' of the body. Therefore every education has to obey physical education. The education of mathematics should be physical education. The education of Chinese classical literature is also to be physical education. The art of drawing pictures and literature, too.[6]

This fact may appear paradoxical in the case of one whose arguments underlay the total acceptance of fascism by many people. However, while his guilt must not be ignored in that it helped diffuse, what he wrote should also be examined as part of the science of oriental medicine and physical philosophy. On this aspect, there seems to be a room to be explored more. If there were not the parallel drawn between the Emperor and the brain-stem sacred point, he could have been talking about the liberating effect of proper physical training, in the same way as traditional practitioners of oriental medicine and the need of the unification of the mind and body. We can also remember the root of bodily democracy in the efforts of the radicals and Pierce Egan's assertion grounded in the notion of 'British Liberty', where sporting or physical activities served to identify 'what we are'.

Therefore an extrapolation must be responsible for this logical leap. If it is disregarded and his analysis was viewed more simply, some of this logical confusion may disappear. Probably the tragedy should be attributed to the fact that "the *topos*" of the Emperor had been located physically and philosophically in a personal-body-mechanism in a Japanese body by Hirata. The mechanism of the physical intervening which he stressed from the view of the psycho-somatics should have been used as far as possible in our striving after peace.

When we consider the military perspective in contemporary times, we recall the Michael Hardt and Antonio Negri's expression—'*bodyless* from the military point of view'—in their *Multitude: War and Democracy in the Age of Empire* (2004). They provide the following description:

Increasingly, U.S. leaders seem to believe that the vast superiority of its firepower, the sophistication of its technology, and the precision of its weapons allow the U.S. military to attack its enemies from a safe distance in a precise and definitive way, surgically removing them like so many cancerous tumors from the global social body, with minimal side effects. War thus becomes virtual from the technological point of view and bodyless from the military point of view; the bodies of U.S. soldiers are kept free of risk, the enemy combatants are killed efficiently and invisibly.

The suicide bomber is the dark opposite, the gory doppelgänger of the safe bodyless soldier. Just when the body seemed to have disappeared from the battlefield with the no-soldiers-lost policy of the high-technology military strategy, it comes back in all its gruesome, tragic reality.[7]

The above description asserts that the bodyless ultimately leads to violence. This idea is similar to Hirata's concept of the training method for the righteous centre of our body, as expressed in the following:

Without the usual training for the righteous centre of our body and devoting yourselves to this purpose, you will not only kill many other people because of owing to your many idle thoughts and much hesitation but you will never enter Nirvana after dying.[8]

4. Conclusion

The structure of military physical education in the modern nation states separated the body and the mind and provided a subjective element to the mind. Even if athleticism, which embodied the idealistic ethic of team spirit as an educational concept in sports, is given an important place in the British Empire, it could not liberate the ideals of British Imperialism such as courage, honour, masculinity, loyalty, and voluntary deeds or self-sacrifice for the British Empire. Marching soldiers aimed at the ultimate amateurism, and they respected the motto of 'fair play'. This ethos justified their courage in falling to bullets.

From '*Pax Romana*' to peace for a civil society, equivalent to bodily democracy:

1. Peace for a community equals peace within a community, which justifies the need for trained physiques among the members.
2. Peace in the modern nation state implies peace at the community level.

3. Therefore, members of the communities train their physiques to promote peace, suggesting that military physical education should be provided in the nation state.
4. In establishing a civil society, individuals should train their bodies based on bodily democracy to bring about peace: a sense of solidarity should be formed collectively with all individuals' bodies, which are autonomically independent as dictated by monism.

It is likely that many countries have a similar military history. Despite this, the mechanics of the media and technologies that were newly developed and supported by globalization served to reintroduce the body into a homogeneous and synonymous world. Under these circumstances, both the young generation and coetaneous adults, irrespective of race and nationality, acquired uniform bodily practices reinforced by the use of the Internet. When it becomes necessary for us to regain the individual rhythm of our respective bodies, it is important that we consider what is required for the philosophy of the body in the context of implementing the motto of 'live'. *Pax Romana*, which originally meant 'peace for a community', has meant 'peace within a community'. This shift to peace in a civil society equivalent to bodily democracy is suggestive. The promotion of peace within a community has justified the need for trained physiques among the members of a community. Peace in a modern nation state effectively implies peace in a community or some communities. A sense of solidarity should be formed through the collective effort of each individual's autonomically independent body, as observed in the historical phase of the body.

Notes

1. Henning Eichberg, "The study of body culture-observing practice" In: *Ido, Ruch dla Kultury/Movement for Culture, Rzeszów* (Poland), 6: 194–200, 2005. cf. Keynote lecture by Henning Eichberg, 8th ISHPES Seminar, 24–27 August 2006, in Ljubljana, Slovenia: "Sport, Nation, Nationalism".
2. Keiko Miyauchi Ikeda, "The Body and Grass-roots Fascism during World War II: 'the topos' of the Emperor in a personal-body-mechanism in Japan", *International Journal of Eastern Sports & Physical Education*, vol.4 no.1, (October 2006), p.97.
3. Friedrich Wilhelm Nietzsche, I- 4 "The Despisers of the body", *Thus Spoke Zarathustr,* written in 1883 and 1885, based on the Thomas Common Translation. MacMillan Company in 1916, printed in Great Britain by The Darwien Press of Edinburgh.

4. DNB's description says that he was born in 1772, but this study accepts J. C. Reid's date. *The Dictionary of National Biography (DNB) Founded in 1882, by George Smith Edited by Sir Leslie Stephen and Sir Sidney Lee, from the Earliest Times to 1900*, vol. IV, published since 1917, the Oxford University Press, pp.560-562; J. C. Reid, *Buck's and Bruisers: Pierce Egan and Regency England*, London, 1971, pp.4-5.
5. Keiko Ikeda, "Pierce Egan's Argument in Defence of Boxing", *Japanese Journal of the History of Physical Education*, vol.11, 1994, pp.1-14. [Japanese]; Keiko Ikeda, *Pre-Victorian Sport: Pierce Egan's "Sporting World"*, Tokyo: Fumaido. Publishing Co., 1996. [Japanese]; Keiko Ikeda, "Traditional Sporting Fancy Made for Modern Sports Ethics: 'Corinthian', 'Paul Pry' and 'Tom & Jerryism'.", G. Pfister ed., *Games of the Past-Sports for the future?: Globalisation, Diversification, Transformation, (ISHPES STUDIES* vol.9), Sankt Augusitn, Academia Verlag, 2004, pp.134-138; Keiko Ikeda, "Sport and Radicals in Pre-Victorian Society of Britain", K.Szikora & G. Pfister eds., *Sport and Politics, ISHPES STUDIES*, vol.9, Semmelweis University Faculty of Physical Education and Sport Science, Budapest, (2002), pp.290-294; Keiko Ikeda, "A Political Analysis of the Historical Development of Sports Writing in Britain from the Early Radicals to the New Left.", in: *International Journal of Eastern Sports & Physical Education*, vol.4 no.1, (October 2006), pp.201-209.
6. Kurakichi Hirata, *Kokumin Taiiku* [*The National Physical Education,* Japanese], Tokyo, 1937, pp.254-255; Keiko Ikeda & Fumie Tsujii, "Ikiru-karada-saiko [Reconsidering 'living body' beyond 'the Culture of Consent'", in: Ikuo Abe, Rie Yamada & Hiroaki Sakakibara eds. *Tayo-na-Shintai-heno-Mezame* [*Awakening for the Multifarious Body: the learning from the history of the discipline of Physical Body,* Japanese], IOM Inc.: Tokyo, 2006, pp.111-112; Ikeda, "The Body and Grass-roots Fascism", pp.91-100.
7. Michael Hardt and Antonio Negri, *Multitude: war and democracy in the Age of Empire,* New York, 2004, pp.44-45.
8. Hirata, *Kokumin Taiiku,* pp.254-255.

References

1. Eichberg, Henning (2005). The study of body culture-observing practice. *Ido, Ruch dla Kultury/Movement for Culture, Rzeszów* (Poland), 6: 194–200.
2. Eichberg, Henning (2006). Keynote lecture. 8th ISHPES Seminar, 24–27 August, in Ljubljana, Slovenia.
3. Ikeda, Keiko (1994). Pierce Egan's Argument in Defence of Boxing. *Japanese Journal of the History of Physical Education*, vol.11, 1-14 [Japanese].

4. Ikeda, Keiko (1996). *Pre-Victorian Sport: Pierce Egan's "Sporting World"*. Tokyo: Fumaido. Publishing Co. [Japanese].
5. Ikeda, Keiko (2002). Sport and Radicals in Pre-Victorian Society of Britain. K.Szikora & G. Pfister eds., *Sport and Politics, ISHPES STUDIES*, vol.9, Semmelweis University Faculty of Physical Education and Sport Science, Budapest, 290-294.
6. Ikeda, Keiko (2004). Traditional Sporting Fancy Made for Modern Sports Ethics: 'Corinthian', 'Paul Pry' and 'Tom & Jerryism'. Pfister, G. ed., *Games of the Past-Sports for the future?: Globalisation, Diversification, Transformation,* (*ISHPES STUDIES* vol.9), Sankt Augusitn, Academia Verlag, 134-138.
7. Ikeda, Keiko (2006). The Body and Grass-roots Fascism during World War II: 'the topos' of the Emperor in a personal-body-mechanism in Japan. *International Journal of Eastern Sports & Physical Education*, vol.4 no.1, 91-103.
8. Ikeda, Keiko (2006). A Political Analysis of the Historical Development of Sports Writing in Britain from the Early Radicals to the New Left. *International Journal of Eastern Sports & Physical Education*, vol.4 no.1, 201-209.
9. Ikeda, Keiko & Tsujii, Fumie (2006), Ikiru-karada-saiko [Reconsidering 'living body' beyond 'the Culture of Consent'. Abe, I., Yamada, R. & Sakakibara, H. eds. *Tayo-na-Shintai-heno-Mezame* [*Awakening for the Multifarious Body: the learning from the history of the discipline of Physical Body,* Japanese], IOM Inc.: Tokyo, pp.93-120.
10. Hardt, Michael & Negri, Antonio (2004) *Multitude: war and democracy in the Age of Empire.* New York.
11. Hirata, Kurakichi (1937). *Kokumin Taiiku* [*The National Physical Education,* Japanese]. Tokyo.
12. Nietzsche, Friedrich Wilhelm (1883 and 1885). I- 4 The Despisers of the body, *Thus Spoke Zarathustr* (based on the Thomas Common Translation in 1916). MacMillan Company in printed in Great Britain by The Darwien Press of Edinburgh.
13. Reid, J. C. (1971). *Buck's and Bruisers: Pierce Egan and Regency England.* London.
14. Smith, George, edited by Sir Stephen, Leslie & Sir Lee, Sidney (1917). *The Dictionary of National Biography* (DNB) *Founded in 1882 from the Earliest Times to 1900.* vol. IV, the Oxford University Press, 560-562.

PERCEPTIONS OF PARENTAL AUTONOMY SUPPORT AND CONTROL, AND ASPIRATIONS OF STUDENT ATHLETES IN SINGAPORE

EUGENE CHEW

Physical Education and Sports Science, National Institute of Education, Nanyang Technological University, Singapore

JOHN WANG

Physical Education and Sports Science, National Institute of Education, Nanyang Technological University, Singapore

Parents are significant others who exert strong influence on young adolescents. This study explores and examines the relationships between perceived parenting dimensions and various psychological-social variables; vis-à-vis basic psychological needs satisfaction, sport motivation, self-perceptions, and life aspirations of student athletes in Singapore. Two hundred and five student athletes (111 males and 94 females) aged 14 to 20 years old responded to the questionnaires. No gender differences were found. Both mother's and father's perceived parenting dimensions of involvement, autonomy support, and warmth correlated highly to student athletes' satisfaction of basic psychological needs of relatedness, autonomy and competency. Comparison of these parenting dimensions showed that mother's involvement and warmth were perceived to be higher than those of the father's. Cluster analysis yielded three distinct groups with characteristic perceived parenting dimensions and psychological needs satisfaction. In comparison, Cluster 1 (labeled Cluster A-A) has average scores for parenting dimensions and psychological needs satisfaction for both parents. Cluster 2 (labeled Cluster L-L) has low scores while cluster 3 (labeled as Cluster H-H) has high scores for both sets of variables. The results from the analyses of the effect of the three clusters on the key variables showed that student athletes with high perceived parental involvement, autonomy support and warmth and reported that their basic psychological needs are highly met, when compared to the other two clusters, had significantly higher autonomous motivation, higher self-perceptions, and rated the importance of, and the likelihood of achieving, intrinsic aspirations higher. These findings are in congruence with the self-determination theory and supports previous studies' findings that involved and autonomy-supportive parenting is linked to higher intrinsic aspirations.

1. Introduction

Youths today live in a world that is vastly different from the world that most of their parents experienced when they were young. Some sociologists view that the changes brought about by globalization are not restricted to economics alone, but are seen in the sphere of politics, culture and personal life (Giddens, 2006). Together with technological advancements, youths today are open to a wider social environment.

The advent of the internet and all its associated technological devices such as email (e.g., Gmail, Yahoo, Hotmail), voice-over-internet-protocol (e.g., Skype), blogs, and social networking community (e.g., Facebook, Friendster) enable effortless communication with diverse people beyond geographical and time constraints. Societal changes brought about by globalization and other forms of modernization place added strain on youths to remain purposeful in their personal lives and also maintain their psychological well-being. In Singapore, the scenario is no different. Singapore aims to be a global city and has kept pace in developing its economy to remain competitive worldwide. The city-state is modern, technologically advanced, and has embraced globalization, constantly gearing itself to both attract and generate wealth. Immersed in such a socio-economic environment, it is not unexpected that youths in Singapore aspire to become rich and famous.

2. The content of life aspirations and well-being

In examining the content of one's life goals or aspirations, Kasser and Ryan (1996) classified intrinsic aspirations as those that are oriented toward inherent growth and satisfying activities and are congruent with the primary psychological needs of autonomy, competency and relatedness proposed by the Self-Determination Theory (SDT) (Deci & Ryan, 1985), while extrinsic aspirations are connected to attaining recognition and external rewards. Researchers (Kasser & Ryan, 1993, 1996; Sheldon, Ryan, Deci, & Kasser, 2004) report that people valuing extrinsic life aspirations such as wealth, fame and image (as opposed to intrinsic life aspirations such as personal growth, meaningful relationships and community contributions) to be associated with lower well-being.

Similar findings were found by Ryan, Chirkov, Little, Sheldon, Timoshina and Deci (1999) when they studied both American and Russian samples. In another study by Williams, Cox, Hedberg and Deci (2000), adolescents' risk behaviors (use of tobacco, alcohol, marijuana, and having sexual intercourse) were significantly predicted by their relative extrinsic life aspirations. Sheldon et al. (2004) show that the content of one's goals (extrinsic or intrinsic), and the motives (autonomous or controlled) for pursuing them, affect psychological well-being. In addition, results of their study indicate that people's choice of extrinsic life aspirations causally affects their subsequent well-being.

Deci and Ryan (1985) pointed to the dangers associated with being overly focused on external rewards. They argued that while the quest of extrinsic rewards *per se* is neither positive nor negative, the incessant pursuit of it might distract people from engaging in intrinsically satisfying activities, and interfere with the development of the congruent self. Sheldon and Kasser (1995), in proposing a model of personality integration draws on the concept of organismic integration described in the SDT and theorized that congruence, as part of personality integration, has to do with how goals connect with organismic needs. In other words, goals that are pursued for self-determined reasons and that involve intrinsically satisfying activity promote organismic congruence. Results from their study supported their presuppositions. In the light of these findings and given the backdrop of strong societal influence on extrinsic and material pursuits, it is important to ask: "How can parents, as key significant others in the lives of youth, influence the development of adolescents today? What forms of parenting are associated with promoting positive child outcomes?"

3. Past studies, and approaches to examining parenting and child outcomes

Researchers have conceptualized their investigations of parenting and child development in various ways. While some have examined parental attitudes, others have explored parental behaviors and parent-child relationships with respect to child correlates (Maccoby & Martin, 1983).

3.1. *Studies based on Baumrind's typology of parenting styles*

Many studies focus on the socialization effects of parenting styles on adolescent development. Baumrind's (1966, 1967) conceptualization of three prototype configurations of parental control –authoritative, authoritarian, and permissive – are widely used in many of the cited studies (e.g., Baumrind, 1971; Chen, Dong, & Zhou, 1997; Dornbusch, Ritter, Leiderman, Roberts, & Fraleigh, 1987; McBride-Chang & Chang, 1998). Results of these studies typically show that authoritative parenting style is linked to better academic performance, adaptive social behaviors, and other positive adolescent outcomes.

3.2. *SDT-based studies examining specific dimensions of parenting style*

Investigators have also based their studies on the SDT (Deci & Ryan, 1985) framework when investigating the links between parental influence, and the child's motivation and psycho-social constructs. According to the SDT, human beings are endowed with innate tendencies that seek to satisfy the three basic psychological needs of autonomy, competence, and relatedness. The social environment plays an important part in that it can either facilitate or impede optimal motivation by supporting or thwarting the fulfillment of the basic psychological needs. Social contexts that enable the satisfaction of these needs are theorized to promote optimal health and psychological well-being. Therefore, one of the critical roles of parents is to facilitate the fulfillment of these needs.

Ryan and Deci (2000) highlighted that when the basic psychological needs of autonomy, competence and relatedness are satisfied, both self-determined motivation and psychological well-being are enhanced. Positive adolescent outcomes are found to be associated with motivation that is highly self-determined. For example, research studies typically show that children with self-regulated motivation, when compared to externally-controlled regulated actions, have enhanced performance (Deci & Ryan, 1991), higher self-esteem (Deci & Ryan, 1995) and general well-being (Ryan, Deci, & Grolnick, 1995).

SDT recognizes that there are activities that do not hold intrinsic interest or appeal to individuals. Thus, it differentiates between intrinsic motivation and non-intrinsic motivation (i.e. extrinsic motivation and amotivation) (Deci & Ryan, 1985). In facilitating the internalization and integration of extrinsic motivation and in enhancing intrinsic motivation, SDT emphasizes the relevance and role of significant others in promoting the desired or requested behavior. Internalization is more likely when significant others in the social context provide suitable support for feelings of relatedness. Perceived competency and the experience of autonomy or sense of volition facilitate internalization and integration of a value or regulation associated with a particular extrinsically motivated behavior. The process of internalization entails different styles of regulation (external regulation, introjected regulation, identified regulation and integrated regulation). Parents are key significant others in the lives of adolescents and therefore play critical roles in this process by supporting autonomy, and providing interpersonal involvement and warmth. Instead of focusing on parenting style which is a constellation of parenting characteristics, researchers have advocated disaggregating the components of parenting style and looking at specific aspects or dimensions of parenting in relation to child correlates (Grolnick & Ryan, 1989). Using this dimensional approach, it is possible to explore each distinct dimension's relative and independent effects on child's outcomes. Parenting dimensions that are closely akin to aspects of Baumrind's authoritative parenting style as well as relevant to the fulfillment of SDT's basic psychological needs of autonomy, competence, and relatedness were examined by researchers. For example, parental involvement, autonomy support, provision of structure, and relatedness are parenting dimensions that are studied by investigators (e.g., Furrer & Skinner, 2003; Grolnick, Kurowski, & Gurland, 1999; Grolnick & Ryan, 1989; Grolnick & Slowiaczek, 1994; Joussemet, Landry, & Koestner, 2008). These studies are mainly in the school socialization and academic achievement context.

3.3. *Parental autonomy support*

Numerous SDT-based studies have collectively maintained the autonomy-supportive role that parents play in promoting adaptive and most favourable child outcomes (Grolnick, Deci, & Ryan, 1997). For example, Grolnick and Ryan (1989) found that children who perceived that their parents are more autonomy-supportive are positively related to the children's self-determined motivation, academic achievement and grades, competence and school behavioral adjustments. Chirkov and Ryan (2001) showed that students of autonomy-supportive parents tended to be more autonomously motivated and are better adjusted.

3.4. *Parental involvement*

Parental involvement refers to the provision of resources in supporting the child's endeavors. It includes intangible resources such as taking interest in the child's activities and devoting time in learning experiences and participating in the child's school activities (Grolnick & Slowiaczek, 1994). Grolnick and Ryan (1989) showed that for third- to sixth- grade children, maternal involvement is positively related to the children's self-regulated motivation and competence in classroom situations.

A later study by Grolnick, Ryan and Deci (1991) also showed similar findings. Children who perceived both their parents as more involved and more autonomy-supportive showed higher autonomous regulation in school, higher perceived competence, and greater control understanding of who or what is responsible for their school outcomes. These variables in turn predicted children's performance. Longitudinal studies also link parental involvement to enhanced children's academic performance (e.g., Keith et al., 1993; Steinberg, Lamborn, Dornbusch, & Darling, 1992). Other studies show that the positive effect of parental involvement on children's academic achievements seems to be linked to the children's perceived competence (e.g., Grolnick & Ryan, 1989; Grolnick et al., 1991; Grolnick & Slowiaczek, 1994).

3.5. *Parenting and relatedness*

Relatedness, one of the three primary psychological needs according to SDT, is analogous to what Harlow (1958) contend as necessary for optimal development of the individual – the need to experience warmth and affection in their interpersonal contact. This sense of relatedness (Ryan et al., 1995) allows intrinsic motivation to thrive and bolsters healthy psychological growth. Studies show that adolescents who reported strong relatedness to their parents are associated with being autonomously motivated and engaged in school; as well as having a greater sense of well-being (Learner & Kruger, 1997; Ryan, Stiller, & Lynch, 1994).

3.6. *Studies on parental influence in the sports domain*

The study of parental influence and adolescent development in the sports domain is relatively new when compared to research done in other domains. Few studies (e.g., Gustafson & Rhodes, 2006; Sallis, Prochaska, & Taylor, 2000) have examined parental support in motivating higher sports outcomes. Many of these studies show that there are significant correlations between parental support and higher physical activity levels. Lewis and Rook (1999), on the other hand, show that there are potential pitfalls to parental influence. When family members exert pressure on their loved ones to be involved in sporting activities, the person may respond in the opposite direction. This could happen when the person perceives that she is being controlled by others. Parental pressure is reported to predict a decreased enjoyment of basketball (Brustad, 1988). It appears that it is not the mere presence or absence of parental influence that determines if the sport-related outcomes are positive but rather the *nature* of the parental influence that is the determining factor.

3.7. *Parenting and life aspiration*

Mothers who showed high levels of autonomy support, involvement and warmth are found to be more likely to promote relatively stronger intrinsic life aspirations (Kasser, Ryan, Zax, & Sameroff, 1995). Some studies show that uninvolved and controlling parenting is associated with the children having more extrinsic life aspirations (Kasser et al., 1995; Williams et al., 2000). The present study aimed to enhance our understanding of parental influence on adolescents' outcomes. Specifically, using the SDT framework, the current study examined autonomy-supportive versus controlling parenting dimension on student athletes' life aspirations.

4. Method

4.1. *Participants and procedure*

Two hundred and five student athletes (111 males and 94 females) aged 14 to 20 years old from six schools participated in the study. Student athletes are students who are in the school training squads of the various sports preparing for the yearly National Inter-Schools Competitions. The questionnaires were administered by the teachers-in-charge of the training squads with instructions from a researcher. Respondents were told that their participation is voluntary and that their responses will be kept confidential. They were told that there were no right or wrong answers and were encouraged to answer the questions honestly.

4.2. *Measurement*

4.2.1. *Perception of Parents Scale*

The student athletes' *perceptions of parental autonomy-support, involvement* and *warmth* were measured using the Perception of Parents Scale developed by Robbins (1994). The reliability coefficients for perceptions of maternal autonomy-support, involvement and warmth (α = .82, α = .78 and α = .82 respectively), and for perceptions of paternal autonomy-support, involvement and warmth (α = .81, α = .82 and α = .85 respectively) for the present sample were satisfactory.

4.2.2. *Basic Needs Satisfaction in Relationships Scale*

The Basic Needs Satisfaction in Relationships Scale (La Guardia, Ryan, Couchman, & Deci, 2000) was used to assess the extent of the fulfillment of their basic psychological needs in their relationships with their parents. Three questionnaire items measure each of the *basic psychological needs of autonomy, competency* and *relatedness*. La Guardia et al. (2000) found reliabilities of ratings for mother and father, were satisfactory. Both confirmatory factor analysis and Chi-square analyses conducted by the researchers showed that a three-factor model provided adequate fit and was significantly more appropriate. For the present sample, the Cronbach's alphas for ratings of the basic needs satisfaction of autonomy, competency and relatedness for mother were .82, .74 and .83 respectively, and for father were .75, .77, and .83 respectively.

4.2.3. *Perceived Locus of Causality Scale*

To measure the student athletes' *sport motivation*, the Perceived Locus of Causality (PLOC) Scale developed by Goudas et al. (1994) assessing different types of motivational orientations was used. Based on an original scale developed by Ryan and Cornell (1989), this PLOC scale was also cross-culturally validated by Wang, Hagger and Liu (In Press) across collectivistic Singapore and individualistic Britain. It has four subscales measuring intrinsic regulation, identified regulation, introjected regulation and external regulation. Cronbach's alphas for external regulation, introjected, regulation, identified regulation and intrinsic motivation for this study were .66, .66, .53 and .84 respectively. The subscale scores were weighted according to the simplex structure of the scale and then added together to form one single score (RAI = 2x Intrinsic + 1x Identified + (-1)x Introjected + (-2)x External). The Relative Autonomy Index (RAI) represents the continuum of locus of causality or degree of autonomy in their self-regulation. Higher positive scores indicate greater perceived autonomy. In assessing amotivation as part of this continuum, an amotivation subscale adapted by Goudas et al. (1994) from the Academic Motivation Scale (Vallerand et al., 1992) was included in the PLOC Scale. Cronbach's alpha for the present sample was .59.

4.2.4. *Physical Self-Perceptions Profile*

The student athletes' self-perceptions of *general self-worth (GSW)*, *physical self-worth (PSW)* and *sport competence* were assessed using selected items from the Children's Physical Self-Perceptions Profile (C-PSPP) scale (Whitehead, 1995) developed from Fox and Corbin's (1989) Physical Self-Perception Profile (PSPP). The reliability, construct and concurrent validity of the C-PSPP was demonstrated by Whitehead (1995). In this present study, the reliability coefficients for sport competence, PSW and GSW were $\alpha = .69$, $\alpha = .85$ and $\alpha = .86$ respectively. For all of the aforementioned measures, subjects responded on a 7-point Likert scale (1 = not true at all, 4 = somewhat true, 7 = very true).

4.2.5. *Aspiration Index*

In examining the *aspirations* of the student athletes, the Aspiration Index (Kasser & Ryan, 1996) was employed. The Aspiration Index, and adaptations of it, are used extensively by researchers investigating the relationships pertaining to extrinsic aspirations and intrinsic aspirations with various constructs (e.g., Grouzet et al., 2005; Kasser & Ryan, 1993; Kasser & Ryan, 1996; Kasser et al., 1995; Ryan et al., 1999; Sheldon et al., 2004; Williams et al., 2000). They were asked to rate on three 7-point Likert subscales on the importance of the aspiration, the likelihood it will happen in the future, and how much the aspiration was attained. Extrinsic aspirations (wealth, fame, image) scores and intrinsic aspirations (personal growth, meaningful relationships, community contributions) scores for each of the dimension (importance, likelihood, attainment) were calculated by computing the mean of the corresponding subscale scores (e.g. Importance of extrinsic aspiration score = mean of the subscale scores of importance of wealth, importance of fame and importance of image). In this present study, satisfactory reliability coefficients for the importance subscale ($.80 \leq \alpha \leq .92$), likelihood subscale ($.81 \leq \alpha \leq .91$), and attainment subscale ($.78 \leq \alpha \leq .88$) were indicated.

5. Results

5.1. *Descriptive statistics*

Table 1 shows the means, standard deviations and ranges for the key variables for the overall sample. Generally, the student athletes perceived higher maternal involvement and warmth than paternal involvement and warmth, and that higher basic psychological needs (autonomy, competency, relatedness) satisfaction were derived from mothers than fathers. In comparing the student athletes'

Table 1 Descriptive statistics for key variables for the overall sample (N=205)

	Mean	SD	Range		
Mother Involvement	5.17	0.96	2.50	-	7.00
Mother Autonomy-support	4.78	0.98	1.22	-	7.00
Mother Warmth	5.33	5.17	1.83	-	7.00
Father Involvement	4.55	1.16	1.00	-	7.00
Father Autonomy-support	4.71	0.99	1.00	-	7.00
Father Warmth	5.00	1.15	1.33	-	7.00
Mother Autonomy Satisfaction	5.02	1.36	1.00	-	7.00
Mother Competency Satisfaction	4.99	1.18	1.00	-	7.00
Mother Relatedness Satisfaction	5.16	1.29	1.00	-	7.00
Father Autonomy Satisfaction	4.81	1.36	1.00	-	7.00
Father Competency Satisfaction	4.88	1.22	1.00	-	7.00
Father Relatedness Satisfaction	4.63	1.43	1.00	-	7.00
Relative Autonomy Index (RAI)	10.86	4.04	-2.00	-	18.00
Amotivation	1.73	0.99	1.00	-	6.67
Sport Competence	4.32	0.98	1.83	-	7.00
Physical Self-Worth (PSW)	4.70	1.24	1.00	-	7.00
General Self-Worth (GSW)	5.23	1.12	1.17	-	7.00
Intrinsic Aspirations Importance	5.92	0.76	3.47	-	7.00
Intrinsic Aspirations Likelihood	5.40	0.88	3.27	-	7.00
Intrinsic Aspirations Attainment	4.21	0.98	1.53	-	7.00
Extrinsic Aspirations Importance	4.28	1.27	1.47	-	7.00
Extrinsic Aspirations Likelihood	4.07	1.18	1.27	-	6.93
Extrinsic Aspirations Attainment	3.20	1.07	1.00	-	6.53

hierarchical self constructs (Fox & Corbin, 1989), the global or general self-worth (apex level) was highest followed by physical self-worth (domain level) and then sport competence (sub-domain level). High level of Relative Autonomy Index (RAI) indicated that the student athletes were on the whole highly autonomous in their sport pursuits. To determine significant differences between male and females, a MANOVA was conducted with sex as the independent variable and all measured and computed variables as dependent variables. No sex difference was found.

Table 2 shows the inter-correlations between all variables examined. All maternal and paternal parenting dimensions of autonomy-support, involvement, and warmth were positively correlated with their corresponding psychological needs (autonomy, competency, relatedness) satisfaction as perceived by the student athletes.

Parenting dimensions of both parents, and the basic psychological needs satisfaction by both parents were positively correlated with global self-worth. Intrinsic Aspirations Attainment was positively correlated to sport competence, physical self-worth and global self-worth. Extrinsic Aspirations Likelihood and Extrinsic Aspirations Attainment were also positively linked to sport competence.

5.2. *Cluster snalysis*

To identify subgroups of student athletes based on parenting dimensions and basic psychological needs satisfaction, an agglomerative hierarchical cluster analysis using the Ward's method was conducted. The cluster analyses were performed on variables for parenting dimensions of both parents (mother autonomy-support, mother involvement, mother warmth, father autonomy-support, father involvement, father warmth), and psychological needs satisfaction (mother autonomy satisfaction, mother competency satisfaction, mother relatedness satisfaction, father autonomy satisfaction, father competency satisfaction, father relatedness satisfaction). All the variables were first standardized.

Cluster analyses yielded three distinct clusters with characteristic parenting dimensions and psychological needs satisfaction. Table 3 shows the cluster means, standard deviations and z scores of the three clusters, and Figure 1 shows their cluster profiles.

Table 2 Inter-correlations for key variables for the overall sample

	1	2	3	4	5	6	7	8	9	10	11	12	13	14
1. Mother Involvement	1.00													
2. Mother Autonomy-support	.69**	1.00												
3. Mother Warmth	.77**	.77**	1.00											
4. Father Involvement	.46**	.36**	.41**	1.00										
5. Father Autonomy-support	.31**	.31**	.31**	.73**	1.00									
6. Father Warmth	.44**	.38**	.53**	.73**	.78**	1.00								
7. Mother Autonomy Satisfaction	.53**	.71**	.61**	.20**	.16*	.27**	1.00							
8. Mother Competency Satisfaction	.60**	.70**	.70**	.32**	.30**	.36**	.71**	1.00						
9. Mother Relatedness Satisfaction	.76**	.69**	.78**	.31**	.26**	.40**	.71**	.72**	1.00					
10. Father Autonomy Satisfaction	.29**	.31**	.35**	.53**	.70**	.68**	.42**	.37**	.40**	1.00				
11. Father Competency Satisfaction	.32**	.28**	.38**	.54**	.65**	.69**	.32**	.52**	.39**	.75**	1.00			
12. Father Relatedness Satisfaction	.44**	.40**	.49**	.72**	.69**	.79**	.38**	.45**	.56**	.75**	.73**	1.00		
13. Relative Autonomy Index (RAI)	.26**	.16*	.21**	.11	.08	.17*	.09	.15*	.21**	.14*	.19**	.15*	1.00	
14. Amotivation	-.24**	-.24**	-.18*	-.11	-.04	-.07	-.10	-.15*	-.12	.02	-.05	-.10	-.55**	1.00
15. Sport Competence	.01	.06	.08	.23**	.25**	.26**	.01	.11	.03	.14	.22**	.20**	.24**	-.18**
16. Physical Self-Worth (PSW)	.23**	.19**	.22**	.34**	.26**	.32**	.17*	.25**	.22**	.20**	.28**	.27**	.26**	-.25**
17. General Self-Worth (GSW)	.31**	.34**	.34**	.35**	.36**	.46**	.28**	.31**	.30**	.40**	.43**	.42**	.31**	-.30**
18. Intrinsic Aspirations Importance	.18**	.21**	.27**	.15*	.21**	.23**	.13	.20**	.17*	.19**	.18**	.16*	.37**	-.22**
19. Intrinsic Aspirations Likelihood	.19**	.20**	.27**	.15*	.17*	.23**	.16*	.24**	.18**	.15*	.20**	.19**	.34**	-.21**
20. Intrinsic Aspirations Attainment	.22**	.14*	.23**	.25**	.20**	.30**	.12	.20**	.17*	.14*	.23**	.20**	.20**	-.16*
21. Extrinsic Aspirations Importance	-.02	-.03	.02	.06	.03	.05	-.05	-.02	-.02	.00	.00	.01	-.17*	.14*
22. Extrinsic Aspirations Likelihood	.04	.03	.08	.09	.05	.11	.03	.04	.03	.04	.09	.07	-.06	.05
23. Extrinsic Aspirations Attainment	.04	-.01	.07	.11	.04	.15*	-.02	-.01	.01	.02	.09	.04	-.04	.03

*p < .05; **p < .01

Table 3 Cluster means, standard deviation and z scores for the 3 cluster solutions

Variable	Cluster 1 (n = 116)			Cluster 2 (n = 37)			Cluster 3 (n = 52)		
	Mean	SD	Z	Mean	SD	Z	Mean	SD	Z
Mother Involvement	4.99	.80	-.19	4.46	.95	-.73	6.07	.58	.94
Mother Autonomy-support	4.56	.82	-.23	4.11	.95	-.69	5.76	.51	1.00
Mother Warmth	5.22	.79	-.11	4.43	1.12	-.90	6.21	.53	.88
Mother Autonomy Satisfaction	4.76	1.11	-.19	3.94	1.44	-.79	6.36	.59	.98
Mother Competency Satisfaction	4.68	.86	-.26	4.13	1.27	-.73	6.28	.54	1.10
Mother Relatedness Satisfaction	4.98	1.02	-.14	4.03	1.43	-.88	6.38	.54	.95
Father Involvement	4.52	.84	-.02	3.27	1.10	-1.10	5.52	.89	.84
Father Autonomy-support	4.68	.76	-.03	3.60	.83	-1.12	5.57	.69	.87
Father Warmth	5.00	.85	.00	3.52	.90	-1.29	6.06	.59	.92
Father Autonomy Satisfaction	4.73	.99	-.06	3.13	.98	-1.23	6.17	.75	1.00
Father Competency Satisfaction	4.77	.87	-.09	3.42	.97	-1.20	6.16	.57	1.05
Father Relatedness Satisfaction	4.58	1.06	-.03	2.82	.96	-1.26	6.01	.82	.97

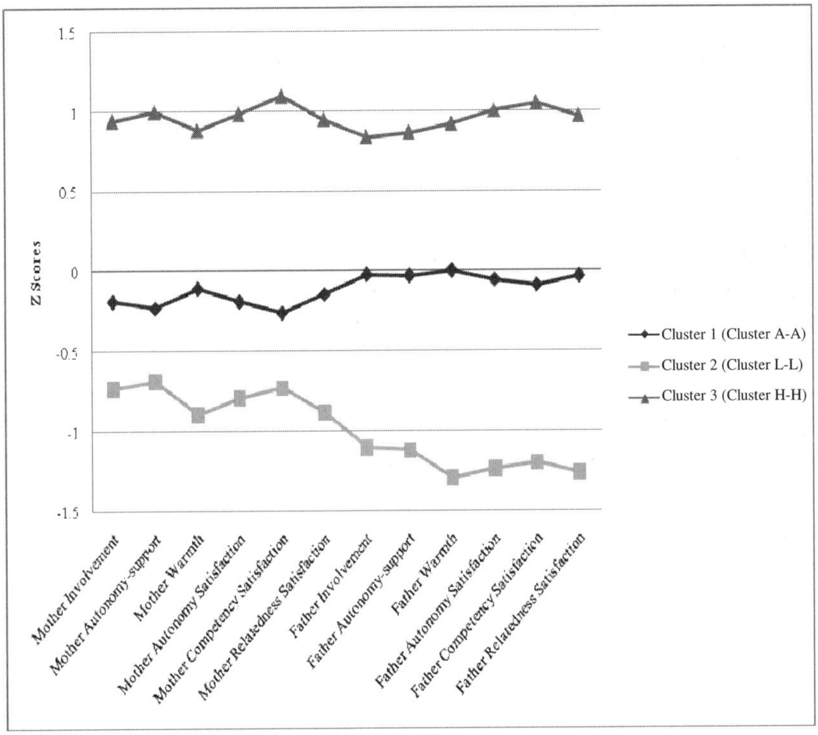

Figure 1: Cluster profiles of the three parenting dimensions-psychological needs satisfaction cluster types

In comparison, Cluster 1 (labeled Cluster A-A) has average scores for parenting dimensions and psychological needs satisfaction for both parents. Cluster 2 (labeled Cluster L-L) has low scores while Cluster 3 (labeled as Cluster H-H) has high scores for both sets of variables.

To examine how these three clusters differed in their motivational orientations (RAI and amotivation), self constructs (global self-worth, physical self-worth, and sport competency), and aspirations (intrinsic and extrinsic), two one-way MANOVAs were conducted. In the first MANOVA, the RAI, amotivation, global self-worth, physical self-worth, and sport competence were used as the dependent variables. Significant differences, with large effect size, were found in the three clusters, Wilks's $\Lambda = .79$, $F(2,202) = 5.10$, $p < .05$, $\eta^2 = .11$. The follow-up ANOVAs revealed that except for sport competence, significant differences exist for all dependent variables ($p < .05$). Post-hoc tests using Tukey's HSD indicated the following comparisons with significant differences (all $p < .05$). Cluster H-H registered significantly higher RAI and global self-worth than the other two clusters. This cluster also showed significantly higher physical self-worth than Cluster L-L. However, amotivation of Cluster H-H was significantly lower than Cluster A-A.

A second MANOVA was conducted to investigate how the three clusters differed in each aspect of importance, likelihood and attainment of their intrinsic and extrinsic aspirations. There were significant differences in the three clusters, Wilks's $\Lambda = .87$, $F(2,202) = 2.29$, $p < .05$, $\eta^2 = .07$, with medium effect size. Follow-up ANOVAs indicated that only Intrinsic Aspirations Importance, Intrinsic Aspirations Likelihood, and Intrinsic Aspirations Attainment showed significant differences (all $p < .05$). Post-hoc test employing Tukey's HSD showed that Cluster H-H was more likely to place higher importance on intrinsic aspirations, and also more likely to indicate higher likelihood of achieving intrinsic aspirations than the other two clusters. Attainment of intrinsic aspirations was also deemed higher by Cluster H-H than Cluster L-L.

6. Discussion

Higher satisfaction of the basic psychological needs derived from parents who were perceived to be autonomy supportive, more involved and showed greater warmth, together with the positive correlations of these factors with global self-worth, suggest the salience of these parenting dimensions in promoting psychological well-being. In this aspect, mothers were found to be more influential than fathers. Also evident was that student athletes with high perceived parental involvement, autonomy support and warmth and reported that their basic psychological needs were highly met (Cluster H-H), had higher autonomous motivation, global self-worth and physical self-worth.

These findings are in congruence with the SDT's assertion, and support previous findings in the academic domain, that the fulfillment of basic psychological needs promotes autonomous functioning and psychological well-being. The high level of RAI found in Cluster H-H suggested a more organismically congruent self (Ryan, 1993). This was further supported by these student athletes registering higher importance, likelihood and attainment of intrinsic aspirations which concurs with what was theorized (Sheldon & Kasser, 1995) and supported by previous findings (Kasser & Ryan, 1996; Kasser et al., 1995) that organismic congruence occurs when intrinsic goals align with primary organismic needs. This is contrary to what would be expected that youths in affluent, materialistic, and modern Singapore would value extrinsic aspirations strongly.

7. Conclusion

On the whole, findings in this study suggest that student athletes with perceived parental autonomy-support that was also characterized by involvement and warmth facilitated a more autonomously motivated, positive and congruent self. Such individuals were also less likely to seek extrinsic forms of recognition or worth such as wealth or fame as they tended to pursue intrinsic life aspirations. This is of importance to youth development in the light of previous findings, which indicate that subscribing to intrinsic aspirations is positively associated with well-being (Kasser & Ryan, 1996), and that individuals' choice of life goals appear to causally affect their subsequent well-being (Sheldon et al., 2004).

References

1. Baumrind, D. (1966). Effects of authoritative parental control on child behavior. *Child Development, 37*, 887-907.
2. Baumrind, D. (1967). Child care practices anteceding three patterns of preschool behavior. *Genetic Psychology Monographs, 75,* 43-88.
3. Baumrind, D. (1971). Current patterns of parental authority. *Developmental Psychology Monographs,* Part 2, 1-103.
4. Brustad, R. J. (1988). Affective outcomes in competitive youth sport: The influence of intra-personal and socialization factors. *Journal of Sport & Exercise Psychology, 10,* 307-321.
5. Chen, X., Dong, Q., & Zhou, H. (1997). Authoritative and authoritarian parenting practices and social and school performance in Chinese children. *International Journal of Behavioral Development, 21*, 855-873.
6. Chirkov, V. I., & Ryan, R. M. (2001). Parent and teacher autonomy-support in Russian and U.S. adolescents: Common effects on well-being and academic motivation. *Journal of Cross-Cultural Psychology, 32*(5), 618-635.
7. Deci, E. L., & Ryan, R. M. (1985). *Intrinsic motivation and self-determination in human behaviour*. New York: Plenum.
8. Deci, E. L., & Ryan, R. M. (1991). A motivational approach to self: Integration in personality. In R. Dienstbier (Ed.), *Nebraska Symposium on Motivation: Vol. 38. Perspectives on motivation* (pp. 237-288). Lincoln: University of Nebraska Press.

9. Deci, E. L., & Ryan, R. M. (1995). Human autonomy: The basis for true self-esteem. In M. Kemis (Ed.), *Efficacy, agency, and self-esteem* (pp. 31-49). New York: Plenum.
10. Dornbusch, S. M., Ritter, P. L., Leiderman, P. H., Roberts, D. F., & Fraleigh, M. J. (1987). The relation of parenting style to adolescent school performance. *Child Development, 58*, 1244-1257.
11. Fox, K., & Corbin, C. B. (1989). The physical self-perception profile: Development and preliminary validation. *Journal of Sport & Exercise Psychology, 11*, 408-430.
12. Furrer, C., & Skinner, E. (2003). Sense of relatedness as a factor in children's academic engagement and performance. *Journal of Educational Psychology, 95*(1), 148-162.
13. Giddens, A. (2006). *Sociology* (5th ed.). Cambridge: Polity Press.
14. Goudas, M., Biddle, S., & Fox, K. (1994). Perceived locus of causality, goal orientations, and perceived competence in school physical education classes. *British Journal of Educational Psychology, 64*, 453-463.
15. Grolnick, W. S., Deci, E. L., & Ryan, R. M. (1997). Internalization within the family: The self-determination theory perspective. In J. E. Grusec & L. Kuczynski (Eds.), *Parenting and Children's Internalization of Values: A Handbook of Comtemporary Theory* (pp. 135-161). New York: John Wiley & Sons, Inc.
16. Grolnick, W. S., Kurowski, C., & Gurland, S. T. (1999). Family processes and the development of children's self-regulation. *Educational Psychologist, 34*(1), 3-14.
17. Grolnick, W. S., & Ryan, R. M. (1989). Parent styles associated with children's self-regulation and competence in school. *Journal of Educational Psychology, 81*(2), 143-154.
18. Grolnick, W. S., Ryan, R. M., & Deci, E. L. (1991). The inner resources for school acheivement: Motivational mediators of children's perceptions of their parents. *Journal of Educational Psychology, 83*, 508-517.
19. Grolnick, W. S., & Slowiaczek, M. L. (1994). Parents' involvement in children's schooling: A multidimensional conceptualization and motivational model. *Child Development, 64*, 237-252.
20. Grouzet, F. M. E., Kasser, T., Ahuvia, A., Dols, J. M. F., Kim, Y., Lau, S., et al. (2005). The structure of goal contents across 15 cultures. *Journal of Personality and Social Psychology, 89*(5), 800-816.
21. Gustafson, S. L., & Rhodes, R. E. (2006). Parental Correlates of Physical Activity in Children and Early Adolescents. *Sports Medicine, 36(1),* 79-97.
22. Harlow, H. F. (1958). The nature of love. *American Psychologist, 13*, 673-685.
23. Joussemet, M., Landry, R. e., & Koestner, R. (2008). A Self-Determination Theory perspective on parenting. *Canadian Psychology, 49*(3), 194-200.

24. Kasser, T., & Ryan, R. M. (1993). A dark side of the American dream: Correlates of financial success as a central life aspiration. *Journal of Personality and Social Psychology, 65*, 410-422.
25. Kasser, T., & Ryan, R. M. (1996). Further examining the American dream: Differential correlates of intrinsic and extrinsic goals. *Personality and Social Psychology Bulletin, 22*(3), 280-287.
26. Kasser, T., Ryan, R. M., Zax, M., & Sameroff, A. J. (1995). The relations of maternal and social environments to late adolescents' materialistic and prosocial values. *Developmental Psychology, 31*, 907-914.
27. Keith, T. Z., Keith, P. B., Troutman, G. C., Bickley, P. G., Trivette, P. S., & Singh, K. (1993). Does parent involvement affect eight-grade students achievement?: Structural analysis of national data. *School Psychology Review, 22*, 474-496.
28. La Guardia, J. G., Ryan, R. M., Couchman, C. E., & Deci, E. L. (2000). Within-person variation in security of attachment: A self-determination theory perspective on attachment, need fulfillment, and well-being. *Journal of Personality and Social Psychology, 79*, 367-384.
29. Learner, D. G., & Kruger, L. J. (1997). Attachment, self-concept, and academic motivation in high-school students. *American Journal of Orthopsychiatry, 67*, 485-492.
30. Lewis, C. E., & Rook, K. S. (1999). Social control in personal relationships: Impact on health behaviour and psychological distress. *Health Psychology, 18*, 63-71.
31. Maccoby, E. E., & Martin, J. A. (1983). Socialization in the context of the family: Parent-child interaction. In E. M. Hetherington (Ed.), *Handbook of child psychology: Vol. 4. Socialization, personality, and social development* (4th ed., pp. 1-102). New York: Wiley.
32. McBride-Chang, C., & Chang, L. (1998). Adolescent–parent relations in Hong Kong: Parenting styles, emotional autonomy, and school achievement. *The Journal of Genetic Psychology, 159*, 421-436.
33. Robbins, R. J. (1994). *An assessment of perceptions of parental autonomy support and control: Child and parent correlates.* Unpublished Doctoral Dissertation, Department of Psychology, University of Rochester, 1994.
34. Ryan, R. M. (1993). Agency and organization: Intrinsic motivation, autonomy, and the self in psychological development. In J. Jacobs (Ed.), *Nebraska Symposium on Motivation: Vol. 40. Development perspectives on motivation* (pp. 1-56). Lincoln: University of Nebraska Press.
35. Ryan, R. M., Chirkov, V. I., Little, T. D., Sheldon, K. M., Timoshina, E., & Deci, E. L. (1999). The American Dream in Russia: Extrinsic aspirations and well-being in two cultures. *Personality and Social Psychology Bulletin, 25*(12), 1509-1524.

36. Ryan, R. M., & Cornell, J. P. (1989). Perceived Locus of Causality and Internalization: Examining Reasons for Acting in Two Domains. *Journal of Personality and Social Psychology, 57*(5), 749-769.
37. Ryan, R. M., & Deci, E. L. (2000). Self-determination theory and the facilitation of intrinsic motivation, social development, and well-being. *American Psychologist, 55*(1), 68-78.
38. Ryan, R. M., Deci, E. L., & Grolnick, W. S. (1995). Autonomy, relatedness, and the self: Their relation to development and psychopathology. In D. Cicchetti & D. J. Cohen (Eds.), *Developmental psychopathology: Theory and methods* (pp. 618-655). New York: Wiley.
39. Ryan, R. M., Stiller, J., & Lynch, J. H. (1994). Representations of relationships to teachers, parents, and friends as predictors of academic motivation and self-esteem. *Journal of Early Adolescence, 14*, 226-249.
40. Sallis, J. F., Prochaska, J. J., & Taylor, W. C. (2000). A review of correlates of physical activity of children and adolescents. *Medical Science Sports and Exercise, 32*(5), 963-975.
41. Sheldon, K. M., & Kasser, T. (1995). Coherence and congruence: Two aspects of personality integration. *Journal of Personality and Social Psychology, 68*(3), 531-543.
42. Sheldon, K. M., Ryan, R. M., Deci, E. L., & Kasser, T. (2004). The independent effects of goal contents and motives on well-being: It's both what you pursue and why you pursue it. *Personality and Social Psychology Bulletin, 30*(4), 475-486.
43. Steinberg, L., Lamborn, S. D., Dornbusch, S. M., & Darling, N. (1992). Impact of parenting practices on adolescent achievement: Authoritative parenting, school involvement, and encouragement to succeed. *Child Development, 63*, 1266-1281.
44. Vallerand, R. J., Pelletier, L. G., Blais, M., Brière, N. M., Senecal, C., & Vallieres, E. F. (1992). The academic motivation scale: a measure of intrinsic, extrinsic, and amotivation in education. *Educational and Psychological Measurement, 52*, 1003-1017.
45. Wang, C. K. J., Hagger, M. S., & Liu, W. C. (In press). A cross-cultural validation of perceived locus of causality in physical education and sport contexts. *Research Quarterly for Exercise & Sport.*
46. Whitehead, J. R. (1995). A study of children's physical self-perceptions using an adapted physical self-perception profile questionnaire. *Pediatric Exercise Science, 7*, 132-151.
47. Williams, G. C., Cox, E. M., Hedberg, V., & Deci, E. L. (2000). Extrinsic life goals and health risk behaviors in adolescents. *Journal of Applied Social Psychology, 30*, 1756-1771.

INVESTING IN HUMAN CAPITAL: POLICY LEADERSHIP AND STRUCTURAL ALIGNMENT OF COACH EDUCATION IN SINGAPORE

EUGENE CHEW

Physical Education and Sports Science, National Institute of Education, Nanyang Technological University, Singapore

The Organisation for Economic Co-operation and Development (OECD) established that human capital development is one of the essential inputs that contribute significantly to the economic and human well-being of a nation. Investing in human capital is therefore a necessity for industry development and economic growth. The sports industry is an emerging industry sector. In Asia-Pacific market alone, experts projected a 29% growth in the sports market from US$13.7 billion in 2006 to US$17.7 billion in 2011. As Singapore positions itself to capture this potential market through government's support and investment in developing the sports sector mainly through infrastructure development and sports events programming, it is critical that ample attention be paid to the development of human capital. Industry development requires more competent manpower in various disciplines. Sports coaching is an identified area for human capital to be developed. This article examines the policy and structural changes that affect coach education in Singapore. Together with an environmental scan of coach education in a few leading countries, it explores ways to provide more avenues as well as relevant approaches for professional development of coaches. The chapter concludes with a call for careful attention to be given to the following: (i) Leadership in national-level sports policy on coaching development and coach education; (ii) Alignment and synergy in sports policy and educational policy in supporting further development of human capital in the sports coaching; (iii) The role of tertiary educational institutions in providing avenues for professional development of coaches; and (iv) Further professional development of coaches at higher education level should pay attention to the approach to be adopted and be both relevant and contextualized to the coaching practice.

1. Introduction

According to the Organization for Economic Co-operation and Development (OECD), investing in human capital is necessary for economic growth (Healy, 2001). Human capital development and social capital development are viewed as part of the essential inputs that contribute to the human and economic well-being of a nation. Human capital is defined as the knowledge, skills, competencies and attributes embodied in individuals that facilitate the creation of personal, social and economic well-being. The OECD's review of studies on the effect of the impact of human capital on growth in the Gross Domestic Product (GDP) suggests that a country's commitment to devote resources to education, especially higher education, have a positive effect on the nation's economic growth.

The sports industry is an emerging industry sector in Singapore. The sports industry contributed about 0.49% (or S$680m) to the GDP in 1998 In 2001, arising from the recommendations of Committee on Sporting Singapore Report, the government of Singapore set the direction for the GDP contribution of the sports industry to be doubled by 2010 (Ministry of Community Development Youth and Sport, 2001). The recent Sporting Culture Committee Report anticipates that the sports sector will contribute S$2 billion to the Gross Domestic Product (GDP) by 2015 (Ministry of Community Development Youth and Sports, 2008). To support this anticipated growth, ample attention needs to be paid to developing competent human capital.

This chapter focuses on the development of human capital in the area of sports coaching in Singapore. It provides background information on the nation's policy and structural changes that have influenced the development of coach education. Together with an environment scan of the coach education framework in a few selected countries, it explores ways in which continual professional development of coaches can be achieved in Singapore; and further considers how the educational development of coaches can be made more relevant and beneficial for practicing coaches.

2. An emerging industry sector in Singapore

According to industry figures, the growth in global sports market is expected to increase from US$96 billion in 2006 to US$124 billion by 2011. Asia-Pacific market alone, experts projected a 29% growth from US$13.7 billion in 2006 to US$17.7 billion in 2011 (Economic Development Board, 2008). Major cities in countries such as the United States of America, Australia, China, Korea, Japan, and middle-eastern cities such as Dubai, Doha, and Abu Dhabi (ITP Digital, 2007, February 7), are constantly transforming their sporting landscape to capture a piece of the global sports market. Singapore is doing likewise. The country recognizes the value of the sports market and has identified the sports industry as a sector that could contribute to the growth of the Singapore economy. The Singapore Sports Council (SSC) is working with the Economic Development Board to identify and promote potential growth areas in the sports sector (Singapore Sports Council, 2007).

In recent years, as a strategy to jumpstart the sports industry, the Singapore Sports Council has supported the staging of marquee events. Staging prominent international sports events in Singapore will also showcase Singapore as a vibrant, global city suitable for foreign business investments. This strategy is in line with the recommendations of the Committee on Sporting Singapore Report in utilizing sporting events to position Singapore as a global city (Ministry of Community Development Youth and Sport, 2001).

The Singapore government further fuels the growth in sports by hosting the Singtel FORMULA 1 (F1) Singapore Grand Prix in 2008, building a Grade 2 FIA-approved permanent race track at Changi capable of hosting races other than F1 (Singapore Sports Council, 2007, October 26), as well as the inaugural Youth Olympic Games in 2010. Its commitment to sports development is apparent in its willingness to invest in sports over two consecutive periods of five years - S$500m from 2001 to 2005, and S$300m from 2006 to 2010 (Singapore Sports Council, 2005, 2006) In addition, at least another S$1.87b is committed to build the Singapore Sports Hub which is expected to be completed by 2011 (Singapore Sports Council, 2008, January 19). The recent Sporting Culture Committee Report estimated that an additional government investment of S$39.8m (2008-2010) and S$36.6m (2011-2015) should be made for implementing the recommendations stated in the Report (Ministry of Community Development Youth and Sports, 2008). Vibrancy in the sports industry is expected to be buttressed by the directions set forth in the Sporting Culture Committee Report.

3. Developing sports human capital in Singapore

While Singapore targets the sports sector as an area for economic growth, Singapore needs to seriously consider developing sufficient and effective human capital to support the potential growth in the sports industry. Having good quality and competent manpower, besides hardware or infrastructure (e.g. new sports hub, new race track at Changi, integrated resorts), should be given ample attention and priority. This is necessary to attract foreign sports investment, provide sports related product and services, and generate business activities in Singapore. This need for more competent manpower for Singapore to achieve the National Sports Vision is also articulated in the Sporting Culture Committee Report. In response the changing and anticipated demands of the sports industry sector, the Singapore Sports Council has also announced plans to enhance manpower capabilities. The upcoming new sports hub and more sizeable sports events and programmes are expected to require more and better trained manpower support (Singapore Sports Council, 2007, October 23). The Singapore Sports Council will work with tertiary educational institutions to increase the number of sport-related courses.

In an effort to provide strategic leadership in human capital development in the sports sector, the Singapore Sports Council collaborated with the Singapore Workforce Development Agency (WDA) in commissioning a study that will identify manpower needs in the sports industry and map out a manpower development plan (Singapore Sports Council & Singapore Workforce Development Agency, 2007). Sports coaching is identified by the SSC-WDA study as one of the key areas that needs further development.

Coaching is central to sports development. High quality of coaching at every level of sports involvement, from participation sports to competitive sports, will contribute to the enjoyment of sports as well as to the achievement of the sporting vision and objectives established by the Singapore government. Sports coaching services constitute an important touch point for consumers of sports.

4. Educating coaches in Singapore

Traditionally, coaches in Singapore were probably former athletes who gained their knowledge and experience from their own coaches, or individuals who have a background in physical education or have attained coaching certifications from the Singapore Sports Council and their National Sports Associations. Some would have a combination of these training and experiences.

4.1. *Coach Education under the purview of the Singapore Sports Council – early years to the present scene*

Training and education of coaches has been undertaken by Singapore Sports Council together with the National Sports Associations of the various sports. Information from the Singapore Sports Council provided a sketch of the policy and structural development related to coaching that have influenced coach education in Singapore (Chew, 2000, 2001, 2002). The account below highlights some of these the key changes.

In 1976, a Coaching Committee was formed to look into the development of coaching courses under the Coaching Plan. These courses were conducted in conjunction with the National Sports Associations (NSAs). The objectives of the Coaching Plan were:

1. to standardize all coaching levels,
2. to stimulate sports associations to develop a coaching scheme, and
3. to improve the quality of coaching.

The Coaching Committee had, over the years, sought to improve the standard of the coaching courses in Singapore. It had also recommended the adoption of the National Coaching Certification Program, developed by the Coaching Association of Canada, for the local courses.

In 1995, there was a revamp of the Coaching Plan and the Coaching Committee was discontinued. Instead, a Technical Committee was formed to look into the curriculum, content and administration of the coaching courses. Under the Technical Committee, the National Coaching Accreditation Programme (NCAP) adopted the National Coaching Certification Program (NCCP) of the Coaching Association of Canada with modifications to include four instead of five levels of certification.

To drive coaching development to a higher level, the Singapore Sports Council felt that greater involvement and advocacy from the stakeholders were needed. While some countries (e.g. Canada, Australia) have coaching associations or councils to steer the professional growth in coaching, Singapore did not have such an equivalent body. In 2000, a Steering Committee on Coach Education and Coaching Development was formed under the Singapore Sports Council to guide the development of coaching and coach education.

The NCAP Elite Level Course (level 4) was launched in 2001 as a pilot course (150 curricular hours) to cater to the further development of elite level coaches in Singapore. At the end of two runs of the course, it was discontinued due to subsequent poor take-up rate and the high level of commitment that was required of practicing coaches.

In 2002, the Coaching Advisory Committee (CAC) was formed. This was in line with the recommendation of the Committee on Sporting Singapore Report to set up a Coaching Council. The CAC currently serves as an advisory board to the Singapore Sports Council and is not yet an autonomous body as was envisaged by the Report. The eventual development of the CAC into a autonomous "professional body managed by the professional (coaches) themselves, with the objective of enhancing the professionalism and standing of the coaching industry" (Ministry of Community Development Youth and Sport, 2001, p. 67) will be a significant milestone for coaching development in Singapore.

The Singapore Sports Council's review of the NCAP was completed in 2007 for subsequent implementation of a competency-based curriculum. This development places coach education in Singapore in line with the competency-based approach undertaken by countries such as Canada, Australia and the United Kingdom. It sets the stage for the mobility, and employability of Singapore-trained coaches across these countries when recognition of the equivalent coaching competencies is established.

The establishment of the National Registry of Coaches (NROC) in 2002 enabled the NCAP certified and accredited coaches to maintain professional networking and support (Singapore Sports Council, 2003). Continuing coach education has also been established as part of the coach education framework for NROC coaches. Coaches are expected to maintain currency of their membership in the NROC through their participation in continuing coach education.

4.2. *Coaching courses offered by educational institutions*

A few educational institutions in Singapore offer sports related diploma or degree programmes. However, none of these institutions offers a programme that specifically specializes in sports coaching. Some of these programmes include a module on sports coaching.

The National Institute of Education (NIE) provides diploma, degree, and higher degree programmes for the professional preparation of physical education teachers. At the moment it does not conduct a programme that specifically prepares one to be a coach. However, there exist a module on the theory and practice of coaching that is taught as part of the Masters of Science (Exercise & Sports Science) programme. This module is aimed at providing understanding of coaching at the elite performance level (National Institute of Education, 2008, June 23).

Republic Polytechnic offers three sports and leisure related diploma programmes. A module on sports coaching is conducted as part of the core discipline modules required for the Diploma in Sports & Exercise Sciences. Students are introduced to the principles of, and applications in, sports coaching (Republic Polytechnic, 2008).

The Nanyang Polytechnic conducts a third year module on the theory and principles of coaching as part of the Diploma in Sports & Wellness Management (Nanyang Polytechnic, 2008 May 4).

4.3. *Coach education in other countries*

4.3.1. *Canada*

Coach education in Canada is largely driven by the Coaching Association of Canada (CAC) which is a not-for-profit amateur sport organization with the mandate to improve the effectiveness of coaching across all levels of the sport system. The influence and reach of the CAC in Canada is pervasive (Coaching Association of Canada, 2005). Since 1974, the CAC works with the various national sport organizations in Canada to offer training and qualifications in coaching for the various sports. The National Coaching Certification Program (NCCP) has five certification levels and is well regard by the coaching and sports community in Canada as the national benchmark for coach education. The NCCP courses have been re-designed to be competency-based.

In its effort to reach out to more people in its delivery of coaching services and coach education programmes, it has established 7 National Coaching Institutes (NCI) across Canada. These NCIs offers development programmes for coaches that lead to the award of a diploma by the NCI which will also enable the coaches to attain Level 4 qualification under the NCCP.

Universities in Canada offer degree-level and masters-level programmes in coaching. The University of Alberta, for example, offers a Degree in Physical Education with a major in Coaching Studies, and also a Masters of Arts with specialization in Coaching with an aim to recognize its strengths in having coaching related expertise. In doing so, the University aligns itself with the federal government recommendations that universities be recognized as an important part of the coach education system in Canada (University of Alberta, 2008).The Master of Arts (MA) degree with specialization in Coaching, provides a linkage between this course and the coach education framework established by the Coaching Association of Canada. The University also indicated that the NCCP Level 4 equivalency will be sought from the Coaching

Association of Canada and that practical coaching experiences with top domestic or international coaches will be an important component of this degree.

The Masters in Kinesiology in Coaching in York University is another example of a degree-level programme. What is particularly interesting is that the University also offers a Coaching Certificate which can be earned in conjunction with the Bachelor of Arts (BA) or Bachelor of Science (BSc) options in Kinesiology and Health Science (York University, 2004).

4.3.2. *Australia*

Coaches and the government of Australia saw the need to enhance the standard of coaching. In 1978, the Standing Committee on Recreation and Sport (SCORS) agreed with the Confederation of Australian Sport (CAS) on the formation of a National Coaching Council to establish the National Coaching Accreditation Scheme (Woodman, 1989). The National Coaching Council was renamed Australian Coaching Council in 1979. For many years since 1979, the Australian Coaching Council was the driving force behind the development of coach education in Australia. Through the National Coaching Accreditation Scheme (NCAS), it aimed to raise standards of coaching and to establish the minimum level of proficiency and training in the appointment of coaches. The NCAS has three levels of certification.

In recent years the work of the Australian Coaching Council has been incorporated into the Australian Sports Commission (ASC). Under the ASC Coaching and Officiating unit, the NCAS remains an integral part and vital part of coach education in Australia. While ASC maintains authority over the course on "Coaching General Principles", it no longer specifies the number of levels of sport-specific courses. Each national sporting organization determines the number of levels and the names of the levels as part of their coach accreditation pathway (Australian Sports Commission, 2007).

In developing coaches, the ASC collaborates with educational and training agencies to organize, promote and conduct courses based on the information provided in the ASC programme curricula. These agencies include State/Territory Coaching & Officiating Centres, National/State Sport Organisations that are accredited to conduct the NCAS, Department of Sport and Recreation, Technical and Further Education (TAFE) institutes, school/college, universities and private service providers. Participants of courses conducted by these training agencies, upon their successful completion, are encouraged to attain an accreditation as part of the NCAS.

At the tertiary education level, the ASC and the Australian Institute of Sports (AIS) collaborated with the University of Queensland to offer a formal coach education pathway for practicing coaches. Coaches who have NCAS qualifications but do not possess qualifications and foundational knowledge in human movement studies are able to pursue further education via the Graduate Certificate in Applied Science (Sports Coaching). This essentially serves as a bridging programme that enables coaches without tertiary educational qualifications to pursue further formal education qualifications (Mallett & Rynne, 2005). Successful completion of this programme will allow coaches to progress to the Graduate Diploma in Applied Science (Sports Coaching) and then the Masters of Applied Science (Sports Coaching).

4.3.3. *Hong Kong*

Prior to 2004, the development of coach education in Hong Kong has been under the direction of the Hong Kong Coaching Committee (HKCC) and was supported by the coach education department of the Hong Kong Sports Development Board (HKSDB). Under the HKSDB, the Coach Accreditation Programme offers training and certification for coaches in Hong Kong. It has three levels of certification. When the Hong Kong Sports Development Board Ordinance was repealed by the Hong Kong government in 2004, the Coach Accreditation Programme continues to be driven by the coach education department that came under the purview of the Hong Sports Institute (HKSI). Currently, the Hong Kong Coaching Committee is a joint committee of the Sports Federation & Olympic Committee of Hong Kong, China and HKSI (Hong Kong Coaching Committee, n.d.).

Opportunities for further updating and upgrading of accredited coaches are made available by the HKCC through the Continuing Coach Education Programme. It consists of international seminars and workshops that are co-organised with National Sports Associations and All-China Sports Federation.

Through an existing collaboration with Beijing Sports University, coaches are able to gain access to the Bachelor of Education in Sports Training programme. This is a five-year, part-time degree programme, and is administered by the HKSI. It provides Hong Kong coaches with an opportunity to gain an academic qualification as well as acquire sport-general and sport-specific knowledge. The first student intake was in September 1999 (Hong Kong Sports Institute, n.d.).

4.3.4. *United Kingdom (UK)*

Sports coach UK, (formerly National Coaching Foundation) is the body that looked into coach education in the UK. The National Coaching Foundation (NCF) was established in 1983 as a sub-committee of the then (Great Britain) Sport Council. It became a Charity in 1989 and was re-branded as "sports coach UK" in 2001(sports coach UK, 2008a).

The Coaching Task Force – Final Report provides us some key information on coach education in the UK (Department of Culture Media and Sport, 2002). Since 1984, NCF has made available generic core courses and resources for coaches from all sports and all levels. Most of the sport-specific coach education courses are run by each National Governing Body (NGB) of the sport. Majority of the NGBs did not adopt the generic materials on sports science, sports medicine and sports pedagogy as there was no requirement for them to do so. As a result, there was inconsistency in the coach education programmes and the qualifications of coaches. Notwithstanding the above observation made by the Coaching Task Force, (Lyle, 2002) noted that the NCF has made significant impact on the development of coaching in the UK, especially in participation coaching and the coaching award schemes run by the NGBs.

The Level 1, 2 and 3 coaching courses were conducted under the NCF. The NCF also launched a Diploma in Professional Studies (Sports Coaching) in 1988 and the Certificate in Sports Coaching in 1993. In the 1990s, the NCF incorporated the National Vocational Qualifications/National Occupational Standards approach to the education and training in their work with the industry lead body to establish industry standards for coaching. (Sports coach UK, 2008b). However, Lyle (2002) asserted that despite the fact that there were at least 26 institutions in UK offering courses in sports coaching at higher national diploma, degree, or Master's degree levels at the turn of the century, the extent of the influence of these higher educational programmes on the practice of sports coaching is felt at the participation level but not at the elite level.

In late 2005, after London won the bid to host the 2012 Summer Olympics, sports coach UK was tasked to develop the UK Coaching Framework. The project was done in collaboration with the national governing bodies of the various sports and the funding agencies. Under the UK Coaching Framework, strategic action areas were identified. Noteworthy for our discussion here is that the UK Coaching Framework is committed to a) developing a UK Coaching System with its unique UK coaching model and coach pathways, b) providing support for the development of coaches including continuous professional development and coaching qualification, and c) developing coaching as a profession by making coaching a professionally regulated vocation through licensing and registration (sports coach UK, 2008c).

5. Educating Coaches – areas for further development

From the foregoing background information and environment scan, we can derive several lessons and venture to take bolder steps towards developing coaches. The role of a central agency in creating synergy among stakeholders is of immense strategic value. This can be facilitated by establishing an overarching coaching framework and a coach education pathway. This central agency can be an association (as in Canada), a government agency (as in Australia), a charity (as in the UK) or a private entity that was evolved from a government agency (as in Hong Kong). The coaching system and the core foundational coach education framework are owned and driven by these central agencies in collaboration with the national sporting organizations of the respective sports. Opportunities for further education, including obtaining formal educational qualifications, are mainly provided by educational institutions.

5.1. *The need for national-level strategic directions and alignment*

In the absence of a coaching association in Singapore, the Singapore Sports Council currently performs this role as the lead agency for coaching development. It is therefore critical that the SSC works with the various government agencies and educational institutions to chart the direction and implement the relevant policies that would pave the way for better aligned human capital development in sports coaching. The government has already set the direction in recommending that the standards of the coaching industry be raised and that the NCAP qualification be made compulsory in the longer run (Ministry of Community Development Youth and Sports, 2008). There is room for the professional preparation of coaches to be made more vigorous and comprehensive. The upgrading of the coach development framework is necessary in lending support to the emerging sports industry and to meet the rising expectations of more sophisticated consumers of sports. It will need the support of all relevant agencies and stakeholders. While the SSC has announced that it will work with institutes of higher learning to provide more sport-related courses, it is crucial that more dialogues and collaborations among these stakeholders take place.

5.2. *The need for commitment through investing in sports coaching*

Singapore needs to seal its commitment to raising the standards of the coaching industry by investing in capacity building. As part of the need to develop human capital discussed earlier, the areas of focus should not be very different from what the UK Coaching Framework has identified for the building the coaching system. Government and private sector investment in sports should focus on building:

1. Capacity for the employment and deployment of coaches
2. Capacity of the National Sports Associations and relevant educational institutions in developing and delivering core foundational coach education courses (under the NCAP structure)
3. Capacity for tertiary educational institutions to cater to the professional development of coaches via higher education programmes at diploma, degree or masters levels.

5.3. *Establishing tertiary education for coaching*

Investment to increase the supply of well-trained professional coaches can be a bold, strategic policy to develop the sports industry. Such a strategy is already practiced in other industry sectors (e.g. financial, biomedical sciences, life sciences) where experts are either courted to come to Singapore with various incentives or vast amount of financial outlay are made to train local experts. The latter necessitates the provision of avenues for attaining professional qualifications.

Leadership in governmental agencies and the local university in Singapore have taken a historically significant step in providing university-level education for developing human capital for the sports industry. In 2009, recognising the need to develop more human resources that would meet the growing sports industry, the Nanyang Technological University has announced the establishment of the Bachelor of Science in Sport Science and Management degree programme (Lin, 2009). This programme is the first degree-level programme offered by a local university in Singapore. While it is not designed specifically to train coaches, it would provide the foundations necessary for the pursuit of a coaching career. Also, graduates from this programme, unlike those graduating from the degree in physical education programme (Bachelor of Science (Education)) who are required to serve a three-year bond in the Ministry of Education as a teacher, can enter the sports industry immediately upon graduation.

Quality formal qualifications and certification is important to establishing professional status. For example, the legal, medical and engineering professions have established its status as a profession through years of academic vigor it its professional preparations. The same would have to happen for sports coaching for it to be accepted as a profession. Lyle (2002) indicated that issues of professional status of coaches "... rested on the nature of formal qualifications and the extent to which these are regulated" (p. 275).

Tertiary educational institutions can be in a unique position to offer continuing education for coaches as they may have the resources and expertise to offer programmes related to coaching. Additional expertise can be augmented through collaborations. For instance, in collaborating with the Australian Institute of Sports (AIS), the University of Queensland is able to tap into the rich coaching experiences and knowledge of the AIS coaches. The ability of the universities/polytechnics in catering for adult learning is another prime consideration in delivering quality continuing education programmes for coaches successfully. Remote access and online course delivery are features that will enable adults to pursue their educational goals whilst maintaining their work and family responsibilities. Resources and technological advances exist in universities or polytechnics. Some of these include internet access and web-based applications, online course delivery platforms (e.g. Blackboard), sports science laboratories, and well-stocked libraries with access to e-databases, e-journals, and e-books. Institutes of higher learning in Singapore such as the Nanyang Technological University and Ngee Ann Polytechnic, already possess such means for course delivery. Given its better economies of scale, universities/polytechnics can acquired new and more effective student/teacher friendly course delivery platforms that would facilitate better online access to lessons, discussions, assessments and student-teacher communications.

Universities pioneering higher education programmes for coaching, such as that offered by the University of Queensland, have found ways to make further education for coaches more accessible and relevant. E-learning and online course delivery allow students who most likely be holding coaching jobs access anywhere around the world. Learning is also made more relevant by integrating what is encountered in coaching practice into the programme structure.

The approach to integrate coaching practice into the programme structure resonates well with the holistic approach to coaching advocated by Cassidy, Jones & Potrac (2004). They stressed the importance for coaching, and also coach education, to take into account the context of the coaching practice. Better learning is achieved when teaching is contextualized. They pointed out that research has shown that coaches consistently failed to make the necessary connections in what they have learnt in discreet units within detached and parallel multi-disciplinary coaching knowledge (e.g. physiology, nutrition, psychology) and apply them to their coaching practice.

From Jones, Armour and Potrac's (2004) work on the life stories of elite level coaches, in structuring higher education programmes for sports coaching one should take into account some of the following key implications:

1. The importance of observing and learning from other coaches, especially more experienced coaches who can act as mentors
2. Currency of knowledge learnt in coaching courses and its relevance to actual coaching practice is important
3. Coaching is about people and dealing with individuals in a social context. People management and the art of coaching need to be developed. It involves knowing how one present himself (impression management) and the use of social power (the ability to get others do what you want them to do).

Likewise, Lyle (2002) emphasized the need to match coach capabilities with the requirements of the practice. He indicated that the principles of coach education and training need to be informed by the coaching process. Professional preparation of coaches involves both formal and informal processes and "can be summarized as follows:

1. teaching and learning of specialized knowledge, values and understanding that underpin the activity;
2. training and practice in the skills-based implementation of practice;
3. initiation/induction into the social and professional mores of the occupation." (p. 275)

Coach education should also build capacities in coaches to move beyond their current practice and knowledge and be able to innovate, to adapt, to experiment, to establish new ways and acquire new knowledge and gain higher level of expertise in coaching (Lyle, 2002). In other words, through the coach education, the coach should acquire the capacity and the necessary learning tools to become an expert and a professional.

5.4. *Delivery approaches to coach education*

As mentioned earlier, the delivery of content knowledge, and more importantly, the application of such knowledge need to be contextualized in coaching scenarios. It "needs to be delivered in an integrated, as opposed to a compartmentalized manner" (Cassidy et al., 2004, p. 183). Cassidy et al (2004) highlighted four ways in which this could be achieved:

1. A critical task-based approach – coaches are given tasks where he needs to acquire needed information, skills and understanding. The role of the coach educator is that of a facilitator of learning.
2. A narrative approach – the coach captures his experience in particular issues/scenarios in writing and then deconstruct his own narratives to analyse what are the factors that influence the coaching process.
3. A problem-based learning (PBL) approach – the learnings as required of by the coach education curriculum is constructed around a carefully designed coaching issues or scenarios. The process of finding a solution to the presented problem facilitates the learning process.
4. Mentoring – this method involves a more experienced coach supervising and monitoring the learning process of a coach with less knowledge, skills and experience. Lyle (2202) advocated a structured approach where the "trainee coach must have available a number of procedures for interrogating the master's practice – stimulated recall, question and answer, critical analysis of practice, simulated examples and joint reflection " (p. 286).

6. Conclusion

The emerging Singapore sports industry is at a juncture where its growth trend needs to be supported by several factors and parallel development areas. Human capital development is one such area that cannot be ignored. To this end, our foregoing discussion on the advances made by other countries, together with our understanding of the development of the coaching industry and coach education in Singapore, allows us to focus on a few things. Specifically, in the development of the coaching industry and coach education, careful attention should be given to:

1. Leadership in national-level sports policy on coaching development and coach education;
2. Alignment and synergy in sports policy and educational policy in supporting further development of human capital in the sports coaching; and
3. The role of tertiary educational institutions in providing avenues for professional development of coaches
4. Further professional development of coaches at higher education level should pay attention to the approach to be adopted and be both relevant and contextualized to the coaching practice. Such programmes should be accessible to practicing coaches via off-site means.

For Singapore, policy leadership in sports coaching, coaching expertise, and tertiary level educational resources do not reside under one particular agency.

The Singapore Sports Council is the leading agency in sports coaching development. Coaching expertise are under the purview of the national sports associations while some tertiary educational institutions are already running sport-related academic programmes and possess sports science expertise and have staff with some coaching expertise. Collaboration among government agencies and educational institutions in charting the future directions for educating coaches for the sports industry is a key factor to the eventual realization of greater professionalism and quality in sports coaching.

References

1. Australian Sports Commission. (2007). *Accreditation*. Retrieved October 1, 2008, from http://www.ausport.gov.au/participating/coaches/education/NCAS
2. Cassidy, T., Jones, R., & Potrac, P. (2004). *Understanding Sports Coaching – The social cultural and pedagogical foundations of coaching practice*. London: Rouledge.
3. Chew, W. C. E. (2000). Coaching and coach education development. Unpublished Paper presented at the 1st meeting of the Steering Committee on Coach Education and Coaching Development. Singapore Sports Council.
4. Chew, W. C. E. (2001). Quality coaching for sporting Singapore - SSC short-term, mid-term and long-term initiatives for the national coaching development plan phase 2. Unpublished Paper presented at the 2nd meeting of the Steering Committee on Coach Education and Coaching Development. Singapore Sports Council.
5. Chew, W. C. E. (2002). National coaching development plan phase 2 - progress update on SSC initiatives. Unpublished Paper presented at the 1st meeting of the Coaching Advisory Committee. Singapore Sports Council.
6. Coaching Association of Canada. (2005). *Overview of CAC*. Retrieved September 27, 2008, from http://www.coach.ca/eng/about_cac/overview.cfm
7. Department of Culture Media and Sport. (2002). The Coaching Task Force – Final Report [Electronic Version]. Retrieved October 1, 2008 from http://www.culture.gov.uk/reference_library/publications/4760.aspx
8. Economic Development Board. (2008). *Industry Sectors - Lifestyle Products and Services*. Retrieved September 27, 2008, from http://www.edb.gov.sg/edb/sg/en_uk/index/industry_sectors/lifestyle_and_sports_businesses.html
9. Healy, T. (2001). *The Well-Being of Nations - The role of human and social capital*. Paris: Organisation for Economic Co-operation and Development.
10. Hong Kong Coaching Committee. (n.d.). *Background*. Retrieved October 1, 2008, from http://www.hkcoaching.com/hk/background.asp

11. Hong Kong Sports Institute. (n.d.). *Sports Coaching: B.Ed. Programme in Sports Training*. Retrieved October 1, 2008, from http://www.hksi.org.hk/hksdb/front/e_sdc1_pst2.html
12. ITP Digital. (2007, February 7). *Sport Tourism in Abu Dhabi*. Retrieved October 1, 2008, from http://www.arabianbusiness.com/property/article/7822-sport-tourism-in-abu-dhabi
13. Jones, R., Armour, K., & Potrac, P. (2004). *Sports coaching culture - from practice to theory*. New York: Rouledge.
14. Lin, X. (2009, February 11). NTU introduces sports degree. *The Straits Times,* p. B16.
15. Lyle, J. (2002). *Sports Coaching Concepts – A framework for coaches' behavior*. London: Rouledge.
16. Mallett, C., & Rynne, S. (2005). *Postgraduate programs in sports coaching*. Paper presented at the Plenary session presentation at the International Council for Coach Education International Masterclass, Limerick, Ireland. Retrieved October 1, 2008, from http://www.icce.ws/conference/Limerick_2005.htm
17. Ministry of Community Development Youth and Sport. (2001). *Report of the Committee on Sporting Singapore*. Singapore: Ministry of Community Development, Youth and Sports.
18. Ministry of Community Development Youth and Sports. (2008). *Sporting Culture Committee Report*. Singapore: Ministry of Community Development, Youth and Sports.
19. Nanyang Polytechnic. (2008 May 4). *Dip in Sport & Wellness Management*. Retrieved September 27, 2008, from http://www.nyp.edu.sg/SBM/sbm_dip_sw.html
20. National Institute of Education. (2008, June 23). *Master of Science (Exercise & Sports Studies)*. Retrieved September 27, 2008, from http://www.pess.nie.edu.sg/ModuleOutline/programmes_moduleoutlines/Degree%20by%20coursework.htm#MES808
21. Republic Polytechnic. (2008). *Diploma in Sports & Exercise Sciences*. Retrieved September 27, 2008, from http://www.rp.sg/courses/shl/dses/course_structure.asp#
22. Singapore Sports Council. (2003). *SSC Quarterly Strategic Review*. Unpublished Report for quarterly review meeting. Singapore Sports Council.
23. Singapore Sports Council. (2005). *Annual Report 04/05 - Harnessing the Past, Leaping into the Future*. Singapore: Singapore Sports Council.
24. Singapore Sports Council. (2006). *Annual Report 05/06 - Going the Distance - Towards 2010*. Singapore: Singapore Sports Council.

25. Singapore Sports Council. (2007). *Annual Report 2006/2007 - Leading the Field*. Singapore: Singapore Sports Council.
26. Singapore Sports Council. (2007, October 23). *Singapore Sports Council gears up for Sports Hub & other major sports programmes & events*. Retrieved September 27, 2008, from http://www.ssc.gov.sg/publish/Corporate/en/news/media_releases/2007_media_releases/ssc_gears_up_for_sports.html
27. Singapore Sports Council. (2007, October 26). *Singapore Government to develop motor sports industry*. Retrieved September 27, 2008, from http://www.ssc.gov.sg/publish/Corporate/en/news/media_releases/2007_media_releases/motor_sports_industry.html
28. Singapore Sports Council. (2008, January 19). *Singapore Sports Hub Consortium led by Dragages Singapore Pte Ltd selected as preferred bidder for sports hub project*. Retrieved September 27, 2008, from http://www.ssc.gov.sg/publish/Corporate/en/news/media_releases/2008/singapore_sports_hub.html
29. Singapore Sports Council, & Singapore Workforce Development Agency. (2007). *SSC-WDA Sports Industry Manpower Survey*. Unpublished Survey.
30. Sports coach UK. (2008a). *History of sports coach UK*. Retrieved October 1,2008, from http://www.sportscoachuk.org/About+Us/Corporate+Information/History+of+sports+coach+UK.htm
31. Sports coach UK. (2008b). *Key waymarks*. Retrieved October 1, 2008, from http://www.sportscoachuk.org/NR/rdonlyres/27A176FF-6865-46EB-A9D3-AD31337C0F9A/0/HistoryofsportscoachUK.pdf
32. Sports coach UK. (2008c). *The UK Coaching Framework* [Electronic Version]. Retrieved October 1, 2008, from http://www.culture.gov.uk/reference_library/publications/4760.aspx
33. University of Alberta. (2008). *Master of Arts with a Specialization in Coaching*. Retrieved September 27,2008, from http://www.physedandrec.ualberta.ca/ma_coaching.cfm
34. Woodman, L. (1989). The development of coach education in Australia. *Sporting Traditions - The Journal of the Australian Society for Sports History, 5*(2), 204-224.
35. York University. (2004). *Coaching Certificate*. Retrieved September 27, 2008, from http://www.yorku.ca/web/futurestudents/programs/template.asp?id=347

MEASUREMENT OF ATTITUDE IN SPORT

DO YOUNG PYUN
Physical Education and Sports Science, National Institute of Education, Nanyang Technological University, Singapore

EUGENE CHEW
Physical Education and Sports Science, National Institute of Education, Nanyang Technological University, Singapore

ALAN CH'NG
Physical Education and Sports Science, National Institute of Education, Nanyang Technological University, Singapore

The objectives of the current chapter are (a) to introduce two measurement techniques of an attitude construct (i.e., direct and indirect measurement), (b) to describe dispositions, advantages, and disadvantages of each technique, and (c) to highlight the trends of these techniques in the sport literature. For the purposes of the study, the authors reviewed and summarized various conceptual studies in measurement theory. While indirect measurements have several advantages, sport researchers are deterred by crucial limitations such as cost, reliability, and validity issues. Therefore, sport researchers have heavily relied on direct measurement techniques such as Likert, Thurstone, and semantic differential scales. These direct scales were examined on how to measure an attitude construct using them and what their advantages and disadvantages are. Considering convenience, reliability, and validity of the direct measurement techniques, sport scholars have preferred Likert scale to measure attitude toward domains of their interest.

1. Introduction

Researchers are often faced with the challenge of how to assess unobserved constructs using precise measurement. Measurement used here is defined as "rules for assessing numbers to objects to represent quantities of attributes" (Churchill & Iacobucci, 2002, p. 401). Churchill and Iacobucci (2002) also pointed out that a researcher's challenge could be figured out when s/he has "the rigour" that rules can be determined and "the skill" to execute the rules (p. 401). A better understating of 'the rigour' and 'the skill' will help researchers to correctly measure a domain they are interested in. Basing on an in-depth literature review, this chapter addresses several measurement issues in assessing attitude, a construct which is frequently studied in the sport context. Attitude has been defined differently by several theorists. Most of these definitions recognise the role that either one or all of the three components of (a) cognition, (b) affects, and (c) behaviour play in one's attitude toward a particular object. Rokeach (1968) defined an attitude as "a relatively enduring organisation of beliefs around an object or situation predisposing one to respond in some preferential manner" (p. 112). Aiken (2002) viewed attitude as "learned cognitive, affective, and behavioural predispositions to respond positively or negatively to certain objects, situations, institutions, concepts, or persons" (p. 3). According to Fishbein (1967), attitudes may be defined as "learned predispositions to respond to an object or class of objects in a favourable or unfavourable way" (p. 257).

There are various techniques developed to measure sport consumers' attitudes toward a certain object. The methods for measuring a person's attitude generally fall into two categories: indirect and direct measurements. With an indirect method, a person's attitude is measured without the person knowing it whereas with a direct method, a subject is asked to give a self-report of his or her attitude (Petty & Cacioppo, 1981). Petty and Cacioppo (1981) explained that indirect measurements usually include instruments such as disguised self-reports, behavioural indicators of an attitude, and physiological indicators of an attitude. On the other hand, common direct measurements are observations, interviews, and questionnaires. Questionnaires often utilize a Thurstone scale, Likert scale, semantic differential scale, or a single item scale (Petty & Cacioppo, 1981). The following sections describe detailed characteristics of each of indirect and direct measurement techniques, with particular focus on Thurstone, Likert, and the semantic differential scales which are popular attitude-scaling procedures used in sport research.

2. Indirect measurement of attitude

When a respondent recognises that his/her attitude is being assessed, this awareness negatively influences the efforts to measure an attitude (Dawes, 1972). This bias resulting from respondents' unwillingness in providing accurate information about their attitudes to researchers is one of most widely recognised disadvantages of direct measurement (Petty & Cacioppo, 1981; Shaw & Wright, 1967). Campbell (1950) asserted the necessity of developing attitude measures that will not elicit reactive responses (as cited in Dawes, 1972):

> In the problem of assessing social attitudes, there is a very real need for instruments which do not destroy the natural form of the attitude in the process of describing it. There are also situations in which one would like to assess 'prejudice' without making respondents self-conscious or aware of the intent of the study. (p. 120)

With indirect measurement, respondents do not deliberately distort their responses because researchers disguise the purpose of a study or do not reveal the true purpose(s) immediately (Lemon, 1973). Indirect measurements are used as a useful way of detecting relatively large differences in affects between respondents (Petty & Cacioppo, 1981). The most frequently used techniques in indirect measurements of attitudes are disguised self-reports, behavioural indicators of attitudes, and physiological indicator of attitudes. As indicated in the Table, unique advantages of these measurement techniques are (a) a complementary way to reduce the obtrusive effects which can be derived from indirect measurement (disguised self-reports), (b) an effective way in particularly assessing political attitudes in a certain country where people may be afraid to reveal their true opinions (behavioural indicators of attitudes), and (c) a best measure in the human body's natural physiological responses to attitudinal stimuli (physiological indicator of attitudes; Churchill & Iacobucci, 2002; Huges, 1974; Lemon, 1973; Petty & Cacioppo, 1981).

However, there is a question as to whether indirect measurements are ethical (Dawes, 1972; Kidder & Campbell, 1970; Lemon, 1973). Kidder and Campbell (1970) criticized the use of disguised measurement techniques noting that their use raises important ethical questions about the rights of respondents to be aware of the true purpose of the instruments to which they are subject. In the case of behavioural and physiological indicator of attitudes, other than reliability issues associated with these instruments, the cost of using these techniques are so expensive that researchers sometimes cannot afford them (Petty & Cacioppo, 1981). Due to these shortcomings, indirect techniques have received little attention from sport scholars. Therefore, when considering the use of indirect measurements a researcher should "weigh up these considerations carefully before he commits himself to measurement of this type, and should exercise their own good sense, and pay due regard to possible abuses in their use" (Lemon, 1973, p. 121).

3. Direct measurement of attitude

In studies of attitudes in the sport context, researchers prefer the direct self-report measurement techniques because it is assumed that the direct scales are superior to the indirect scales in terms of reliability and validity (Lemon, 1973; Petty & Cacioppo, 1981; Stevens, 1966). Against the view of respondents' deliberate transmissions of their incorrect attitudes in direct measurements, Petty and Cacioppo (1981) argued that this disadvantage is not problematic in attitude research because "most attitude research does not deal with highly sensitive issues, and in many studies the subjects' attitudinal responses are kept anonymous" (p. 22). Thus, they suggest that there is little reason to conclude that indirect measurements misrepresent respondents' attitudes. Another advantage of using direct measurement is the precision or sensitivity of scales; direct measurement scales are better at "pinpointing relatively small differences in attitudes that may exist between subjects" (Petty & Cacioppo, 1981, p. 22). Advantages and disadvantages of each scaling method are described in the Table. More detailed descriptions of the Thurstone scale (Thurstone, 1928), Likert scale (Likert, 1932), and the semantic differential scale (Osgood et al., 1957), that are commonly used in direct measurement techniques are presented below.

3.1. *Thurstone scale*

While working on scaling human perceptions of sensory stimuli such as light and sound, Thurstone (1928) realized that people could rank opinion statements in terms of their favourableness toward some objects just as people can rank noises in term of loudness. The steps in constructing a Thurstone scale to measure an attitude are summarized below (Petty & Cacioppo, 1981; Thurstone, 1928):

1. Development of a Thurstone scale begins with collecting a list of 100 to 150 belief statements from several groups of people who are asked to write out their opinions on an issue and from the literature.
2. Editing collected statements for a list of about one hundred brief statements of opinion.
3. Two or three hundred subjects as judges are asked to arrange the statement in eleven piles ranging from opinions most strongly affirmative to those most strongly negative.
4. Only those statements that result in a consistent sorting by the judges are retained; whenever there is much disagreement among the judges' rating, the item is eliminated.

5. The researcher allocates "a scale value" to statements that are retained corresponding to the median category to which the judges have assigned it; each statement is assigned a scale value such that it is rated higher than its value by half the judges and lower than this value by the other half.
6. Based on the criteria of selecting a high degree of agreement among the judges on their appropriate category, the researcher finally selects a final set of items (around 20 items) that range all along the favourable-unfavourable continuum.
7. In order to measure an attitude, the researcher asks each subject to check all items with which he or she personally agrees in the final statement pool. The attitude score is the median of the scale values of the statements that the person endorses.

Through these steps, an attitude can be measured by a Thurstone scale. In comparison to other scales, although constructing a Thurstone scale is a rather difficult and tedious process, especially in assembling an item pool, it represents a fairly precise estimate of respondents' attitude toward an object a researcher seeks for (Likert, 1932; Petty & Cacioppo, 1981).

As described in the steps, the final series of attitude items contains carefully selected statements of belief about an object with "different evaluative weight" from a negative evaluation to a positive evaluation, also including a neutral evaluative aspect (Fishbein, 1967, p. 264). Respondents simply check their agreement or disagreement with each statement (Thurstone, 1928). In order to obtain an attitude score, the researcher computes the mean or median score of the evaluative weights that each agreed statement contains (Thurstone, 1928). In Thurstone's scale, an attitude measure, thus, can be obtained based on very restricted range of belief statements which have strength (respondents' agreement) and evaluative aspects (judges' evaluative range from 1 to 11; Fishbein, 1967). Even though a Thurstone scale is highly recognised as a precise estimate of attitude, it is generally not recommended for use in marketing research because of it is a time consuming technique, expensive, and disliked by respondents due to a lot of reading (Huges, 1967; Huges, 1971).

3.2. *Likert scale*

The Likert scale is to date the most widely used tool to measure attitudes in the sport context because it is easy for researchers to construct and to interpret, and simple for respondents to answer (Schiffman & Kanuk, 2002). As with a Thurston scale, the researcher starts with a large set of statement items.

However, with a Likert scale the researcher simply decides which items indicate favourableness to the attitude object rather than giving these items to judges (Fishbein, 1967). Edward and Kenney (1967) also indicated that constructing a Likert scale is less time consuming and less laborious than Thurstone scales. The steps in constructing a Likert scale are summarized as follows (Likert, 1932):

1. A large number of opinion statements related to the attitude object are collected (i.e. this step is similar to Thurstone's procedure)
2. A large sample of subjects rate the extent of their own agreement with each statement on a five- or seven-point scale
3. Since the scale supposes that each of the items measures the same underlying attitude, any items that do not correlate highly with the total score (obtained by summing the responses to the individual items) are removed from the pool
4. The subject's final attitude score is obtained by summing the responses to the items that remain

The principal benefit of the Likert scale has been that it provides the researcher the option of considering the responses to each statement separately, or of combining the responses to produce an overall, summated scales (i.e., this scale is often called a summated scale) (Schiffman & Kanuk, 2002).

Unlike the Thurstone scale, the Likert scale does not contain a neutral evaluative aspect in the items (Fishbein, 1967). The key point is that the Likert scale should fall at one or the other extreme direction of favourableness or unfavourableness (e.g., 1 or 11 on the Thurstone continuum) in order to measure an attitude (Edwards & Kenney, 1967). Belief statements that indicate neither favourableness nor unfavourableness should be deleted from the final item pool (Fishbein, 1967). Thus, a researcher should carefully select attitude items which do not have different meanings for different people (Fishbein, 1967).

3.3. *Semantic differential scale*

The semantic differential scale is one of the most ubiquitous techniques in direct measurement of attitudes (Dawes, 1972). The semantic differential scale was originally designed to investigate the underlying structure of words (Churchill & Iacobucci, 2002; Osgood et al., 1957). This measurement technique was later adapted to measure attitude toward a wide variety of people, objects or issues.

It is found that the responses to the bipolar scales tended to be correlated and that three basic uncorrelated dimensions could be found to explain most of the meaning we assign to different words: "evaluation" (e.g., "good-bad, sweet-sour, or helpful-unhelpful"), "potency" (e.g., "powerful-powerless, strong-weak, or deep-shallow"), and "activity" ("fast-slow, alive-dead, or quiet-noisy"; Churchill & Iacobucci, 2002, p. 382; Osgood et al., 1957). The first dimension, *evaluation*, corresponds to what we consider an attitude (Petty & Cacioppo, 1981). Thus, Osgood et al. (1957) stated that attitudes could be measured by having subjects rate an attitude object on bipolar adjective pairs that represented the evaluative dimension of meaning. However, a validity issue can be questioned during the development of scales. When a researcher measures an attitude toward a certain object, s/he should carefully select appropriate adjective pairs in relation to that object so that different respondents may not have different meanings on those items, as is the case with the Likert scale (Fishbein, 1967). For example, when a researcher attempts to measure attitude toward a certain sports team, s/he uses a previously reported attitude scale adjective pairs such as "dirty-clean" (Fishbein & Raven, 1962, p. 36). In this situation, respondents may not connect this adjective pair with their attitude toward the team. Respondents may also have difficulty of understanding what "dirty" and "clean" mean in relation to the sports team. Thus, one important matter to consider with the use of semantic differential scales is to focus on developing samples of adjective pairs instead of using basic adjective pairs so that a score could be generated for the attitude object (Churchill & Iacobucci, 2002).

Some sport scholars use different scales to directly measure respondents' attitude toward an object. Fishbein and Raven (1962, p. 36) provided a valid and reliable scale to measure attitudes which could be obtained by having the subject judge the concept on a series of bipolar probabilistic scales (e.g. "impossible-impossible", "false-true", "existent-nonexistent", "probable-improbable", and "unlikely-likely" for belief scales; "harmful-beneficial", "wise-foolish", "dirty-clean", and bad-good" for attitude scales).

4. Conclusion

The chapter described three broadly used indirect attitude measurement scales. Due to the several aforementioned limitations involved with the indirect measurement techniques, attitudes can be often directly measured by the semantic differential scales in that respondents are asked to check their overall attitude toward an object (Fishbein & Ajzen, 1974). In contrast, attitudes can be inferred from the evaluating a responses to belief statements using Thurstone and Likert scales. Comparing the three scales a Likert scale is easier than a Thurstone scales because unlike the Thurstone scales, the Likert scale can be accomplished with the same set of people (Petty & Cacioppo, 1981). In spite of simple procedures, the Likert scales have equivalent reliabilities with Thurstone's scales (McNemar, 1946; Poppleton & Pilkington, 1964). When the semantic differential scales are applied to sport studies, scholars sometimes fail to develop appropriate items related to the interest of research, especially, when a study explores the attitude of a new construct. This failure raises questions regarding validity of the resulting semantic scales (Churchill & Iacobucci, 2002). As a result, the Likert Scale is considered as the most popular form of attitude scales (Edwards & Kenny, 1946; Petty & Cacioppo, 1981; Schiffman & Kanuk, 2002), and many researchers in sport also depend on the Likert Scale to measure consumers' attitude toward objects such as sports teams, sponsorship, or advertising through sport. It should be noted that when measuring consumers' attitude, researchers should use very restricted range of belief statements that reflect the evaluative dimension of concept.

References

1. Aaker, D. A., Kumar, V., & Day, G. S. (2000). *Marketing research* (7th ed.). New York: John Wiley & Sons, Inc.
2. Aiken, L. R. (2002). *Attitudes and related psychosocial constructs: Theories, assessment, and research.* Thousand Oaks, CA: Sage Publications, Inc.
3. Cacioppo, J. T., & Sandman, C. A. (1981). Psychophysiological functioning, cognitive responding, and attitude. In R. E. Petty, T. M. Ostrom, & T. C. Brock (Eds.), *Cognitive responses in persuasion*. Hillsdale, NJ: Erlbaum.
4. Campbell, D. T. (1950). The indirect assessment of social attitudes. *Psychological Bulletin, 47*, 15-38.
5. Churchill, G. A., & Iacobucci, D. (2002). *Marketing research: Methodological foundations* (8th ed.). Mason, OH: South-Western.
6. Dawes, R. M. (1972). *Fundamentals of attitude measurement.* New York: John Wiley & Sons, Inc.
7. Di Vesta, F. J. (1966). A developmental study of the semantic structures of children. *Journal of Verbal Learning and Verbal Behaviour, 5*, 249-259.
8. Edwards, A. L., & Kenney, K. C. (1967). A comparison of the Thurstone and Likert Techniques of attitude scale construction. In M. Fishbein (Ed.), *Readings in attitude theory and measurement.* New York: John Wiley & Sons, Inc.
9. Fishbein, M., & Ajzen, I. (1974). Attitudes towards objects as predictors of single and multiple behavioral criteria. *Psychological Review, 81*(1), 59-74.

10. Fishbein, M., & Raven, B. H. (1962). The AB scales: An operational definition of belief and attitude. *Human Relations, 15*, 35-44.
11. Fishbein, M. (1967). A consideration of beliefs, and their role in attitude measurement. In M. Fishbein (Ed.), *Readings in attitude theory and measurement.* New York: John Wiley & Sons, Inc.
12. Hughes, G. D. (1967). Selecting scales to measure attitude changes. *Journal of Marketing Research, 4*, 85-87.
13. Hughes, G. D. (1974). The measurement of beliefs and attitudes. In R. Feber (Ed.),
McGraw-Hill, Inc.
14. Kidder, L. H., & Campbell, D. T. (1970). The indirect testing of social attitudes. In G. Summer (Ed.), *Attitude measurement.* Chicago: Rand McNally.
15. Lemon, N. (1973). *Attitudes and their measurement.* New York: John Wiley & Sons, Inc.
16. Likert, R. (1932). A technique for the measurement of attitudes. *Archives of Psychology, 140*, 5-55.
17. McGrath, J., & McGrath, M. E. (1962). Effect of partizanship on perceptions of political figures. *Public Opinion Quarterly, 26*, 236-248.
18. Osgood, C. E., Suci, G. J., & Tannenbaum, P. H. (1957). *The measurement of meaning*. Urbana, IL: University of Illinois Press.
19. Petty, R. E., & Cacioppo, J. T. (1981). *Attitude and persuasion: Classic and contemporary approaches.* Dubuque, IA: Wm. C. Brown Company Publishers.
20. Rokeach, M. (1968). *Beliefs, attitudes, and values: A theory of organization and change.* San Francisco: Jossey-Bass.
21. Schiffman, L. G., & Kanuk, L. L. (2002). *Consumer behavior* (7th ed.). Upper Saddle River, NJ: Prentice Hall, Inc.
22. Shaw, M. E., & Wright, J. M. (1967). *Scales for the measurement of attitudes.* New York: McGraw Hill.
23. Stevens, S. S. (1966). A metric for the social consensus. *Science, 151*, 530-541.
24. Tanaka, Y., Oyama, T., & Osgood, C. E. (1963). A cross cultural and cross concept study of semantic space. *Journal of Verbal Learning and Verbal Behaviour, 2*, 392-405.
25. Thurstone, L. L. (1928). Attitude can be measured. American *Journal of Sociology, 33*, 529-554.

		Strength	Weakness
Direct Procedure	Thurstone Scale	• A precise estimate of where a person stands on the underlying attitudinal dimension.	• Difficult to construct and administer • Many judges (e.g., 200~300), considerable time, effort, and money required
	Likert scale	• Easier to construct than the Thurstone scale with the same set of people. • Equivalent reliability with and high correlation with Thurstone.	• A total score does not reflect a unique attitude since the total can be derived in many different ways (e.g., the total score does not explain differences of each scores of items)
	Sematic differential scale	• Equivalent reliability with Thurstone and Likert scales. • A good consistency of the mass of a cross-cultural study (Tanaka, Oyama, & Osgood, 1963) • The use of relatively disguised ways to measure an attitude (MaGrath & McGrath, 1962) • The stability of the evaluation-potency-activity framework across different age groups (Di Vesta, 1966) • In overall, a good performance in reliability and validity tests • Allow subjects to express the intensity of feelings toward an object	• Very restricting in situations where respondents are not familiar with an attitude object • Adjectives may not exactly represent an attitude object (Osgood et al., 1957)
	One-item Rating scale	• Much easy to construct	• Not as reliable as the Thurstone, Likert, and semantic differential scales
Indirect Procedure	Disguise self-reports	• Complementary way to reduce the obtrusive effects of indirect measurement	• Ethical problem: misleading subjects for the purpose of the study • Difficult to devise a suitable procedure
	Behavioural indicators of attitudes	• Particularly useful in assessing political attitudes in a country where people may be afraid to give their true opinions to interviewers	• Somewhat expensive • Unrepresentative behaviours may be observed
	Physiological indicator of attitudes	• A "perfect" measure in the human body's natural physiological responses to attitudinal stimuli (Cacioppo & Sandman, 1981)	• Elaboration preparation and expensive equipment • Inconsistent reliable results

Source: Summarized and cited from Churchill and Iacobucci (2002); Huges (1974), Lemon (1973); Petty and Cacioppo, (1981).

PROVISION OF PSYCHOLOGICAL SERVICES TO TAIWANESE ATHLETES FOR THE OLYMPIC AND ASIAN GAMES

TSUNG-MIN HUNG

National Taiwan Normal University, Taiwan

The use of sport psychology to harness and bring out the best in athletes in major competition is not new. In Taiwan, the model employed for the provision of sport psychology services is creative in that it draws upon expertise that resides in universities with sport science capability. Stages in sport psychology service provision and athlete engagement are described. Sport specific examples include the monitoring of heart rate and EEG in pistol shooting, and heart-rate in archery in competition and non-competition settings are used as entry point evidence base for the sport psychologist to work on, on an individualized basis. Other non-intervention approaches like sleep deprivation and project adventure are also described.

1. Introduction

The application of psychological knowledge and skills to enhance athletes' performance has been documented for decades, but it is not until the late 1990s that psychological services were formally introduced to the top athletes in Taiwan. These services were started by the Sport Affair Council (SAC), a ministry-level administrative body in the central government of Taiwan. A sport science team was organized at the National Training Center (NTC) to support the athletes and coaches in preparation for major international competitions such as the Olympic Games and the Asian Games.

The sport science team consists mainly of experts from several sports. The chapter will focus on the general aspects of sport psychology services provided in Taiwan over the last few years. Specifically, I will describe the facilities, service content and general practice of sport psychology services at the NTC. An introduction of the sport psychology service administered to athletes in preparation for the 2004 Athens Olympic Games is detailed elsewhere (Hung,

Lin, Lee, & Chen, 2008; Hung, Tan, & Shiang, 2009; Postolache, Hung, Stiller, Soriano, Montes, & Rosenthal, 2005).

2. Structure of service provision

With regard to the structure of the sport science team, the director for the entire team was appointed by the SAC. There are five division directors to cover the areas of conditioning, exercise physiology and biochemistry, nutrition, sport biomechanics, and sport psychology. Each division director recruits a few faculty members to share the workload, with four or five members recruited for the Olympic Games and a few more for the Asian Games.

Model countries such as the USA, Australia, and Hong Kong employ full time sport psychologists to help their athletes. However, there is currently no full time sport psychologist working at the NTC. Instead, the sport psychologists are faculty staff from the major universities in Taiwan that have sport related departments. These psychologists work part-time with their students to provide services at the NTC. Although it is more desirable to employ full time sport psychologists in order to maximize the quality of service, the use of part time experts is an interim arrangement which still produces some positive outcome.

The services provided to the preparation for the 2004 Athens Olympic Games can be used to illustrate how sport psychology has been applied to help athletes in Taiwan (as Chinese Taipei). These services were considered as the most sport science-involved Olympics in Taiwan's history. A total of eight sport psychologists were appointed by the NTC to help the athletes from several key sports, which are considered as potential medal winners at the 2004 Olympics.

Cooperation between the sport psychologists and the sport team started about a year and a half prior to the Games, the sport psychologist usually visiting the athletes at least once a week. Additionally the assistants, working under the supervision of a sport psychologist, spent even more time with the athletes. The sport psychology service provided to these athletes was not intended to be an academic endeavour; rather, a client-centered approach was adopted throughout the sessions.

The service content was similar to most sport psychology services employed by other countries. The service started with an orientation session attended by the NTC administrative personnel as well as the entire sport science team, coaches, and athletes. The orientation is significant because it sets the atmosphere for successful cooperation between sport science experts and the sport team. This general orientation session is then followed by several orientation sessions specific to each sport science discipline. During the discipline-specific sessions, both the sport psychologist and the assistants meet with the sport team members.

3. Stages in service provision

Lessons learned from past experiences suggest that winning support from the coaches is pivotal to successful sport science work. Strong efforts were devoted to educate the coaches about the effectiveness of the sport psychology intervention in enhancing athletic performance. Supporting materials related to the sport psychology services were also provided. Key psychological constructs such as motivation, attention, arousal, and anxiety are introduced, and preliminary communication between the sport psychologist and the sport team members is initiated. The rapport-building stage is followed by the preliminary diagnostic stage.

Information relevant to athletes' cognitive, emotional, and behavioral states, in and out of their sport, is gathered from their coaches, teammates, and other supporting staff such as the trainer and administrator. The sport psychologist and assistants spend time on on-site observation during training and competitions to better understand the behaviour of the athletes. In addition, several in-depth interview sessions are used to understand athletes' psychological strength and weaknesses. Although psychological inventories such as the Athletic Psychological Skills Inventory (APSI; Chiu & Chi, 2001), the Chinese version of the Task and Ego Orientation in Sport Questionnaire (TEPSQ; Chi, 1993) and the Chinese version of the Sport Competition Anxiety Test (SCAT; Lu, 1990) are typically used in research, these self-report tools are used in complement, with the diagnosis based mainly on the results of the in-depth interview.

In addition to the traditional self-report approach to understanding athletes' psychological states, psycho-physiological variables such as heart rate and EEG which are associated with concentration and other psychological states are also measured. For example, Figure 1 demonstrates the measurement of EEG and heart rate during pistol shooting.

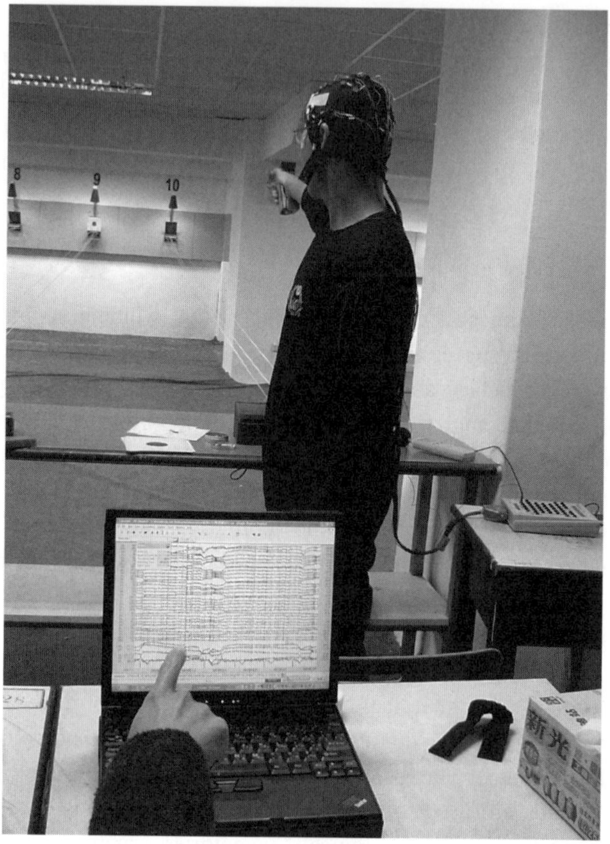

Figure 1: Measurement of heart rate and EEG during pistol shooting

In the intervention stage, psychological skill training is introduced to both coaches and athletes. The intervention consists of typical and non-typical psychological skill training programs. For the typical training, relaxation techniques such as progressive muscle relaxation, breathing, and imagery are introduced and practised on a regular basis.

Sleep deprivation and project adventure constitute the non-typical intervention activities. Sleep deprivation is designed to reduce the impact of insomnia due to competition stress. Figure 3 shows the record of sleep quality by an electronic device.

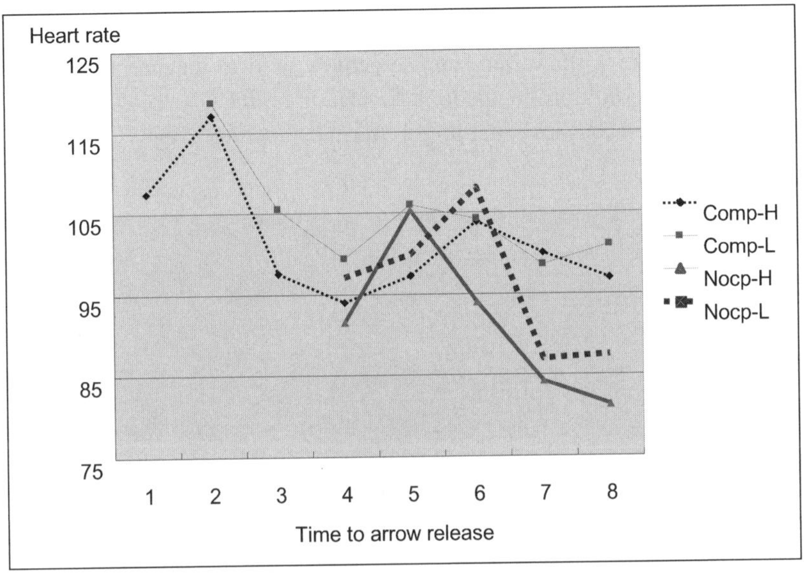

Figure 2: Shows the differences in the temporal dynamic of heart rate for a top archer between high and low scores under competition and non-competition conditions

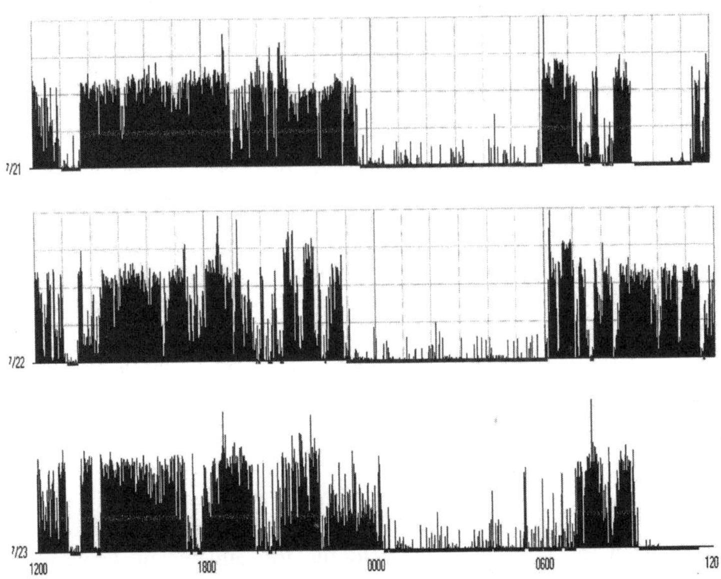

Figure 3: Record of quality of sleep by an electronic activity monitoring device

Project adventure is an outdoor activity used for team building and individual exploration. Figure 4 shows an example activity used to toughen the athletes' mental quality. In addition, competition simulation for the Olympics is employed to help athletes and coaches better prepare for the important event.

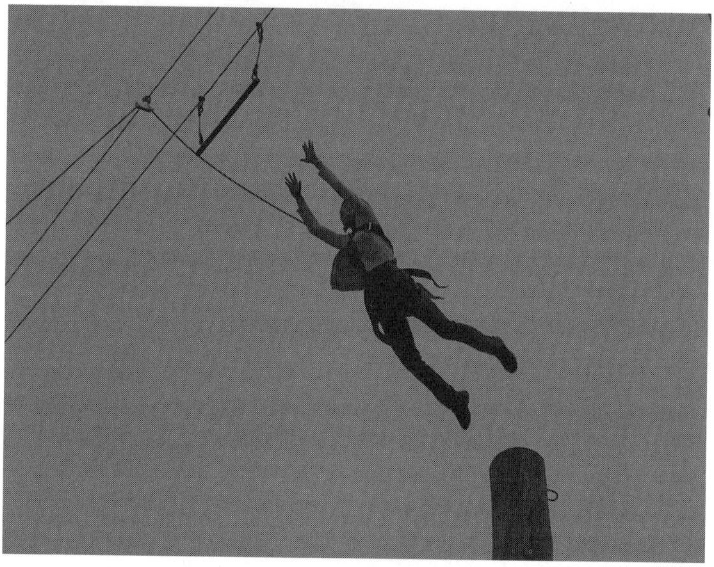

Figure 4: Activity used to challenge athletes' psychological limits

On-site services are also provided during important international competitions. Typically the services are provided at the later stage of the entire process to make this service effective, with the sport psychologist traveling with the team for some of the important competitions. The main purpose of the on-site service is to not only provide a comprehensive package to cover every aspect of the competition but also to evaluate the effectiveness of the psychological skills training provided before the competition. Moreover, new psychological issues arising from the competition can be uncovered and dealt with more efficiently when the sport psychologist is on-site.

4. Conclusion

Service provision in sport psychology to the top athletes in Taiwan mostly parallel those practised in other countries. However, the service is not provided in a constant manner in that there is a limited period of time that is available before a major competition for the sport psychologist and the team to work together. The time constraint poses a challenge for both parties and more creative solutions are needed so that more positive results of such interventions can be harvested for competitions. Information from this chapter may be helpful to countries facing with similar challenges to incorporate sport psychology services for athlete preparation for major international competitions.

References

1. Chi, L. (1993). A revision of Chinese task and ego orientation in sport questionnaire: Analysis of validity and reliability. *Bulletin of National College of Physical Education and Sports, 4*(1), 175-185.
2. Chiou, Y., & Chi, L. (2001). The development of the athletic psychological skills inventory. *Psychological Bulletin for Sport and Exercise Psychology of Taiwan, 1,* 21-45.
3. Hung, T., Lin, T., Lee, C., & Chen, L. (2008). Provision of Sport Psychology Services to Taiwan Archery Team for the 2004 Athens Olympic Games. *International Journal of Sport & Exercise Psychology, 6(3),* 308-318.
4. Hung, T., Tang, W., and Shiang, T. (2009). A case study of integrated sport sciences for an Olympic archer, *Journal of Medical and Biological Engineering* (in press).
5. Lu, J. (1990). A study on sport competition trait anxiety in collegiate athletes. *Bulletin of Physical Education, 12,* 45-70.
6. Postolache, T. T., Hung, T., Stiller, J. W., Soriano, J. J., Montes, F., & Rosenthal, R. N. (2005). Sports chronobiology consultation: From the lab to the arena. *Clinics in Sports Medicine, 24,* 415-456.

JAPANESE CHALLENGES FOR ENVIRONMENTAL PROTECTION IN THE OLYMPIC MOVEMENT

JUNKO TAHARA

Faculty of Physical Education, Kokushikan University, Tokyo, Japan

In Japan, large-scale initiatives for the protection of the environment were adopted for the Sapporo Winter Olympic Games in 1972, more than 20 years earlier than the declaration by the International Olympic Committee (IOC) for environmental protection when hosting the Olympic Games. The downhill ski events were held on Mount Eniwa but the course was a part of a special nature reserve. The Olympic Games Organizing Committee and the Japanese Olympic Committee, in accepting the demands of the local nature conservation association, dismantled all of the downhill course facilities after the Games. Afforestation was pursued over fifteen years, after the Winter Olympic Games with the aim of restoring the forest to its original state. These environmental conservation experiences in Sapporo were put to good use again in the Nagano Winter Games in 1998. However, the problem of raising the starting point of the men's downhill ski course to a higher elevation was a strong point of contention in the Nagano Olympics. The problem gave rise to intense strife between the peoples. However, the internal contradictions and conflicts between conservationists and Olympic Game protagonists for the protection and management of nature over the years were clarified and contributed to further progress made toward protection of the environment.

1. Introduction

Recently in the sports world, there is a mounting awareness that there should be responsible behavior towards conservation in the global environment. Whether it involves the clearing of forestlands for the construction of sports facilities or in the generation of large quantities of waste, sports have more than a small impact on the environment. Conversely, changes in the environment also have an impact on sports. In this discourse, I would like to present an overview of the global environment and sports, and how Japan has addressed this issue.

The following are environmental challenges that we face:

1. Global warming
2. Destruction of the ozone layer
3. Acid precipitation
4. Reduction of wild flora and fauna species

5. Reduction of forestlands
6. Global-scale desertification
7. Marine contamination
8. Trans-boundary movement of hazardous waste

The prevention of global warming with rising temperatures in the atmosphere and oceans and the occurrence of climatic changes due to human activities is a major issue. Some sports may be negatively affected because of rising sea-levels due to global warming. For example, it may no longer be possible to play beach volleyball if the oceans eventually rise and cover the beaches. It is gradually becoming difficult to engage in skiing, bobsledding and other sports of the Winter Olympics without using artificial snow, as global warming affects the natural climate in winter, where once snowfall was abundant. There is therefore urgency and a need to reduce, if not prevent global warming so that sporting pursuits that are widely enjoyed by mankind can continue.

2. Environmental initiatives of the IOC

The reason why the IOC first began to place importance on environmental issues is because Juan Antonio Samaranch, the IOC President at that time, called for active efforts to deal with environmental conservation during the early 1990s. This was prompted by increasingly serious global warming, acid rain, desertification and other forms of environmental destruction in many parts of the world (Tokyo 2016 Bid Committee, 2008c). Samaranch asserted that the environment would be added as a pillar to the Olympic Movement.

At the Olympic Congress held in Paris in 1994, the theme of Sport and the Environment was taken up as an agenda and a Sport and Environment Commission was established under the IOC (Tokyo 2016 Bid Committee, 2008c). Provisions for environmental conservation were added to the Olympic Charter in 1995. Article 2-13 of Chapter 1 states that the mission and role of the IOC is ‘to encourage and support a responsible concern for environmental issues, to promote sustainable development in sport and to require that the Olympic Games are held accordingly.”

Furthermore, the IOC World Congress on Sport and Environment is also convened every other year starting in 1995. The IOC adopted the Olympic Movement Agenda 21 at the World Congress on Sport and Environment held in 1999 based on Agenda 21, an action plan for environmental conservation adopted at the UN Conference on Environment and Development (Earth

Summit) held in Rio de Janeiro in 1992 (Tokyo 2016 Bid Committee, 2008c). This set forth the principles of environmental conservation and guidelines for action in the sports world. It spells out the basic approach to environmental conservation activities through sports as well as methods for the practical application of those activities by athletes, coaches, organizations, corporations and others involved in sport.

3. Sapporo Winter Olympics 1972

In Japan, we faced a significant environmental issue more than 20 years before the IOC became fully committed to environment conservation. The downhill ski courses for the 1972 Sapporo Olympics were constructed by clearing forestland on Mount Eniwa for the Olympic Games and, after the conclusion of the Games, all of the related facilities were removed and the restoration of the forestland was promoted through afforestation.

Mount Eniwa has an elevation of 1,320m and is located in the suburbs of Sapporo, some 30 km south of the centre of the city. It was furthermore selected for the downhill ski competition because it was able to provide the standard elevation for men's and women's ski courses that were required by the International Ski Federation rules. The Organizing Committee explained to the IOC that the distance from the Olympic Village to Mount Eniwa could be covered in 30 minutes by vehicle upon the completion of a new road. The committee proposed a so-called "compact Olympics" with relatively short distance movement for the athletes and associated officials.

These courses were located in the special protection area of the National Park, so the Hokkaido Nature Conservation Society expressed as a condition that, after the Olympic Games, the affected area would be restored as much as possible to its original state by entirely removing the facilities constructed for the ski courses and replanting the forestland that had been cleared. The Olympic Organizing Committee accepted this condition and, based on that, asked for and received the approval for facility construction for the Olympic Games from the Ministry of Health and Welfare.

At that time, the Association's trustees, acting as individuals, presented the case before the general meeting of the International Union for Conservation of Nature and Natural Resources (IUCN) with the idea of moving the courses, if possible, to a more convenient location, which would resolve the problem of nature protection. That would also facilitate ease of use of the facilities by many people after the Olympics and the funds invested in the facilities would not be wasted. They succeeded in obtaining the signatures of virtually all of the representatives from around the world on a document opposing damage to the natural environment in the vicinity of Mount Eniwa. The petition letter was sent to the IOC President Avery Brundage (Ide et al. 1966). The letter made an appeal to the IOC to advise the Japanese Olympic Committee (JOC) to search for a new location for the downhill courses in a more suitable area and in turn recognize and actualize the harmony of the Olympic Winter Games and the protection of nature and the environment. However, the petition was not successful and the location for the Olympic Winter Games remained unchanged.

The construction of the Mount Eniwa downhill courses was a difficult undertaking, which required the use of explosives to level the surface of the mountain and included the installation of concrete blocks to prevent collapses on the steep mountain slopes. Besides the ski courses for men and women, which were from 2800m to 2100m in length, a total of 38 facilities were constructed that included two cable cars, lifts, management headquarters, lodging facilities, heliport and other structures. It was reported that trees were cleared from approximately 2,900m^2 of forestland, 6 tons of explosives were used and the total cost of the construction of the Olympic Winter Games facilities amounted to ¥834 million.

The downhill courses were finally completed after overcoming numerous difficulties and the Sapporo Winter Olympic Games were launched. The downhill ski competition was conducted for a period of four days. After the Olympics, all of the facilities on Mount Eniwa were removed and the area was re-forested as the process of restoration began. The restoration project, which continued over a period of fifteen years after the Games, was completed in 1986 at a cost of ¥240 million.

There are newspaper articles dealing with the conditions of the restoration of the Mount Eniwa downhill courses more than twenty years after the conclusion of the Olympics (Hokkaido Shinbun, 1992, et al). All of the articles report that Aka-ezo-matsu (red spruce, Picea glehnii) trees were planted instead of the original Ezo-matsu (spruce, Picea jezoensis) because saplings of that species were no longer available on the market.

The final report of the restoration project issued by the Japan Amateur Sports Association evaluates the project in this manner: "This is the sole example of success in forest restoration in Japan. Issues of harmony with the surroundings and assimilation will be resolved with the passage of time." The newspapers, however, stated that "even though the restoration project is completed, it would be difficult to call it restoration. It is more like a plantation." Harsh comments were also heard that it would take 100 years for the area to return to its original state. What messages and lessons can be distilled from the experiences of the Sapporo Olympic Games? The downhill courses were constructed on Mount Eniwa for geographical convenience, which contributed in part, to the success of the Games. A significant lesson learnt was huge cost, enormous work and time required to restore the environment once it is disrupted. Perhaps the legacy of the Games was the strong awareness of the protection of nature was engraved in the hearts of the people.

4. Nagano Winter Olympics 1998

"Coexistence with beautiful and abundant nature" was advocated as the ideal to be achieved at the time of the Nagano Winter Olympics in 1998, and various measures were taken to protect the environment (Tokyo 2016 Bid Committee, 2008c). In the development of the competition facilities in Nagano Olympics, efforts were made to use existing facilities as much as possible and, even when newly constructed, the clearing of forests was reduced to a minimum and seedlings were planted to restore the forest after the conclusion of the Olympic Games (Tokyo 2016 Bid Committee, 2008a). In addition, the use of chemicals for hardening the snow (snow hardening agent) was reduced on the cross-country ski course and the condition of the snow was maintained by laying tatami mats under the snow (Tokyo 2016 Bid Committee, 2008a). Care was also taken to avoid imposing a burden on the National Park located within the ski competition area when setting up the ski courses (Tokyo 2016 Bid Committee, 2008c).

"Dove balloons" were released during the opening ceremony rather than real doves, the symbol of peace. The dove balloons were made of material that gradually decomposes into water, carbon dioxide and other substances when exposed to ultraviolet rays (Tokyo 2016 Bid Committee, 2008c). In addition, the dishware used at the Olympic Village was made of a mixture of apple and paper pulp (Tokyo 2016 Bid Committee, 2008a). Besides that, the introduction of hybrid, natural gas and other vehicles that had minimal impact on atmospheric contamination and other environment-friendly elements were evident everywhere, in event management, demonstrating a strong stance of environmental conservation to those attending the Olympic event (Tokyo 2016 Bid Committee, 2008a).

However, the Nagano Olympics, too, had an issue that had to be addressed. The problem of raising the starting point of the men's downhill ski course to a higher elevation erupted immediately prior to the start of competition. Many people remember this problem as a symbol of the problem of nature conservation in the Nagano Olympics. It all started with a request from the

International Ski Federation (FIS) to raise the starting point initially planned at an elevation of 1,680m to 1,800m at the site of the Happo-One downhill ski course in the Northern Alps. The request was made at the time of the field survey in 1993, five years prior the Olympics, due to the desire to further enhance competition among the skiers. In response, the Nagano Olympics Organizing Committee (NAOC) continued to consistently deny the request. Since the 1,680m elevation had basically been approved by the IOC Executive Board, it was thought that it would be implemented essentially as planned. However, the confrontation abruptly became more serious when the FIS emphatically demanded that the starting point be moved to the higher elevation in a mere five months prior to the Olympics. The arguments at the time for and against raising the starting point can be summarized as indicated (Togashi, 2004a):

The reasons for supporting the higher starting point included:

1. There were opinions expressing dissatisfaction with the short skiing time and that the athletes would not have time to fully demonstrate their skills (about 1 minute 30 seconds, some 10-15 seconds shorter than most past competition records).
2. There was a desire to provide the highest possible competitive conditions worthy of the Olympics as a special event.
3. It is a fact that its establishment as a legitimate ski slope had thus far been tolerated and it would be possible to use it in the competition without violating any laws.
4. It is a short-term competitive event on the snow and, if appropriate care is taken, there would be little fear of deterioration of the natural environment.

The reasons for not supporting the high starting point included:

1. Even if it is not raised, the course design satisfies the FIS rules and it would sufficient for the competition.
2. From the beginning when it was decided that Nagano was to be the ski venue of the Olympic Games, the starting point was set at a location outside of the National Park at an elevation of 1,680m. A fundamental agreement has been reached among the concerned parties, with the exception of the FIS, not to raise the starting point any higher.
3. Happo-One is known for its unique topography, wild flora and fauna, and it is a special area with a natural environment that requires protection.
4. If the starting point was raised any higher, it would not be possible to avoid the continued development of skiing and new facilities in the National Park (class 1 special zone) and there are also legal problems. The Olympic Games cannot be considered as an exception.

There was the tendency to give top priority to the Olympics, which is epitomized by the view that "anything is okay as long as it's the Olympics". The opposite viewpoint was an absolute adherence to principles expressed where "even the Olympics cannot be treated as an exception." These opposite viewpoints became a source of conflict and tension among its supporters. The controversy culminated about two months prior to the start of the Olympic Games with an official announcement that the starting point was to be elevated to 1,725m, about halfway between the previous 1,680m and 1,800m points, with neither side coming to terms with the other in the debate (Togashi, 2004a). As points of agreement by those involved when proceeding with the task, a portion of the national park would be crossed by the short jump, no construction work would take place in the park, the use of snow hardening agents would be prohibited and other conditions were imposed (Togashi, 2004a).

Further, this happened because internal contradictions came about due to the establishment of national park boundaries without taking into account the continuity of natural ecosystems as well as the promotion of the utilization of nature with priority over protection (Togashi, 2004a).

The debate surrounding the issues of protection and utilization of Happo-One continued after the Nagano Olympic Games, while, at the same time, public projects to restore the damage and volunteer conservation activities by the local residents commenced (Togashi, 2004a). There were also sites in the village that were designated as new natural monuments with protection promoted more than ever (Togashi, 2004a). During winter, the use of the ski was also restricted by the company management (Togashi, 2004a).

Even though the controversy surrounding the issue of the starting point for the ski competition in the Winter Olympic Games at Nagano led to great strife among the peoples, awareness of environmental considerations and the conservation of nature was heightened and this led to further strengthening of protection and nature management over the years.

5. Initiatives in Tokyo

The Tokyo Metropolitan Government advocates the goal of "reducing the volume of greenhouse gas emissions in Tokyo by 25 % by 2020" as part of its "Tokyo's Big Change - The 10-Year Plan" formulated in 2006 (Tokyo Metropolitan Government, 2007). The following goals are advocated in the 2008 program for implementing the "Tokyo's Big Change - The 10-Year Plan" and activities have commenced (Tokyo Metropolitan Government, 2007).

1. Greening of school playgrounds to nurture healthy children
2. Ensuring a rich abundance of greenery in Tokyo through the development of umi-no-mori (sea forests), doubling roadside trees, etc.
3. Passing on the precious greenery of Tokyo to the next generation through forest revitalization, etc.
4. Developing a movement through the Green Tokyo Fund
5. Forming urban districts with no power poles
6. Creating beautiful cityscapes

The installation of lawns will aroused much enthusiasm for physical exercise among the children and the lawns will also reduce injuries. In addition, that will also reduce the ground surface temperature by 8.3° C and will also reduce dust pollution (Tokyo Metropolitan Government, 2007). Tokyo is engaged in bidding activities for the 2016 Olympic Games and has set forth its commitment to making it the most environmentally-friendly Olympics by greening the whole city.

6. Conclusion

The Olympic Games has the potential for causing unforeseen destruction of nature and impacting the environment in ways that cannot be anticipated in meeting the needs and requirements of the Games. In terms of nature conservation, it is necessary to conduct comprehensive environmental impact assessments overall, including the development of transportation networks linking venues and other related facilities, and alterations to nature and to the local communities (Togashi, 2004b). In spite of the short-term nature of the Olympic festivities, most of its impact on nature is not transient. We must not forget that, in the Olympics today, in the shadow of that brilliant stage where athletes strive to win medals, there is a considerable burden on the environment that gradually emerges over a long period of time in a diversity of forms (Togashi, 2004b). We must remember that, not infrequently, people speak of nature conservation just as if it had been accomplished by drawing attention to the efforts made (Togashi, 2004b). Measures implemented by humans consist of some aspects that are well done, some that are not necessarily done well and yet others the outcome of which will become apparent sometime in the future (Togashi, 2004b). In order to give life to experience gained through the Olympics, it is important to conduct proper assessments on the impact on the environment and to reduce any dire consequences as much as possible. The global environment will not be improved solely through the activities of specific individuals or countries. Therefore the Olympic Movement has an important role to play in raising the global awareness and be in the forefront of environmental protection. That is indeed an Olympic Spirit worth preserving and propagating.

References

1. *Hokkaido Shinbun* (Hokkaido Newspaper) June 4, 1992.
2. *Asahi Shinbun* (Asahi Newspaper) April 1, 1989 and July 3, 1989.
3. *Hokkai Taimusu* (Hokkai Times) June 17, 1996.
4. Ide, A. et al. (1966). Letter to the Avery Brundage dated September 2, 1966. International Olympic Committee.
5. Togashi, H. (2004a). Legacy of the Debate over the Starting Point in the Nagano Olympics Men's Downhill Ski Competition. In: Kondo Y. (Ed), Supotsu Rini no Tankyu (In Pursuit of Sports Ethics), Taishukan-Shoten, pp. 70-80.
6. Togashi, H. (2004b). To what Extent did the Nagano Winter Olympics Protect the Environment? In: Kondo, Y. (Ed), Supotsu Rini no Tankyu (In Pursuit of Sports Ethics), Taishukan-Shoten pp. 62-70.
7. Tokyo 2016 Bid Committee (2008a). *Minnna-wo Musubu Orinpikku – Yume-Kando-Mirai* (The Olympic Games Uniting Our World – Aspiration, Inspiration, Anticipation -) (Olympic Reader for Elementary School Students), Tokyo Metropolitan Government, Japanese Olympic Committee, and Tokyo 2016 Bid Committee. pp. 36-39.
8. Tokyo 2016 Bid Committee (2008b). *Sekai-wo Musubu Orinpikku* (The Olympic Games Uniting Our World – Enthusiasm, People, Sports), (Olympic Reader for Junior High School Students), Tokyo Metropolitan Government, Japanese Olympic Committee, and Tokyo 2016 Bid Committee. pp. 36-39.
9. Tokyo 2016 Bid Committee (2008c). *Mirai-wo Musubu Orinpikku* (The Olympic Games Uniting with the Future – Courage, Earth, Symbiosis -), (Olympic Reader for Senior High School Students), Tokyo Metropolitan Government, Japanese Olympic Committee, and Tokyo 2016 Bid Committee. pp. 36-39.
10. Tokyo Metropolitan Government (2007). Basic Policies for the 10-Year Project for Green Tokyo. http://www.chijihon.metro.tokyo.jp/actionplan/2.pdf